Care of the Ophthalmic Patient

A Guide for Nurses and Health Professionals

Edited by

John P. Perry

Director of Nursing at Manchester Royal Eye Hospital, UK.

and

Andrew B. Tullo

Consultant Ophthalmic Surgeon, Manchester Royal Eye Hospital, UK.

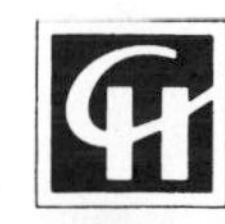

CHAPMAN & HALL

London · Glasgow · New York · Tokyo · Melbourne · Madras

Published by Chapman & Hall, 2–6 Boundary Row, London SE1 8HN, UK

Chapman & Hall, 2–6 Boundary Row, London SE1 8HN, UK

Blackie Academic & Professional, Wester Cleddens Road, Bishopbriggs, Glasgow G64 2NZ, UK

Chapman & Hall GmbH, Pappelallee 3, 69469 Weinheim, Germany

Chapman & Hall USA, 115 Fifth Avenue, New York NY 10003, USA

Chapman & Hall Japan, ITP-Japan, Kyowa Building, 3F, 2-2-1 Hirakawacho, Chiyoda-ku, Tokyo 102, Japan

Chapman & Hall Australia, Thomas Nelson Australia, 102 Dodds Street, South Melbourne, Victoria 3205, Australia

Chapman & Hall India, R. Seshadri, 32 Second Main Road, CIT East, Madras 600 035, India

Distributed in the USA and Canada by Singular Publishing Group Inc., 4284 41st Street, San Diego, California 92105

First edition 1990

Reprinted 1993

Second edition 1995

Typeset in 10.5/12 pt Palatino by EXPO Holdings, Malaysia

Printed in Great Britain at the Alden Press, Oxford

ISBN 0 412 59290 8 1 56593 334 6 (USA)

A catalogue record for this book is available from the British Library

Library of Congress Catalog Card Number: 95-067611

∞ Printed on permanent acid-free text paper, manufactured in accordance with ANSI/NISO Z39.48-1992 and ANSI/NISO Z39.48-1984 (Permanence of Paper).

Contents

Contributors

Janet Bott, formerly Ward Sister, Manchester Royal Eye Hospital

Peter Cole, formerly Ophthalmic Optician, Manchester Royal Eye Hospital

Valerie M. Darbyshire, Henshaws Society for the Blind, Manchester

Deirdre Donnelly, formerly Research Sister, Manchester Royal Eye Hospital

Robert Doran, Consultant, Leeds General Infirmary

Gordon Dutton, Consultant, Western Infirmary, Glasgow

Josephine Duvall-Young, Consultant, High Wycombe General Hospital

Andrew Elliott, Consultant, Manchester Eye Hospital

David Etchells, Consultant, Frimley Park Hospital, Surrey

Jane Fox, Sister, Casualty Department, Bristol Eye Hospital

Janie M. Grabham, Senior Nurse (Theatres), Manchester Royal Eye Hospital

Efty Joannadu, formerly Tutor, Moorfields Eye Hospital

Meg Johnson, formerly Sister, Manchester Royal Eye Hospital

Patrick W. Joyce, Staff Ophthalmologist, Southport

Pat Lapworth, formerly Clinical Teacher, Moorfields Eye Hospital

Brian Leatherbarrow, Consultant, Manchester Royal Eye Hospital

Rowena McNamara, Orthoptic Teacher, Leeds General Infirmary

Janet Marsden, Sister, Manchester Royal Eye Hospital

S. Jane Merchant, Executive Director of Nursing and Quality, Central Manchester Healthcare Trust

Tim Ossei Berkoh, Clinical Teacher, Moorfields Eye Hospital

Karen Partington, formerly Research Sister, Manchester Royal Eye Hospital

John Perry, Director of Nursing, Manchester Royal Eye Hospital

Michael Raines, Consultant, Royal Victoria Hospital, Blackpool

Grant Raymond, Consultant, Flinders Medical Centre, Adelaide, Australia

Ian Rennie, Senior Lecturer, Royal Hallamshire Hospital, Sheffield

Mary Rowell, formerly Director of Education, Moorfields Eye Hospital
John Sandford-Smith, Consultant, Leicester Royal Infirmary
John Storey, formerly Principal Optometrist, Manchester Royal Eye Hospital
Gail Thomas, Sister, Manchester Royal Eye Hospital
Andrew Tullo, Consultant, Manchester Royal Eye Hospital
Steve Vernon, Senior Lecturer, Queen's Medical Centre, Nottingham
Linda Whittaker, Tutor, Manchester College of Midwifery and Nursing
Pamela C. Williams, formerly Social Worker, Manchester Royal Eye Hospital

Preface

While this book is primarily compiled for nurses who care for patients with eye disease, it will be useful to other health professionals who are also interested in the holistic care of such patients, e.g. opticians, orthoptists, social workers and junior medical staff.

The second edition has been revised to take account of recent dynamic changes in medical treatments, and clinical management and the influences of health and social policy. The subspecialty developments of vitreous and retina, oculoplastic and orbital treatments in particular have been developed within the text.

Since we are aware of the need to produce a book that is easily used as a reference text, the layout has been improved to easily distinguish text, illustration and nursing care plans.

The developments of day surgery are discussed at length to show planning, implementation and audit of this service, its effect on patients and the need for a multidisciplinary approach. The role of the multidisciplinary team in providing an emergency specialist service is covered in relation to Nurse Practitioner developments (a 30-year full circle). Speculation as to the future role of the specialist nurse within the multidisciplinary team is included where innovative developments are thought possible. The effects of the Patients' Charter are discussed where appropriate, and a whole new chapter has been incorporated to highlight the requirements for quality and professional standards.

The care is presented as a systematic approach to common actual and potential problems. Typically, a problem is identified, with a desired outcome and the nursing interventions possible to achieve this. Evaluation has not been included as this is dependent on an identified time limit for outcomes to be achieved, which is individual to each patient.

The book is split into Part One, which considers the holistic needs of patients who have visual problems and takes a patient-centred approach to the management of patient's needs, and Part Two, which is based on a medical model, where each section of the eye is studied separately: the applied physiology of that part of the eye; the more common conditions affecting it; the possible medical management of the condition and the nursing care of the patient. The list of medical conditions is not exhaustive; only a general guideline of medical management is given as far as it influences nursing care. A list of widely available books for further reference to ocular pathology and medical management is given in the Appendix.

The specialist knowledge and skills required to nurse children with ophthalmic disease have been discussed where appropriate throughout the book; in many instances the basic principles can be applied to caring for such children. General aspects of nursing children in hospital or the community have been omitted as these can be found in other appropriate publications.

While the editors are aware that patients and nurses may belong to either gender, throughout the text, the former is referred to as 'he' and the latter as 'she', in order to maintain consistency.

John Perry
Andrew Tullo
Manchester, April 1995

Acknowledgements

We are very grateful to the following for their help and support in producing this book: Ms Christine Ruttledge for word processing; Richard Neave for all the artwork; and the Clinical Imaging Department, Manchester Royal Eye Hospital, for all the photographs.

Part One

Principles of Ophthalmic Patient Care

1 Introducing the Visually Impaired Person

Janet Bott

Chapter Summary

Anyone for whom this book has been written is likely to meet the shortsighted individual who is happily unaware of his problem until, perhaps in early teens, a first pair of spectacles provides the kind of vision his chums have enjoyed for years. When those same friends first reluctantly put on reading glasses in their forties our myope may still be happily reading without glasses. Such events are normal, but may go hand in hand with serious threats to vision.

Our reader will meet children with a need for spectacles and patches to aid their developing vision and to prevent squint. In the elderly the threat to sight from age-related degeneration of the retina or from glaucoma is common. Some of the elderly are unlucky enough to be afflicted by both these major problems. Our reader will meet the occasionally tragic case where, despite dramatic medical advances, a young diabetic may become entirely blind. It is more likely, though, that you will come across the astonished octogenarian whose sight is restored to normality by modern cataract surgery.

The expressions 'visually impaired', 'visually disabled' and 'visually handicapped' are widely used to describe people who do not see well. Each expression does, however, have a subtly different meaning. Woods (1975) classified **impairment** as a 'disturbance of the normal structure and functioning' of the eye, **disability** as 'loss or reduction of functional ability and activity consequent upon impairment', and **handicap** as the 'disadvantage in more social terms consequent upon impairment and disability'. The relationship between the three categories cannot be assumed. This must be borne in mind in the following text, where the term 'visual handicap' has been used to imply a varying classification. For instance, a child in the 1950s in the UK with a slight refractive error would have had minimal disability but would have been handicapped by the stigma attached to the wearing of spectacles.

A person who is born with a visual handicap will have different physical and psychological problems, at different stages of their life, when compared to someone who has an acquired visual handicap. How a child overcomes his handicap depends largely on the family and how much time is given to teaching things other babies and children learn for themselves. The child who has never seen anyone walking has no idea how to move his legs, what posture to adopt, what to do with his head or even where to place his hands in relation to the rest of his body. An abnormal gait often leads people to believe that mental handicap accompanies the visual loss.

More centres are now available to help train visually handicapped children from an earlier age and expert advice is more readily available to advise parents. Many of the developmental problems can be overcome with the correct help.

Behavioural problems in visually handicapped children are usually a result of lack of stimulation. These may present as body rocking, head banging, swaying or abnormal hand waving. These should cease when the child is given something interesting to do.

As the majority of visually handicapped people in Britain are elderly, it may seem to many that visual handicap is less of a tragedy when it is part of 'old age'. Coupled with ill health or other failing senses in the elderly, however, it could be seen as an even greater tragedy as it may signal the loss of independence. As we age, learning Braille may prove to be beyond us, as may safe mobilization with a dog or long cane.

A person who has suffered visual loss goes through the same stages of grief as someone who has suffered a bereavement. They may refuse to believe their blindness is permanent, and waste a great deal of time seeking help elsewhere. Anger may be projected on to the family, doctors or nurses in an attempt to apportion blame for the condition. They may become depressed and withdraw from their family and surroundings. All of these emotions must be recognized as normal. They must be given the opportunity to talk about feelings without being put down. Rehabilitation cannot begin until the final stage, that of acceptance, has been reached.

Friends and relatives should allow the person to develop at their own rate, and not be too hasty to step in and do things for them. With an over-willing family it is easy for a newly visually handicapped person to become apathetic, allowing others to do everything for them. This will make it harder in the long term for them to regain independence.

A person, young or old, should be allowed to make mistakes providing they are in no danger. To lessen the chances of knocking something over accidentally it is helpful if any unnecessary articles in a room are removed and any ornaments are pushed to the back of a table or shelf.

It is a common belief that the blind have special powers, in that the other senses are heightened, or that they possess 'ESP'. Indeed some blind people foster this belief as a way of coping with their handicap. The congenitally, or early blind tend to develop an acute sense of hearing and touch, but these are acquired by practice. They are not inherent to visual loss, neither are any of the other attributes associated with blindness, for example, courage, bravery, patience or cheerfulness. Visually handicapped people, like anyone else, can be moody, impatient and bad-tempered. It does not mean that one person has adjusted well because they are cheerful, and the other has not because they are moody. They may have been like this before their loss. Likewise, someone who has been looked after too well by a relative while sighted should not be expected to rehabilitate to total independence once they have suffered a visual loss, even though they may be physically capable.

The Newborn Child

By about 6 weeks the sighted baby will begin to smile at its parents by imitating them. This may be delayed in a baby with a visual handicap. Parents can 'smile' at their handicapped baby in other ways. Touch is very important: stroking the cheek or head, blowing on the baby's ear or neck are all tactile ways of smiling. Fraiberg (1977), in a study of blind children, found that some visually handicapped babies will smile at 3 months in response to a parent's voice. Talking to the baby is important for the mother, as this is the first way the baby will recognize those close to it. Smell and feel also play an important part in recognition. Fraiberg (1977) also demonstrated that at 8 months some visually handicapped children will display 'stranger anxiety', which was previously thought to depend on visual discrimination of faces.

A sighted child will begin to lift its head and eventually sit up as it takes an interest in its surroundings. Visually handicapped children need to be encouraged by being propped up on a pillow or against a chair, and also by being pulled up from a lying position by the hands as a form of game. It is difficult for a child with little or no vision to maintain its balance. This has to be learnt as they discover where the floor is in relation to their body in different positions.

It has been estimated that 90% of the information reaching our brains does so through the ability to see. A baby starts to crawl by going towards something, either a toy that has rolled out of reach or the arms of its mother. Once a toy rolls out of the reach of a visually handicapped child, it ceases to exist for the child. Parents can help by trying to attract the child with toys that make a noise, by calling him, or by letting him smell food. Before doing this, they have to show the baby how to move his legs to obtain forward movement, by holding his feet and moving his legs. This is a long, laborious process, but with great rewards at the end.

A majority of visually handicapped children prefer to crawl backwards so that it is their bottoms that come into contact with obstacles rather than their heads. When old enough, a baby walker will help the child discover its surroundings and also protect against knocks.

A baby's first plaything is its body. When dressing, parents should tell the child what is happening. 'The jumper goes over your head, your arms down the sleeves.' Games such as 'This little piggy' and 'Round and round the garden' can help. Toys need not be expensive — balls containing bells are ideal. Rattles or squeaky toys can be hung over a cot where the baby will touch them accidentally, though care should be taken not to have the string so long that it can wrap itself round the baby. A rattle needs to be placed in the baby's hands and shaken to teach the baby what it does. Toys can also be made by putting articles in a pot that can be sealed. Books on toys are available from the Royal National Institute for the Blind (RNIB).

When feeding the baby, its hands should be placed on the bottle or breast to feel the source of its food. When solids are introduced, the baby's hands should be moved from plate to mouth to encourage self-feeding.

If it is still uncertain that the baby has any vision, the parents should be encouraged to try and stimulate the baby's visual potential. This can be done by shining a light on the baby's face and moving it from left to right and up and down. If the baby appears to follow the light, brightly coloured objects can be substituted. Care should be taken not to use anything that makes a noise, or a false result may occur as the baby turns its head in the direction of the noise. Until the child begins to explore, the usual safety precautions for a baby apply.

THE TODDLER

Before speaking to a child, its name should be mentioned to gain its attention, especially if there are other children within hearing. Visitors must be told to talk to the child before touching it, as this can be very frightening. Where possible, the mother should talk to the child no matter what she is doing, as this is the only way the child will know she is still there. If she has to leave the room she must tell the child, and reassure it that she will still be able to hear should the child want her. If a family has a pet, a bell should be placed on its collar so the child will know when the pet has come into the room.

The child will now be exploring its surroundings either by crawling or walking while holding on to things. This is a time of danger and fear for both the child and its parents. More care has to be taken than with a sighted child. Loose rugs or mats should be removed or fixed down. Doors should be wedged open or firmly closed to prevent trapped fingers and bumped heads. If the child has been left alone in a room, care should be taken by anyone entering in case the child is behind the door. Fires should be covered by a guard. Floor-standing ornaments should be removed or cornered off so the child cannot reach them. Wires or flex should be fixed down to the floor or walls and dangerous articles should be well out of reach.

Excessive background noise should be avoided, as this can be confusing for the child. A ticking wall clock can be a good way of locating something else nearby. A musical toothbrush and hairbrush can make the acts of grooming more fun to learn for the child and a musical potty can aid in toilet training.

Play should be as normal as possible, although a visually handicapped child will need to be shown what to do with a toy several times. Other children should be encouraged to visit, and mother and child can attend a playgroup. Most groups, if asked, will provide an area where the visually handicapped child can play alone until it has become used to the extra noise and bustle.

Mealtimes should be fun, but they will also be very messy. If possible the floor around the child's chair should be covered. A lot can be learnt at mealtimes about different textures as well as about hand to mouth coordination. The child should be allowed to explore as much as is reasonably possible.

It should be remembered that all children need discipline, and visually handicapped children are no exception. They should not be forgiven things because of their handicap. Not only will this cause resentment among other children in the family, but it will cause the child to have a double handicap, the second one being bad manners and selfishness.

As with the baby, any residual vision should be encouraged by the use of brightly coloured objects, mirrors and torches.

The Schoolchild

Local Education Authorities (LEAs) are responsible for assessing the needs of a visually handicapped child. They will then make a statement as to how they intend to meet these needs. Parents have access to this information and may appeal if they wish. Help and advice is offered to parents by the Advisory Centre for Education. Some LEAs provide pre-school education for children over 2 years of age with visual handicap.

The final choice of school will depend on the degree of visual handicap, and whether other handicaps are present, although attitudes are now changing (p. 34). Schools for the blind are few, so many children will need to board. The children study the same subjects and take exams as fully sighted children do. The schools provide advice to the child on what employment is available. They have staff trained specially to deal with subjects such as Braille, and a vast array of aids for children with some vision. Their major disadvantage are that children may have to board and that the only children they come into contact with are also visually handicapped.

Normal schools have the advantage that the child can live at home and mix with sighted children, but they lack equipment and staff.

Vocational Assessment Centres can bridge the gap between school life and work. They offer encouragement in going out, dressing and grooming, at the same time assessing the child for skilled or manual employment.

The Teenager

As with all teenagers, this is a very sensitive age. If the child has been educated at a residential school, he/she may not have many friends who are sighted and this can present a problem during the school holidays. Communication can be a problem due to lack of eye contact. Family and friends should be made aware of any potential problems and, if possible, these should be discussed and ways of overcoming them worked out. Above all, children must be allowed continued independence provided they are in no danger.

The child should have learnt by now how to become mobile with a stick or long cane but may feel self-conscious about venturing out into the 'sighted' world alone. Talking books, Braille books and music will feature strongly in helping to keep the visually handicapped teenager amused, but the whole holiday should not revolve around these activities. It is important to maintain contact with a peer group.

Eve Gardiner of Max Factor has an interest in problems regarding make-up for the visually handicapped of all ages, and has written a guide to basic make-up techniques, free on request. To help with choice of clothes and colours, the RNIB have produced eight different-shaped buttons to represent different colours. Tidy habits will make life a lot easier.

ADULTHOOD

EMPLOYMENT

Visually handicapped individuals who are on the blind or partially sighted register may also register as disabled with the Manpower Services Commission. This makes them eligible for special facilities and gives them an advantage in finding employment, as all employers with 20 or more in their work force have to employ 3% disabled people. Suitable types of employment include light engineering, audio typing, telephony, computer programming, physiotherapy, social work, solicitors and many others. The Employment Services Division may pay for taxis to or from work, or to the nearest bus stop if public transport is not available locally.

For the more severely handicapped, sheltered workshops, run on a factory-type basis, offer employment. The basic wage is reasonable, but to be eligible people must be reasonably independent.

LOW VISUAL AIDS

Some hospitals have low visual aid clinics to which referral by an ophthalmologist is usually required. These clinics have a variety of aids, from spectacle magnifiers to monocular telescopes, to help people use what little vision they have left. Some hand-held magnifiers can be heavy and bulky, in which case a stand magnifier may be of more use.

ORGANIZATION IN THE HOME

Visually handicapped people with some vision may need a little help in arranging their home to make maximum use of available daylight or existing lighting facilities.

Windows should be kept clean and curtains well drawn back, to allow as much natural light into the room as possible. Light-coloured walls and ceilings will help to reflect light and large, light shades will allow more light to be distributed from the bulb.

Anglepoise lamps are useful for directing extra light for close work. A large variety of aids are available from the RNIB for use around the home.

In the kitchen reversible chopping boards can be used to make use of contrasting colours, e.g. white potatoes can be cut on the black side of the board while beetroot can be cut on the white side. Contrasts can also be used when laying a table or setting a meal out on a plate. Non-slip mats and plate guards are useful. Braille discs are available for washing machines and irons, from the manufacturers or the RNIB. A rotary-type washing line is useful, as it allows the person to stand still while hanging out the washing.

Templates are available for writing cheques or addresses, and some banks will send out their monthly statement in Braille if requested. Most shops nowadays allow guide-dogs and, when asked, will provide an assistant to help with shopping.

If medications are required, the RNIB will provide, free of charge, a dispenser to screw on to medicine bottles which will measure out 5 ml. Most chemists can provide labels in Braille to stick on medicine bottles.

Couples embarking on the road to marriage may want advice on genetic counselling, especially if both partners are visually handicapped, which is often the case.

Leisure

Radios are available, where needed, on long-term free loan from the British Wireless for the Blind Fund, and talking books can be obtained from the British Talking Book Library, post free. A minimum reduction in the television licensing fee is available for those registered as blind.

More clubs and associations are opening their doors to people with a visual handicap. The types of hobby they pursue depend on the degree of visual handicap: for instance, a person with tunnel vision can play pool as well as any sighted person, but with a little extra concentration and effort. Other hobbies include fishing, swimming, dancing, climbing, walking, drama and gardening, to name but a few.

Old Age

For a person who has been visually handicapped for some time, it is likely that old age will not present any extra problems that have not already emerged. However, those whose visual handicap has arrived at the onset of old age will need a lot of help. Initially, the social worker will arrange an assessment to see how the person can cope at home. It will be decided with the person and their family how much help they will require, or if sheltered accommodation will be needed. If a telephone is needed for someone living alone, the cost may be met by the local authority. A home improvement grant may be available. The social worker can arrange home help, meals-on-wheels or transport to a day centre luncheon club. Safety devices may be installed in the home, such as rails by the toilet or bath, and bath mats.

Usually, assessments are carried out at 6-monthly intervals, although the family and patient are usually in possession of the social worker's phone number, if any problems arise. More elderly visually handicapped are now being looked after in their own home with help.

To summarize, with adequate support and positive motivation, persons of any age can lead a relatively independent life in their own environment. As will be seen later, problems are created for visually handicapped persons when they are removed to an alien and possibly hostile environment such as hospital (see Chapter 7). Here some of their independence may be lost, and their personal safety may be put at risk.

References

Fraiberg, S. (1977) *Insights from the Blind*, Souvenir Press, London.

Gardiner, E. (undated) Max Factor leaflet, supplied on request.

Woods, G. E. (1975) *The Handicapped Child*, Blackwell Scientific Publications, Oxford.

2 ASPECTS OF COMMUNITY CARE

John Perry

CHAPTER SUMMARY

INTRODUCTION

The present social policy in the UK is aimed at increasing all aspects of medical care in the community rather than in hospital. The Medical Research Council in 1982 showed that the older the age group, the higher the incidence of ocular pathology, as shown in Table 2.1.

Table 2.1 Incidence of eye disease

Age group (years)	Incidence of serious eye disease (%)
52–64	9
65–74	32
75–84	78

As people live longer, the number of people in the community with ophthalmic conditions is increasing. Therefore, the Community Nursing Team is more likely to find itself caring for patients who have defective vision.

The primary source of such patient referrals is the ophthalmic units. The trend in earlier mobilization from improved microsurgical techniques has led to earlier discharge of patients from hospital following eye surgery. Given the predominantly elderly age group of these patients and their shorter stay in hospital, there is a need to ensure that patients are able to comply with the prescribed treatment when they return home and there is, therefore, an increased need to refer to the primary care services.

THE ROLE OF THE COMMUNITY NURSE

The frequency of the prescribed treatment on discharge can be anything from every 2 hours to once daily. With an already excessive workload, it is unrealistic to expect the community nurse to instil all the drops prescribed to patients in their home. Therefore, the role of the community nurse is that of supervisor/mentor, initially visiting daily and slowly withdrawing as competence in self-care develops. In many instances, where elderly patients are unable to instil their own medication, the help of relatives, friends or neighbours may be utilized. The hospital nurse should be aware of the needs of patients on discharge and prepare patients to instil their own medication prior to going home (or friends or relatives, if necessary). It is essential that the level of competence a patient has reached on discharge, or the number of carers who will be helping, is communicated to the community nurse in order to help her plan her workload and identify priorities. She, in turn, needs a sound knowledge of the more common ophthalmic conditions, their treatment and nursing care. A basic knowledge of the actions of topical medication is necessary, as some drugs have to be instilled at specific time periods to be maximally effective, e.g. in glaucoma therapy.

As the general public assume that all nurses have a good knowledge about everything, they will look to the community nurse for advice and reassurance concerning any problems they have. The community nurse should, therefore, have a knowledge of the likely visual outcome of any surgery and when the ultimate visual result is likely. Many patients expect an instant return of good vision after surgery and the community nurse will probably have to reassure patients that this takes time, and support them and their carers for the first few weeks following surgery.

With the shorter hospital stay some complications following surgery may not become apparent until the patient's return home. Where the community nurse is visiting, the patient will usually bring his problems to the nurse's attention. The nurse must, therefore, be able to make an examination of the eye and be able to identify grossly abnormal findings, such as hyphaema, hypopyon, leaking wound, corneal oedema and prolapsed iris, any of which can occur after intraocular surgery, especially if the eye is rubbed or knocked. The nurse should know which problems need to be referred immediately to the ophthalmologist or to the general practitioner and be able to make an accurate report of the examination findings in order to take advice from colleagues. In considering the care the community nurse is required to give to the patient, the care plan opposite may be useful.

When considering a patient's ability in instilling medication following surgery, Donnelly (1987) pointed out that patients who had instilled eye medication prior to their operation did not find the procedure any easier following

Problem	Goal	Nursing intervention
Difficulty in instilling medication due to lack of confidence and practice of the skill.	The patient or carer will develop the skill and confidence to instil medications.	1. Assess the present level of ability to instil medication. 2. Advise the patient on how to improve the skill. 3. Praise and reassure the patient as to his abilities. 4. Gradually withdraw support as confidence and skill develop. 5. Where the patient is unable to master the skill, identify, train and support other carers, e.g. family or neighbours.
Potential complications, following surgery, of infection, inflammation or injury.	The patient will make a satisfactory recovery and complications will be prevented, or detected in the early stages and treatment given.	1. Ensure the patient is aware of hygiene when instilling medication. 2. Advise the patient of difficulties in perception of depth and the possible injuries that can occur when bending forward, hairwashing or carrying very heavy items,e.g. shopping. 3. Procure the help of other carers, voluntary or statutory, when activities of living are compromised by the restrictions. 4. Examine the eye on each visit. Refer patient for appropriate help if there are any abnormal findings or patient complains of severe pain or sudden reduction in vision.

surgery and still required support and reassurance on discharge home. The large majority of patients referred to the community nursing service will have had a cataract extraction. A test for glasses usually occurs at 6–8 weeks following surgery by which time medication is discontinued. The patient's need for community nursing care will vary with each individual and be influenced by whether it is the first or second eye operated on and the amount of family or neighbourly support.

Specialist Ophthalmic Nursing Skills

Felinski (1989), in a study of the skills and knowledge of community nurses in the Central Manchester Health Authority, revealed a higher percentage of nurses who felt unprepared to meet the needs of ophthalmic patients in the community. Given that ophthalmology is considered a minor specialty in most general nursing schools, clinical experience in an ophthalmic unit is a privilege of the few, and present district nurse training does not intend to develop clinical knowledge; it could be suggested that

Felinski's findings be applied on a wider scale unless in-service training is facilitated by employing authorities. In many instances, community nurses, who find themselves ill equipped to deal with a large ophthalmic workload, have developed their own professional knowledge through contact with local ophthalmic units/wards' nursing staff.

In some health authorities, it has been found beneficial to employ a hospital-based ophthalmic community nurse who is able to give more specialist care to patients in their home, such as regular epilation of lashes, removal of lid sutures and care of bandage contact lenses, to name but a few. In areas where no such service exists, such patients have to make frequent visits to the outpatient department, in many instances enduring long waits, especially when transport is required. Given the present economic climate, the employment of a specialist ophthalmic community nurse may not be financially viable but the author is aware of district nursing students who would be prepared to extend the care they give to ophthalmic patients if they were trained to undertake these new skills.

Advising the Ophthalmic Patient

At the beginning of this chapter it was indicated that many of the elderly have serious eye diseases that affect their vision to varying degrees. Many of these people may be clients/patients of a health visitor or district nurse for other reasons and the members of the community nursing team may find it necessary to advise the patient and his immediate family where activities of living are compromised by the reduced vision.

Much of this advice may be given by the health visitor or it could be the role of other professionals, such as the social worker. Whoever is giving the advice requires considerable knowledge to be effective.

The patient may be eligible for registration as blind or partially sighted (Chapter 3) and receive the help following from such registration. If this is not possible, the patient may still benefit from some of the items available to help the visually handicapped and the health visitor should be able to help him purchase such items, either locally or by mail from the Royal National Institute for the Blind. The patient could be advised on the use of contrast and light to help him make maximum use of the vision he has. The following points should identify areas where help can be given.

1. Natural Light

Ensure windows are clean and, if net curtains have to be used, that they are clean as well, to allow as much natural light as possible. Net curtains should be discouraged as they filter the amount of light entering a room. The use of ties for other curtains may be useful. Glare from sunlight in a room can be a hazard and window blinds can eliminate this problem.

2. Artificial Light

Shadows cast by lighting can be effectively reduced by fluorescent light, including reading lamps, and reduced running costs make them very beneficial for daytime use. For the safety of visually handicapped people, light switches are best sited so that they can be switched on before entering a room. Outside lights at exterior doors will aid mobility at night and the use of security lights that are automatically activated when approached will help when the person returns home at night.

Wall lights, floor-standing lamps and table lamps can be strategically placed to aid activities, e.g. over a telephone, over a writing table and at the table used to take meals. Lamps can be placed behind chairs used for reading or sewing, on the bedside table or fitted over the bed. Likewise, a light fitted for shaving or applying make-up is advantageous. The light bulbs or tubes should be of the maximum wattage for the particular lamp and the most appropriate lampshade should be used (Fig. 2.1).

3. Contrasts

Colour contrasts are a very effective way of helping a visually handicapped person identify important objects. Doors and door frames should be a contrasting colour to the walls, which should be a light colour to reflect the light. Carpets should also be of a light plain fabric, as patterns can be mistaken for shadows. Steps should have a white edge for easy identification. Other suggestions for contrast are cutlery against table mats, toilet rolls, cooking utensils, e.g. gravy in a white enamel saucepan, dark razors to contrast with shaving cream and contrasting backgrounds for containers and their contents.

A simple home assessment with the patient can highlight many suggestions to help make life easier. It is worth noting that this form of assessment is not necessarily within the remit of just the community nursing team and can also be undertaken by social services or occupational therapists.

Children

The final area of interest in the care of ophthalmic patients in the community is that of children. All children should have some form of visual assessment and, in the pre-school age groups, this is usually undertaken by the health visitor or, in some areas, the community orthoptic service. The over-fives are usually assessed by the school nursing service at periodic intervals.

Health visitors are usually very involved with visually handicapped or blind children and their families, usually in conjunction with social services and specialist teachers. The health visitor's role can be to support the parents, especially with their emotional acceptance of a disabled child. The parents will also have to be taught how to use play in order to maintain the child's development as much as possible (Chapter 1). Where visual loss is caused by a hereditary disease, support has to be given to the family following genetic counselling.

The whole room is lit by the upwardly directed light from this type of shade, which is suitable for wall lamps
(a)

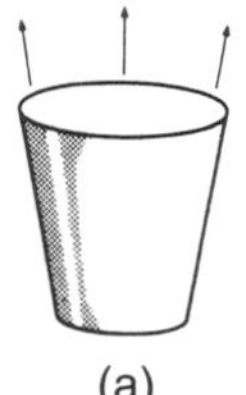

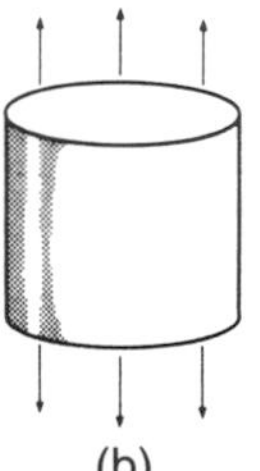

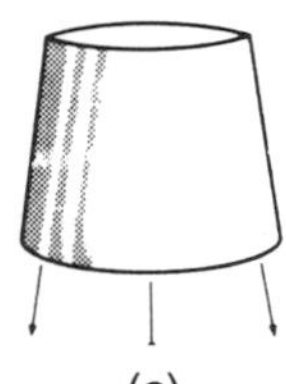

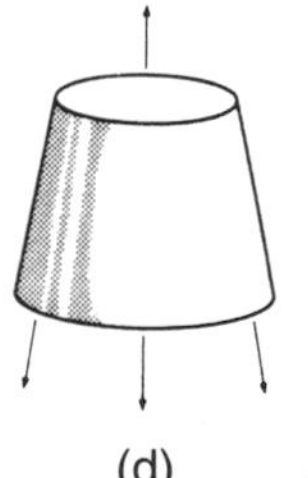

Figure 2.1 Lampshades: useful designs.

Conclusion

The role of the community nursing team in the care of patients with eye disease will increase with the ageing population, current social and health policy and the early discharge of patients. The trend towards day case surgery, especially for cataracts, will make considerable demands on community nursing services. Professional accountability and emphasis on quality of care mean that community nurses must be able to meet these demands and nurses should be asking managers, educationalists and specialized units to provide short clinically-based courses to meet this need.

References

Donnelly, D. (1987) Instilling eyedrops: difficulties experienced by patients following cataract surgery. *Journal of Advanced Nursing*, **12**, 235–243.

Felinski, S. (1989) Not seeing eye to eye. *Nursing Times*, **85** (20), 57–59.

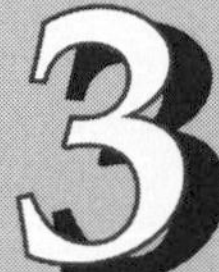

3 Social Aspects of Visual Handicap

Pamela C. Williams and Valerie M. Darbyshire

Chapter Summary

The role of the social worker

Registration procedure

Statutory and voluntary services

The visually handicapped in society

Conclusion

References

Useful addresses

Note
The title 'social worker' has been replaced by 'care manager' since the original writing of this chapter.

This chapter focuses on the social implications of impairment or loss of vision. The first part describes, in general terms, the role of the social worker in a medical setting and then more specifically in an ophthalmic unit. The infinite range of patients' social problems and the nurse's role in the early identification and referral of these problems is discussed. The remaining parts provide a summary of information relating to visually impaired patients. In the procedure for registration as 'blind' or 'partially sighted', the resulting benefits and services are outlined and evaluated. The final section considers the role of the visually handicapped person in society and identifies both positive achievements and negative aspects of disability.

The Role of the Social Worker

The role of the social worker is commonly given scant attention in books and articles written for general nursing staff. In ophthalmic nursing books, the subject almost appears to be taboo. Yet the social worker has a key role to play in the overall health care of hospital patients. Under the new management structure in the National Health Service, units are now being run on a cost-effective basis with the emphasis upon shorter periods of inpatient treatment and, where feasible, an increase in day case surgery. The social worker, in these circumstances, should be available to forge links with services which can support patients on discharge from hospital. This liaison role is only one of a number of tasks undertaken by the social worker which are now outlined in two situations.

The Role of the Social Worker in a Medical Setting

In all areas of medicine and surgery, the social worker's aim is to provide appropriate assistance to each patient referred with social, economic and emotional problems relating to the patient's illness. The kind of assistance offered is wide-ranging, from a simple practical act such as arranging a home help to long-term involvement with the patient and his family in their adjustment to illness, handicap or a terminal condition. The social worker will initially assess whether the referral is appropriate for her particular range of skills, and if so, she will offer help that is tailored as far as resources permit to meet that particular patient's needs.

In contrast to patients' more specific medical conditions, their social circumstances are infinitely variable, depending upon their own ability to cope (personality, intellect, motivation), their family support, housing conditions, financial and employment situations. Although the social worker's objective is to help to improve the patient's quality of life, she also aims to preserve and enhance the patient's ability to be independent. This often entails reinforcing and building on the patient's own strengths and qualities, which can easily become submerged under the grief reactions which normally follow the loss or impairment of any part of the body and compounded often by additional losses – his employment, his role within the family and his self-esteem. Skilled counselling is often required over a period of time and this may be offered by the hospital-based social worker. She tries first to encourage the patient to express his feelings and second to interpret and explain his anxieties and his reactions to his illness, supporting him and his family through the various stages of grieving. This hopefully increases the patient's and his family's understanding of what is happening to him and slowly helps him to adjust to his illness, regain confidence and begin to make plans for the future. In the case of visual impairment, the speed and degree of the patient's adjustment will to some extent be conditioned by his previous attitudes to blindness and expectations of blind people.

The social worker's training in communication skills is of paramount importance in interpreting and conveying information in a medical setting. This task extends far beyond the commonplace communication difficulties between medical staff and the patient and/or his relatives. Enabling communication between members of a family who are under stress, or between the patient, hospital staff and community workers, is a role frequently undertaken by the social worker. She provides a bridge between the institutionalized, protected medical environment and the often harsh realities of the outside world. Skilled communication includes the ability to listen carefully, to make sense of what the patient is saying, especially about how he is feeling, and often to identify an underlying problem which the patient is unable or unwilling to speak about initially. Ideally this should be achieved in a relaxed atmosphere and in privacy; both these conditions are difficult to achieve on a hospital ward.

The social worker's skills at handling interpersonal relationships can prove to be of vital importance in bringing the patient, his family and hospital staff towards a greater understanding of each other's point of view. This could make all the difference between a patient accepting or rejecting a course of treatment. It could also help a spouse towards accepting the partner's illness or disability. The social worker needs to be able to relate to people of all ages, social backgrounds and cultures with equal competence. Underlying much hospital social work is the ability to function as the 'enabler', providing the freedom for patients and staff alike to talk openly and in confidence to someone employed within, but not by, the hospital or unit. An important aspect of this neutral position is that the social worker is able to encourage patients to appreciate their rights and to make their own decisions, for instance whether or not to be registered as visually handicapped. It is equally important, and indeed the duty of the social worker in this situation, to ensure that the patient is well informed before reaching such a decision.

On a more practical level, social workers provide information and advice on a wide range of social problems, including housing, domiciliary care, welfare rights, family and personal difficulties. Having identified with a patient that a particular resource or service would meet his needs, the social worker plays an important role in liaising with appropriate community workers to arrange for the patient to be visited at home. It is important to bear in mind that the services required by that patient may not be readily available. Resources provided by both health authorities and social services departments are overstretched, and waiting lists exist in many areas for such basic requirements as commodes, meals-on-wheels and home helps. Caution is essential in order to avoid raising false hopes. The social worker will try where appropriate to contact the patient's family or neighbours in order to establish a support network prior to discharge. This co-ordinating role is of even greater importance when elderly patients have no family support and are totally dependent upon community services. On admission to hospital the patient is thrown int 'foreign' environment and often feels threatened and vulnerable, having been cut off from everything that is familiar. Re-establishing these community links is critical when discharge is being planned and the social worker's knowledge of community services and resources is invaluable. In spite of this, the level of hospital social work support in some parts of the country is being drastically reduced, if not withdrawn altogether, as part of the current effort by some local authorities to reduce spending levels.

The Role of the Social Worker in an Ophthalmic Unit

Here the social worker requires additional specific knowledge of eye disease and visual handicap in all its aspects. Blind people quickly become disillusioned with social workers who do not have this specialist knowledge to draw upon.

Credibility is important in building up a positive relationship between social worker and client: for instance, when dealing with a newly blind patient or the parents of a blind baby, the social worker will strive to gain the patient's confidence by first demonstrating that she has knowledge and experience of the effects of blindness, the rehabilitation skills needed and the services available.

Ophthalmic units vary in size from a small ward in a district general hospital to large teaching eye hospitals. Referrals can be made from any department to the social worker, who is often required to balance the need to respond to an emergency with that of offering longer-term support and counselling to patients who, for instance, have problems in adjusting to their loss of vision. Referrals from the Accident and Emergency Department may concern injuries to children where the doctor or nurses suspects child abuse (non-accidental injury). The social worker has an essential part to play in the ensuing enquiries which may include arranging a case conference after the child's admission to hospital or, in extreme cases, applying to a court or a Justice of the Peace for a Place of Safety Order to ensure that the child is admitted to or remains in hospital. Subsequently the social worker may be involved in court proceedings regarding the child's future care.

Referrals from the ophthalmic children's ward often involve supporting the parents of a child whose eye condition has just been diagnosed and who will be permanently visually impaired. The social worker might also be asked to see a child who shows signs of distress on the ward concerning difficulties at home or at school often related to his visual problems. The social worker is sometimes asked to provide the link between a blind child and his school- or area-based social worker during the child's admission to hospital. Parents commonly experience financial and other difficulties in arranging daily visits to their children or care for other siblings. When a child is referred to a national hospital many miles away for treatment, the social worker will, if appropriate, liaise with a colleague in advance to meet the child and his parents on arrival, in order to provide continuing support in their crisis.

Ophthalmic wards for adults refer patients to the social worker for the whole range of services and support already described but, in addition, refer patients for urgent specialized counselling who have suffered severe or total loss of vision due to trauma, natural causes or, sometimes, following surgery. In some instances, patients who have lost the vision of only one eye require as much help and support as the severely visually impaired in coping initially with that loss. The work undertaken by the social worker frequently extends to the patient's relatives, who suffer similar reactions and emotional responses to those events. The social worker's task includes careful listening and assessing the patient's understanding of the crisis, allowing the patient to express his feelings, giving information and advice, planning and offering counselling on a longer-term basis. With the patient's permission, she may also need to liaise with a great range of people, departments and organizations prior to his discharge (Fig. 3.1).

Not all the social worker's ophthalmic ward referrals, however, are concerned with loss of vision. A considerable proportion of the workload is akin to that of an acute ward on a geriatric unit. Many patients admitted for surgery, especially for cataracts, are elderly and some of these are frail, either physically or mentally, and live alone. Suitable arrangements have to be made for their support on discharge in conjunction with their families or other carers, within the two- or three-day postoperative period. These ophthalmic patients, and younger patients admitted for minor surgery or treatment, should be distinguished from patients of all ages who are faced with sight-threatening conditions and poor prognoses or who are already visually handicapped. The aim of cataract surgery is after all to improve vision. The two groups of patients have different expectations and different needs.

Other referrals come to the ophthalmic social worker from a variety of sources both within and outside the hospital. Doctors in outpatient departments refer patients who appear distressed when registration (as blind or

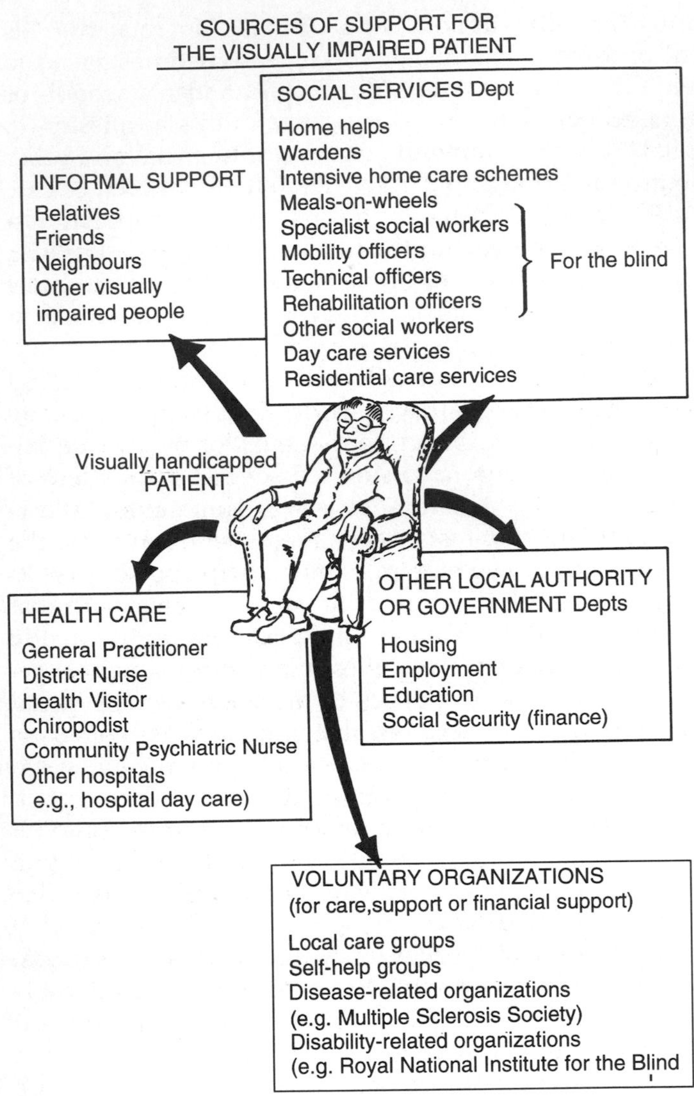

Figure 3.1 Sources of support for the visually impaired patient.

partially-sighted) is discussed or who appear to have difficulty in caring for themselves due to poor vision. From the same source, or from the Accident and Emergency Department, come referrals requesting that emergency care arrangements be made for a dependent relative when an ophthalmic patient needs to be admitted urgently. Opticians refer patients who confide that they are, for instance, burning their fingers while using the cooker or who require a white cane for safer travel. Relatives and other professionals often approach the social worker directly for information and advice of a specialist nature. Where the request concerns a specific patient the social worker would only be able to help if that patient was fully aware of the enquiry.

The Role of the Nurse Regarding Patients' Social Problems

No mention has been made, so far, of the nurse's role in dealing with patients' social problems. Some professionals feel that their particular contribution to the patient's care is so clearly defined that no other professional should encroach upon their territory. There is no 'right' or 'wrong' person to help a patient who is clearly in distress and needs to talk. The nurse is trained to deal with the patient's anxiety on admission to the ward or on the day he is going to theatre. If, in addition, he needs to unburden himself of some particular worry in the middle of the night or while in the bath, then the 'right' person is the one who is on hand at the time. In this, the nurse also needs to be an attentive listener. The nurse's role at this stage is to be able to determine whether the patient could be helped by the social worker and if so, whether he would agree to being referred. Identifying problems at an early stage is an important task for the nurse but the real skill is in knowing if and when to refer to another worker. The nurse should gain sufficient general knowledge of visual handicap from the remaining parts of this chapter to be able to answer straightforward queries or to give general advice. She should therefore be better informed in order to decide what should be referred to the social worker and what could be dealt with by ward staff.

Patient Support Services

The time of registration can be extremely traumatic for the patient and though medical and nursing staff may be concerned for the individual they do not always have adequate time to discuss the implications of registration fully. At such times the patient needs to talk to someone who understands the problems and can offer advice and information on services as well as provide access to counselling if required. In a number of hospitals around the country advisory services have been set up by voluntary societies in partnership with the hospital. Henshaw's Society for the Blind provides such a service at the Manchester Royal Eye Hospital.

This service is complementary to the service provided by the social worker. Patients value the opportunity to discuss their problems in this way and a great number of worries and concerns can be addressed at an early stage.

Registration Procedure

Most people imagine that 'blind' people live in a world of total darkness and that partially sighted people can see very little. In fact there are many varied degrees of vision within the categories of 'blindness' and 'partial sight', and much confusion in the minds of the general public in distinguishing between the two groups.

The statutory definition of blindness is 'so blind as to be unable to perform any work for which eyesight is essential'. Though there is no legal definition of partial sight, it is deemed that persons may be registered partially sighted if they are 'substantially and permanently handicapped by defective vision caused by congenital defect, illness or injury'.

The registration document BD8 is completed by a consultant ophthalmologist if the patient agrees to be registered. There is a choice about this and some people may not wish to be registered, seeing registration as a sort of stigma. The idea of being on a register held by the 'authorities' or being 'known to Social Services' is seen by some as a disadvantage. If a person does not wish to be registered then that is his choice and should be respected. It should not, however, prevent him from obtaining services that will be helpful to him. The patient's right to self-determination is of great importance.

The BD8 form was revised in 1990 and now consists of five parts. Parts 1–4 comprise the main registration document and Part 5 is for statistical purposes only. After the BD8 has been completed a copy is held by the consultant, further copies of the form are distributed to the patient's GP, the local Social Services Department, and the final copy is available to the patient. Part 5 is sent to the Office of Population Censuses and Surveys.

There are no great financial benefits to be derived from registration and, contrary to popular belief, there is no such thing as a 'blind person'. Registration as a blind person does not give any automatic right to any financial assistance. For those blind people who pay income tax there is an additional personal allowance and details of registration should be sent to the local Inspector of Taxes in order to claim extra allowance. Social Services Departments will normally provide a letter confirming date of registration for this purpose. A very small reduction is allowed on the price of a TV licence – currently £1.25. Travel concessions are available in most areas with free passes for local travel.

However, the details of such concessions may vary from area to area and need to be checked out locally. Car parking concessions via the Orange Badge Scheme can be obtained through Social Services Departments.

The British Wireless for the Blind Fund provides radios/cassette players for registered blind people. Certain items for blind people can be sent through the post free of charge by using an 'Article for the Blind' label (available via resource centres or from the Royal National Institute for the Blind – RNIB). The benefits listed so far only apply to people who are registered blind.

People who are registered blind or partially sighted are eligible for membership of the Talking Book Library, administered by the RNIB. Books are recorded on special cassettes and a playback machine is provided. Cassettes are delivered to the individual's home via the postal service. A similar postal service using standard cassettes is offered by the 'Calibre' library. In some areas of the country local authority libraries provide taped material that may be borrowed by people who are visually impaired. In addition, talking newspapers are available in many areas, providing regularly recorded local news on standard cassettes. Registration as blind or partially sighted is a qualification for Severe Disablement Allowance, but only if all other criteria are met.

Similarly, people who are registered blind or partially sighted may qualify for Disability Living Allowance, which comprises a care component and a mobility component. There is also a Disability Working Allowance for those people who are working at least 16 hours per week but whose earning capacity is limited by illness or disability. People who are registered may qualify for higher rates of income support and housing benefit and possibly a rebate against Council Tax. Individuals should be advised to contact their local Benefits Agency for further information.

The range of services available through the Social Services Departments regardless of registration includes home help, domiciliary care, luncheon clubs, meals-on-wheels, day care and social work support.

Under the National Health Service and Community Care Act 1990, Social Services Departments are required to carry out an assessment of individual needs; the wishes and needs of carers are also taken into account and a suitable package of care should be designed to meet the needs of each individual. On receipt of a completed BD8 form Social Services will normally arrange for such an assessment to take place. Sadly, the number of specialist officers is declining and some authorities have little in the way of specialist services. They can now, however, 'purchase' specialist services from a variety of 'providers', ensuring that appropriate care is available, if not from their own resources. For example, local authorities may choose to buy in rehabilitation services from a voluntary society if they have no specialist staff and this arrangement can work very satisfactorily for the benefit of visually impaired people.

Statutory and Voluntary Services

The previous section dealt with registration procedures and outlined some of the benefits and services which may be available to people who are visually impaired. In some instances gaining access to these services can be difficult for the patient, and there is no uniformity of provision. Standards and levels of service will vary from area to area.

Prior to 1970, services for blind and partially sighted people were provided by Welfare Departments of local authorities according to the requirements of the National Assistance Act 1948. However, with the inception of Social Services Departments and a generic form of service provision, services to visually impaired people have been diluted and specialist services are given a low priority (Shore, 1985).

Social work services are often described as inadequate, an opinion borne out by the Social Services Inspectorate report *A Wider Vision* (1988) and the RNIB Needs Surveys (Bruce, McKennell and Walker, 1991; Tobin and Walker, 1992). Over the years since the Blind Persons Act of 1920, various pieces of legislation have influenced the provision of services. Section 29 of the National Assistance Act 1948 required local authorities to provide welfare services for blind and partially sighted people. The Chronically Sick and Disabled Persons Act 1970 placed a duty on local authorities to meet the identified needs of disabled people, including blind and partially sighted people. The Disabled Persons (Services, Consultation and Representation) Act 1986 strengthened their rights to services and took greater account of the needs of carers. Unfortunately, local authority funds are not always sufficient to meet these requirements.

The recently implemented National Health Service and Community Care Act 1990 required local authorities and health authorities to publish their community care plans in order to provide a comprehensive range of care for people in the community.

Social Services Departments are required to undertake full community care assessments to identify individual needs and, in consultation with service users, carers, medical and nursing staff, to find suitable packages of care to meet those needs. When needs cannot be met from their own resources, they are able to purchase from other agencies. This is an opportunity for local authorities to draw on the expertise of those organizations that provide specialist services for visually impaired people.

Some local voluntary societies provide resource centres where visually impaired people can obtain equipment, information and advice relating to all aspects of visual handicap. These resource centres are often the focal point for activities for visually impaired people and are a valuable addition to the services provided by the statutory sector.

There are organizations that cater for the particular needs of people who are both deaf and blind; they are listed below in Useful Addresses.

Traditionally, voluntary organizations have pioneered services for people who are visually impaired as well as supplementing statutory provision. The new legislation affords the opportunity for more joint working and improved services which will enhance the quality of life for visually impaired people.

Rehabilitation Services

For most people the prospect of losing their sight is very frightening. However, it really is not possible to lay down a set of rules for working with people who have a visual impairment because, like everyone else, they are all different, all possessing different skills and talents, all with different personalities. Some will be totally independent and perfectly able to manage while others may need help with almost everything. What is vital is that we, as professionals coming into contact with visually impaired people, do not rely on our imagination with regard to their abilities or disabilities.

The reader will be aware that there are many varied degrees of vision within the definitions of blindness and partial sight. There are also differences between those people who are born blind and those who become blind in later life. So it is important to check with each individual what they can or cannot see; then the appropriate help can be offered.

There is a misconception on the part of some well-meaning sighted people that blind people are endowed with some extra 'sixth sense' and are more cheerful or gifted than the rest of the human race. This of course is not the case. They can be just as difficult as the rest of us – because they are people, not because they are blind.

When thinking in terms of rehabilitation, one has to consider certain points. Each individual's adjustment will depend on his own character, situation and attitude. He will also be greatly affected by the attitudes of those around him. It was Helen Keller who said, 'It is not blindness but the attitude of the seeing to the blind which is the hardest burden to bear'. Those who are born blind grow up without having experienced sight and their concept of the world around them is made up of touch, sound, taste and smell. However, those who lose sight in later life are quite different. They often retain some residual vision which can be used quite effectively, and generally they retain some visual memory, having lived most of their lives as sighted individuals. This visual memory can be used in their rehabilitation programmes.

In order to offer constructive help we need to understand what it is really like to be visually impaired. One way of doing this is to think of a typical day's activities and imagine trying to do all those things without sight. Imagine boiling a kettle, pouring a cup of tea, crossing a room full of furniture, let alone a busy road! All are extremely hazardous when you cannot see.

Rehabilitation training offers practical help from skilled staff to enable visually impaired people to manage their daily lives. Such training can be arranged at a residential centre, at a day centre or in the client's own home, whichever is most appropriate. Rehabilitation officers are able to design, implement and evaluate individual programmes of rehabilitation leading towards greater integration, self-determination and independence for visually impaired people of all ages, and their families.

The overall aim of rehabilitation is to enable visually impaired people to continue performing the tasks they have always done, by simply finding 'other ways'. There is no doubt that visual impairment makes daily life exceedingly difficult, but with the use of special equipment and a simple methodical approach it is possible for people to maintain their independence.

Three of the most important aspects of rehabilitation are mobility, communication and daily living skills.

Mobility

Even moving around your own home can create panic when your sight is diminished. Mobility training sets out to enable the individual to relate to his environment. This means learning to use the other senses more effectively. The degree of mobility which can be achieved, as with all aspects of rehabilitation, depends on physical, psychological and social factors unique to each individual, among the most significant being the person's motivation and immediate goals. The nature of the visual impairment, whether total or partial, is of prime importance – someone with light perception, for example, has a point of reference that a totally blind person does not. Someone who can distinguish shapes or forms can often identify and make good use of visual cues.

Areas covered in mobility training include basic orientation, outdoor and indoor mobility, use of sighted guide and use of appropriate aid, e.g. guide cane, long cane. Occasionally a powerful lens is all the help a person needs. Guide dog training may also be recommended for a younger, physically fit person.

It should be noted that it may take many hours of instruction to enable a person to become independently mobile. Individual contracts are agreed at the onset of training, so it can be a long and arduous process.

Communication

Communication can become a serious problem for the visually impaired person. It is astonishing how much visual information we take in without even noticing. The meaningful expressions and gestures we all use as part of our non-verbal communication are lost, or at best distorted, to a visually impaired person. We receive information via the senses of taste, smell, touch, vision and hearing. If any of the senses are missing or impaired, the quality of the experience is reduced.

In more general terms shop windows, advertising hoardings, books, magazines, newspapers, TV, all sources of visual information are lost to the blind and partially sighted.

Some systems are available which help to compensate for this loss. Rehabilitation officers can teach Braille and Moon, which are systems of embossed print, enabling blind people to read and write; however, only a very small percentage of blind people are Braillists. Typing is a useful skill which is also taught by rehabilitation officers. Talking books are of tremendous value to the visually impaired. Talking newspapers are also available now in many areas, keeping visually impaired people informed of local events. Tape recorders are used by a great many blind people for correspondence and the storage of information. Rehabilitation officers instruct in their use.

Low vision aids prescribed through the Hospital Eye Service and certain local opticians are of great benefit to some people. It is helpful, when meeting someone with visual impairment, to verbalize to avoid confusion. Always address the person by name. Always inform the blind person when you are leaving – a light touch on the arm can be helpful. Be clear in what you say – do not rely on facial expressions and gestures to convey moods or feelings.

Daily Living Skills

By using a variety of aids and gadgets it is possible to help visually impaired people undertake many household tasks.

Rehabilitation officers can offer advice about lighting; appropriately positioned light can improve visual acuity quite markedly, as can careful use of contrast.

It is vital that size, light and contrast are considered when dealing with visually impaired people. It is also extremely important that anyone who comes into contact with visually impaired people realizes that everything must be kept in its place; a change of position of furniture or possessions can be disastrous for someone with failing sight.

It is also important to ensure that visually impaired people are helped to access leisure activities and this is an integral part of the rehabilitation process. Rehabilitation officers liaise with social workers, teachers, consultants, doctors, nurses and appropriate voluntary agencies to ensure that visually impaired people receive services that meet their needs.

There is no stereotype pattern of rehabilitation and many clients find their own solutions. However, with care, guidance, strength, determination and the passing of time, most people can be taught to cope. Of course their problems do not go away, but they become manageable. With appropriate support, facilities and training, visually impaired people can and do lead useful lives, making a valuable contribution to the communities in which they live.

Visually Impaired Children

The RNIB Survey, Vol. 2, *Blind and Partially Sighted Children in Britain* (Tobin and Walker, 1992), estimates that there are around 10 000 children who are visually impaired but in England only about 4500 are registered as such.

When a child is registered as blind or partially sighted his parents and family are also likely to need a considerable amount of support.

As well as the statutory services provided by local education authorities and Social Services Departments, additional provision is available through voluntary societies and various parent support groups.

The Education Act 1981, implemented in April 1983, imposed a duty on local education authorities (LEAs) to provide for children with special needs in 'mainstream' schools. Children with special needs are formally assessed and a 'statement' of special educational needs is prepared, outlining how the LEA will meet those needs. Parents have a right to examine the 'statement' and to express their opinion as to how their child's needs can best be met.

Statements must be renewed every year. Under the Disabled Persons (Services, Consultation and Representation) Act 1986, LEAs and Social Services Departments are required to identify children with disabilities at the age of 14. LEAs must keep school leaving dates of disabled children under review and must notify Social Services of that date 8–12 months in advance. Social Services Departments should then carry out an assessment of a young person's needs for social services within 5 months.

The Children Act of 1989 requires local authority Social Services Departments to keep registers of children 'in need', including children who are blind or partially sighted. This Act has brought their needs into the mainstream of provision of services for children. The Act also requires local authorities to provide help with such things as holidays and day care for children in need and, taking account of parents' and children's wishes, to provide an appropriate package of care.

The Royal National Institute for the Blind offers an educational advisory service and a number of other organizations provide help and support for parents.

Henshaw's Society for the Blind offers a comprehensive information, advice and counselling service for parents via their resource centres in Manchester and Liverpool and their patient support service at Manchester Royal Eye Hospital. The Royal London Society for the Blind runs a parents' support service at Moorfields Eye Hospital.

LOOK is an umbrella organization for parent support groups across the country.

A social worker or rehabilitation officer should be able to advise on local sources of help.

Training and Employment

The Employment Department offers a range of services specifically for people who are disabled and has a commitment to enabling disabled people to achieve their potential with regard to training and employment.

In 1992 the Employment Service was restructured and set up new teams of specialist workers known as placement, assessment and counselling teams (PACT) and nine ability development centres (ADCs).

The Disability Employment Advisers based at local job centres are part of the PACT and work with disabled people who need help in obtaining employment. The Disabled Persons Register is a voluntary register held by the Employment Department as distinct from registers held by local authorities.

'Access to Work' is a new scheme which commenced in June 1994. It includes a range of services for disabled people and their employers and can offer help to unemployed, employed and self-employed disabled people. Access to Work is run by PACT teams and can pay for certain special facilities, as described in the Employment Department group publication *Disabled People and Work*.

Training and Enterprise Councils (TECs) and Local Enterprise Companies (LECs) offer training for disabled people. There are 82 TECs in England and Wales and 22 LECs in Scotland. They can provide advice on job training, starting a business, expanding a business and making career and training decisions. The Job Centre is the starting point to access these specialist services.

The RNIB has five regional employment teams providing support and advice on all employment matters for visually impaired people. The RNIB also has a student support service.

Recreation

Besides the more formal aspects of rehabilitation already discussed, leisure pursuits play an important part in the overall process. Recreational activities for the blind are infinitely varied, according to individual interests and abilities. For the less active elderly person a weekly outing to a local 'blind club' for tea and a chat may prove to be an essential lifeline, especially since many in this group are socially isolated. At the other end of the scale, blind athletes competed successfully in the World Championships and Games for the Disabled, held in Sweden in 1986, gaining 13 gold medals for Great Britain.

The newly blind person would be well advised to try to continue, if at all possible, with his previous interests, if they can be adapted. There are, however, many activities, outdoor and indoor, particularly well suited to the needs of visually handicapped people. Outdoor pursuits include fell-walking, sailing, angling, archery, bowling, gardening, tandem cycling and all manner of sporting activities. Indoor hobbies include music, drama, craft work, woodwork, card games, chess, draughts, dominoes and a variety of other table games, which are available from the RNIB, specially adapted for use by visually handicapped people. However, many well-adjusted independent blind people have virtually no contact with leisure groups organized specifically for the blind, preferring to participate as far as possible on equal terms with their sighted friends and colleagues.

The Visually Handicapped in Society

There is a forceful argument for not writing this section at all! By writing about 'the visually handicapped' as a group there is a danger of perpetuating the attitude that they all have features in common, for instance, 'blind people are cheerful'. By generalizing about 'the visually handicapped' we are indeed stigmatizing them, identifying them as different from the rest of society, while the great majority of visually handicapped people are in fact striving to make their contribution to society in as ordinary and individual a manner as possible. It is hoped, however, that the value of this section will lie in encouraging the nurse to look at some of society's entrenched attitudes towards 'the blind' and to consider her own stance on the subject before encountering her first visually handicapped patients.

One of the most striking and enduring features of the video accompanying the Staff Development Package on Visual Handicap (Welsh Office, 1981) is the interview with the gentleman who pleads with the viewer to treat him as an ordinary person. What appears, on the surface, to be a straightforward and reasonable request in fact conceals wide-ranging prejudices shown by society in general towards disabled people. The International Year of Disabled People 1981 was planned not purely to raise funds or provide ramps to public buildings, though these aims are worthy in themselves. The much wider objective was to increase public awareness of disability and of the very ordinary needs of disabled people; it was intended to incorporate these needs into society's future planning and development, particularly in relation to buildings, as commonplace rather than exceptional. It was hoped that the person in a wheelchair or using a white cane might eventually come to be accepted as a normal member of society who just happens not to be able to walk or see. Alas, 12 months was not long enough to offset centuries of prejudice! In fact, a major part of the 'handicap' endured by disabled people is created by the attitudes of able-bodied members of the community who all too often focus on the disability and fail to see the whole person.

The pathetic image of the blind man selling matches or busking with an accordion is still alive in the minds of too many people today. This image of helplessness and dependency evokes pity and a patronizing attitude, for example, by expressing unwarranted amazement at some ordinary everyday achievement. Sighted people often experience fear and uncertainty in encounters with blind people; fear that they would be unable to cope with such a situation themselves and fear about how to behave in the presence of a blind person. Faced with this, a sighted person may seek ways of avoiding his own discomfort by either shunning the blind person or trying to hide his own embarrassment by overwhelming the blind person with inappropriate help or unnaturally bright and jolly conversation.

Visually handicapped people are as diverse in terms of personality, intellect, occupation, interests and range of social problems as the rest of the population. The only common denominator is their visual disability. As demonstrated earlier, the social worker for the visually handicapped can be presented with any problem across the whole spectrum of social work tasks; statutory child care, financial difficulties, housing problems, domiciliary care and family crises, including divorce, are typical but no different from demands from the sighted population. Neither does visual handicap respect particular social groupings, with patients coming to eye hospitals from all walks of life, from company directors to workers on the shop floor, from the professionally qualified to manual labourers. Visually handicapped people are not bestowed with unreal virtues either! A small number become inmates of HM prisons, while others become addicted to drugs or alcohol. In general terms, the problems of visually handicapped people only reflect problems within society as a whole.

The same principle applies when considering the achievements of blind people in our society. Seen first in terms of employment, blind people are engaged in this country in industry, in commerce and in the professions. In light engineering they undertake assembly work, machine operating and inspection work. In the commercial world they occupy posts from junior typist to managing director. Within professional occupations blind people work in the church, law, social work, teaching, physiotherapy and music (including piano tuning). In recent years the growth of the computer industry has provided an added bonus for the blind people who can be trained to work as computer programmers. Within these work settings, some blind people have achieved success, promotion and acclaim on personal merit while others, working within their own limits, remain in routine occupations with no aspirations for advancement. This situation is not restricted to visually handicapped employees but is applicable to the workforce in general.

There are, however, some visually handicapped people who are outstandingly successful within their own spheres. Some blind musicians have achieved international fame as composers and performers in 'pop', jazz and classical music. Some blind university lecturers and teachers have been acclaimed for their research and expertise in their given areas of study. Some blind people have successfully served their communities as elected local councillors. One notable recent example of such success is David Blunkett who, after the general election of 1987, became the first blind MP to enter the House of Commons for 30 years. He had previously served as Leader of Sheffield City Council and had also been elected to the National Executive of the Labour Party and to the Shadow Cabinet.

Of equal importance, however, are the achievements of the many hundreds of blind people who neither seek nor hope to achieve national fame and who are never likely to become household names. These ordinary members of society may be unobtrusively pursuing their jobs and bringing up families, but equally deserve admiration for their personal achievements in overcoming society's prejudices. There is, for example, a widespread belief that a blind woman could not possibly undertake the role of wife and mother, simply because of her blindness. Yet there are numerous examples in this country of blind parents successfully bringing up children. Parenting skills are rooted in the ability of an individual to provide a secure and stable emotional relationship as well as physical care. Blindness does not prevent a mother from providing love, warmth and security for her child. A well-adjusted blind mother will know when to ask for practical help. Some support from a sighted relative or friend is usually welcomed, if only to match up pairs of socks! The extra effort, concentration and organization required from the visually handicapped person to achieve the same goals as his sighted counterpart should, however, not be underestimated. Some blind people succeed in making their daily routine look easy but frustration, stress and tiredness are often experienced, especially in combining, for instance, a full-time job with parenthood or running a home.

The ophthalmic nurse has a particular responsibility towards her patients and blind people in general to try to counteract the prejudice held by society at large, which inhibits and handicaps their lifestyle, by approaching blind people in an open, non-judgemental manner; by accepting blind people as full and responsible members of society, wanting to play their part; by not patronizing blind people; by helping to educate the general public and increase its awareness of the needs of blind people; by offering practical help as and when required in a manner acceptable to the blind person, this being especially important in the unfamiliar hospital environment. The goodwill and dedication of the ophthalmic nurse in fostering these attitudes are vital elements in the campaign to effect some long-term change in public opinion.

Conclusion

The purpose of this chapter has been to provide an insight into the social problems that may result from visual handicap, an appreciation of the role of the social worker in tackling these problems and a knowledge of the range of services available. This should enable the reader to acquire an overall picture of what can be achieved by blind people while remaining realistic about the limitations of resources available. Nursing and social work staff have a shared objective in trying to promote the interests of visually handicapped patients. A collaborative approach can only serve to improve the standard of patient care.

The opinions expressed in this chapter are based on the writers' experiences in specialist social work and do not necessarily represent the views of their previous or present employers.

References

Bruce, I. McKennell, A. and Walker, E. (1991) *Blind and Partially Sighted Adults in Britain: The RNIB Survey*, Vol. 1, HMSO, London.

Tobin, M. and Walker, E. (1992) *Blind and Partially Sighted Children in Britain: The RNIB Survey*, Vol. 2, HMSO, London.

Shore, P. (1985) *Local Authority Social Rehabilitation Services to Visually Handicapped People*, Royal National Institute for the Blind, London.

Social Services Inspectorate (1988) *A Wider Vision*, HMSO, London.

Welsh Office (1981) Video Accompanying Staff Development Package on Visual Handicap, HMSO, London.

Useful Addresses

British Talking Book Services
Mount Pleasant, Alperton, Wembley, Middlesex HA10 1RR
Tel: 0181 903 6666

The Disabled Living Foundation
380–384 Harrow Road, London W9 2HU
Tel: 0171 289 6111

Guide Dogs for the Blind Association
Alexandra House, 9–11 Park Street, Windsor, Berkshire SL4 1JR
Tel: 01753 855711/7

Henshaw's Society for the Blind
Warwick Road, Old Trafford, Manchester M16 OGS
Tel: 0161 872 1234

National Deaf Blind League
18 Rainbow Court, Paston Ridings, Peterborough PE4 6UP
Tel: 01733 573511

National Library for the Blind
Cromwell Road, Bredbury, Stockport SK6 2SG
Tel: 0161 494 0217

North Regional Association for the Blind
Headingley Castle, Headingley Lane, Leeds, West Yorkshire LS6 2DQ
Tel: 0113 275/2666/7

Partially Sighted Society
Queens Road, Doncaster DN1 2NX
Tel: 01302 68998

Royal National Institute for the Blind
224 Great Portland Street, London W1A 6AA
Tel: 0171 388 1266

Royal National Institute for the Blind School of Rehabilitation Studies
University of Central England, Faculty of Health and Social Studies, Cox Buildings, Perry Bar, Birmingham B4 2SV
Tel: 0121 331 5000

St Dunstan's Working for Men and Women Blinded in the Services
PO Box 4XB, 12–14 Harcourt Street, London W1A 4XB
Tel: 0171 723 5021

The Scottish National Federation for the Blind
PO Box 500, Gillespie Crescent, Edinburgh EH10 4HZ
Tel: 0131 229 1456

SENSE (National Deaf Blind and Rubella Association)
11–13 Clifton Terrace, Finsbury Park, London N4 3SR
Tel: 0171 272 7774

South Regional Association for the Blind
55 Eton Avenue, London NW3 3ET
Tel: 0171 722 9703

Talking Newspaper Association of the United Kingdom
National Recording Centre, Heathfield, East Sussex TN21 8JD
Tel: 01435 866102

Telephone for the Blind Fund
Green Haynes, Dean Oak Lane, Leigh, Surrey RH2 8PZ
Tel: 01293 862472

Wales Council for the Blind
Shand House, 20 Newport Road, Cardiff CF2 1YB
Tel: 01222 473954

4

MODELS FOR OPHTHALMIC NURSING PRACTICE

Mary Rowell

CHAPTER SUMMARY

The purpose of this chapter is to examine the use of models in ophthalmic nursing practice. Before discussing their specific application, however, it is worth considering some general points about the nature and function of models.

Individuals and groups tend to accept many beliefs without question. These beliefs, often taken for granted, are instilled into those who are learning, and presupposed in the forming of further ideas. For this reason, if for no other, it is important that we examine the beliefs which form the 'springboard' for our action. In my view, nursing needs to adopt an eclectic approach. We need to evaluate critically the assumption on which practice is based. The points raised in this chapter are intended to initiate some exploration of the beliefs which underpin our commitment to care in the speciality of ophthalmic nursing. Parts of several models may be useful in building a relevant one for the situation in which we work together to provide informed and sensitive care. It may be that one particular model comes close to our shared conception of what is important for practice; however, commitment to such a model, and its feasibility, will depend upon the following.

1. The model developed, while it may derive support from models already practised, should evolve from the shared beliefs of those people actually concerned with the specific care setting.
2. It should be flexible.
3. The development must take account of the reality of nursing practice within the context in which it is to be used.

It will be important to keep these points in mind while examining current nursing theory.

The Nature of Models

A model by definition provides a representation of reality. An architect presenting a proposal for a building design will produce for consideration a three-dimensional representation of the proposed structure. Models of this sort are made up of small-scale raw materials. A nursing model is similar, in that it provides a representation of reality, but in contrast consists of ideas, assumptions and knowledge. Models of this type are a means by which we can organize these component parts. In developing a model we are enabled to identify important concepts and thus, the model provides a framework for action (Table 4.1).

Working models include concepts that we believe are important in practice. These in turn reflect our values and beliefs. Three essential components may be clearly identified in a model for practice:

1. the beliefs and values which provide the foundation for the model;
2. the goals or aims of the practitioner;
3. the knowledge and skills that the practitioner requires in order to achieve these goals.

Roy (1984) outlines the essential elements of a model for nursing practice as:

1. a description of the nature of the person receiving care;
2. a statement of the goal of nursing;
3. a definition of health;

Table 4.1 Developmental influences on self-care in relation to the requirements for effective living

Life changes	Common requirements for effective living	Life-cycle stages
Poor health/disability	Air	Intra-uterine stages
Oppressive living conditions	Water	Neonatal stages
Terminal illness/impending death	Food	Infancy
Status-associated problems	Elimination	Childhood
Abrupt change of residence or environment	Activity/rest	Adolescence
Education deprivation	Social interaction/solitude	Early adulthood
Problems of social adaptation	Prevention of hazards	Development stages
Failure to establish health individuality	Promotion of normality	Pregnancy
Loss of relatives		Middle age
Loss of jobs or possessions		Old age

4. a specified meaning of environment;
5. a representation of nursing activities.

Why Use a Model?

Each of us, although we may not be consciously aware of it, attempts to give some structure or organization to our diverse ideas. In so doing, we examine and use the relationships which exist between the ideas. This process leads us to form personal models which guide our actions. Very often these personal models are not shared and thus remain implicit.

The concept and subsequent practice of nursing is influenced by many external factors, e.g. social administration, medical technology and public expectation. The care given to the individual is also influenced by the implicit model held by the nurse giving the care.

It is important, therefore, that all those concerned in the delivery of care together identify the concepts which they think are important. In this way, a model of care is made explicit and avoids conflict and confusion for both patients and nurses alike.

McFarlane (1986) stresses the complexity of nursing and suggests that models may have a value for practice in a number of different ways. They may:

1. serve as a tool which links theory and practice;
2. clarify our thinking about the elements of a practice situation and their relationship to each other;
3. help practitioners of nursing to communicate with each other more meaningfully;
4. serve as a guide to practice, education and research.

Types of Model

In recent years there has been an emergence of models in nursing. These models have been used in practice and widely publicized. Models derive from fundamental theories and concepts, and they may be clearly classified according to their specified focus. Models represent differing theories about the nature of the persons receiving care, and views concerning the aims of care, and the nursing activities required to achieve these aims.

Systems Models

The concept of a system is one which will be familiar to nurses. An example in physiology is the respiratory system. Another is a filing system using paper or computer disk.

People may also be described as systems and models of this type make use of general systems theory, as a foundation for the analysis of a nursing situation. The person is viewed as an open system, that is, one which can constantly interact with its environment. Roy, Riehl and Roy (1980) and Johnson (1980), in their development of models for care, view the person as an individual possessing biological, psychological and social systems which are interrelated. The internal systems exist in a state of constant interaction with the external environment and can be affected by stressors which occur within the system or which are external to the system. The person is seen as striving to maintain relative balance both internally and in respect of the external environment. The focus of nursing intervention involves manipulating the relationship between the environmental stimuli and the patient's ability to adapt to one stimulus.

Interaction Models

These models focus on the nature of the nurse–patient interaction. They are based on a theory of symbolism through which people are seen to be able to give meaning to the external stimuli with which they interact. Blumer (1969) outlined three essential elements of this theory.

1. Human beings act towards things on the basis of the meanings that things have for them.
2. The meaning of such things is derived from, or arises out of, the social interaction that one has with one's fellows.
3. These meanings are handled in, and modified through, interpretation processes used by the person in dealing with things he encounters.

On this view the nurse is seen as assisting the patient or client in finding a meaning in a situation of ill health.

Travelbee (1971), Riehl and Roy (1980) and King (1981) have also developed models based on interactionist theory.

Developmental Models

These models emphasize the concepts of growth and change.They recognize defined stages of development and assume a predictable direction through the life span. Such models take account of physical, cognitive, social and moral development. The theory underlying such models may be applied in the following ways.

1. It may provide a basis for the identification of a person's needs with respect to their stage of development. The

risk, it seems to me, is that unless the idea of variables is introduced the model lacks the flexibility essential for individualized care.
2. The use of developmental theory may be extended to assist the nurse and the patient in finding personal development in the nursing and health/illness situation (Peplau, 1952).

Activities of Living, Human Needs and Self-care Models

These have a shared focus on the basis of human needs for life and health as a means by which nursing action is directed. Henderson (1966) and Roper, Logan and Tierney (1990) focus essentially on human needs and activities of living. Orem and Vaughan (1980) develop this concept to apply to the self-care model, which will be described in some detail later in this chapter. Examination of these various types of models may reveal inherent common characteristics.

When assessing the suitability of any given nursing model there is a need to take account of the situation in which the model is to be used and adapted accordingly.

Ophthalmic Nursing: the Setting

Nursing is influenced by changes in society's attitudes of health and illness. It also takes account of new developments for health care and the change in patterns of disease. Ophthalmic nursing has experienced considerable change during the past decade. Some of this change has come about as a result of change within the nursing profession in general, but much has resulted from medical and technological development. We have witnessed, in particular, the refinement of microsurgical technique and advances in the therapeutic use of lasers. For the patient or client these medical and technological developments have brought about the following results:

1. a decrease in the length of hospitalization;
2. more care is delivered on an outpatient basis;
3. an increasing amount of intraocular surgery is being carried out on a 'day care' basis;
4. responsibility for continuity of care has become that of the patient or those who are able to support him at home.

The effect of the above has far-reaching consequences for the delivery of nursing in the ophthalmic setting. The patient returns to his home with an immediate need to adapt within that situation. He may have persisting visual impairment, may be elderly or in some way relatively dependent, or may have accompanying systemic disorder. There may also be influencing factors which derive from the prevailing socio-economic climate. Importantly, the information, teaching and support which the patient requires may be inadequate to ensure that he can manage when he returns home. Greater stress is also placed on the already stretched community nursing resources and often the nurses involved have received inadequate preparation for the specialist nursing practices with which the patient may require assistance.

Amos Griffiths (1981) points out that, despite the responsibility to ensure that patients can manage, evidence suggests that they are not given the opportunity to participate in their own treatment while in hospital but are expected to cope adequately at home. These considerations are important influences on the changing role of the ophthalmic nurse and on her delivery of care. I would suggest that the following factors are important in the present situation.

1. Early assessment of the patient/client's needs is required. This must be carried out comprehensively, and at an early but appropriate time, to ensure that he receives the support that may be required.
2. More emphasis needs to be placed on effective teaching for the patient or those assisting him to ensure that he is adequately supported in self-care.
3. Relevant preparation for community nursing staff involved in assisting the patient should be offered by specialist centres, or by liaison nursing staff experienced in ophthalmic practice.

Because of the changes described above, my contention is that an adaptation of a self-care model for nursing practice is appropriate for ophthalmic patient care.

The final part of this chapter will, therefore, be concerned with a description of one such model, with suggestions for its application to ophthalmic nursing.

The Self-care Deficit Model: Orem

The nursing model described by Orem (Orem and Vaughan, 1980) focuses on the concept of 'self-care'.

Levin, Katz and Holst (1979) define self-care as 'a process whereby a lay person functions on his own behalf in health promotion and prevention, and in disease detection and treatment'.

Orem views the person as a rational, biological organism, affected by his environment. Her model is based on the belief that people have self-care needs and that they have the right to meet these needs themselves whenever possible. Self-care is a predetermined action which has as its aim the meeting of individual needs for effective living.

Orem states that self-care is learned behaviour which derives from an intrinsic curiosity; it is facilitated by teaching and supervision from others and by experience of the process and outcome of self-care measures. The goals of nursing implied within this model are to meet self-care needs as appropriate in the following ways:

1. supporting the patient in meeting his own self-care needs;
2. enabling a relative or friend to be the self-care agent;
3. the nurse acting as the self-care agent.

The knowledge component of Orem's model focuses on those actions which are taken by people in order to function effectively. For the maintenance of health, Orem considers self-care in the following areas is essential:

1. adequate intake of air, water and food;
2. adequate excretion of waste products;
3. a balance between activity and rest, both mental and physical;
4. avoidance and prevention of hazards to life and well being;
5. a balance between social interaction and solitude;
6. promotion of normality, as this relates to the social context and personal potential of the individual.

In so identifying the above areas of need for effective living, Orem provides us with a framework for patient assessment. Orem refers to these areas as 'universal self-care demands' and these may be influenced by developmental factors and life change events. In considering the way in which a person copes with illness, that is, a deviation from a state of health, Orem stresses that, in assessment, three areas should be considered together with the universal care needs. These areas are physical function, structure and behaviour.

Health deviations may challenge existing self-care patterns. The introduction of new self-care practices may be necessary in order to correct the imbalance between the need and the existing ability of that person to meet the need.

Where there is a balance between the need and the person's ability to meet that need, individual self-care is possible. Where the demand implied in need outweighs the ability to meet it, the person has a self-care deficit.

The view of the person within this model centres upon the belief that a need for self-care always exists. Where a self-care deficit occurs, that deficit needs to be met. In a new-born baby, the parent acts as the self-care agent; Orem calls this dependent care – that which is given by another person, a friend or relative for instance.

If the self-care deficit creates a demand which is such that it cannot be met by the individual or by others able to offer care, nursing intervention is required. On this view, the goals of nursing are to help the person in meeting his self-care needs. The assistance provided by the nurse is directed towards the support of life, recovery from ill health resulting from disease or injury, and in developing the ability to cope with, and adapt to, the effects of disability.

Nurses help patients in a systematic way, and Orem identifies five helping methods:

1. acting or doing for another;
2. guiding another;
3. supporting another (physically and psychologically);
4. providing an environment which promotes personal growth and development;
5. teaching another.

The development of self-care actions, or the restoration of existing patterns of self-care, is achieved in stages. Different actions or combinations of helping methods may be required at different stages and these will be determined by the needs in terms of the self-care deficit which the patient has.

The Process of Nursing

Having briefly outlined the main features of the Orem model I will now go on to consider the way in which this theory may be applied in practice.

Assessment

Nursing begins with the assessment of the patient in order to identify his individual needs and problems.

Assessment of problems should be defined in terms of self-care deficit, that is, where the ability of the person and/or others cannot meet the self-care demand. This may occur in any of the identified universal areas of self-care demand. The areas of deficit constitute patient problems for which a plan of nursing intervention will be needed.

As we have seen, the length of hospitalization is short for many ophthalmic patients and much care is given on a routine and urgent outpatient basis. It is, therefore, very important that patient assessment be carried out quickly and thoroughly. Orem's model clearly makes possible such an assessment, as it is equally adaptable to the ophthalmic accident and emergency department as it is to the ward (Walsh, 1985).

There has been much discussion as to whether core plans may be used effectively in ophthalmology. Martin and Glasper (1986) describe a core nursing plan as one which is 'based on an explicit nursing model which deals with particular nursing problems or needs and which are allied to an agreed policy or procedure discussed with medical colleagues. For each problem or need an appropriate range of actions and interventions are prescribed.'

It should be stressed that core plans are not standardized care plans, which aim to make the patient fit into the plan. The emphasis of the core plan is to assist the nurses to focus on a person's individual needs without repeatedly rewriting procedures. While it is not within the remit of this chapter to develop a discussion of the relevance or not of using such plans, the issue may be one which could valuably be considered by ophthalmic nurses. The point which is of practical significance is that, should a unit decide upon the adoption of core nursing plans, the Orem model may be used effectively as the basis for such plans. While a large number of patients receiving ophthalmic care are not otherwise unwell, particularly in terms of illness which is life-threatening, many of our patients require general anaesthesia for surgical purposes. Therefore, assessment of the patient's ability to care for his airway in order to breathe adequately to provide sufficient oxygenation, or to maintain adequate circulation and a safe level of consciousness, is essential. The patient's inability to do so may be defined as a self-care deficit. In this case, we can see the relevance of commencing assessment in Orem's terms of physiological function.

Examination of the eye as well as the more general physical examination constitutes an important part of the care required of the ophthalmic nurse. Orem's logical sequence of assessment, which takes account of physical structure, proves helpful in this respect.

Finally, assessment of behaviour identifies the effects a person's disorder may have on his mental state and lifestyle. For the ophthalmic patient with anxiety, fear, lack of understanding, or visual impairment (temporary or permanent) appropriately planned nursing intervention is necessary. Assessment based upon universal self-care demands and health deviancy helps to provide a clear indication of the way in which the person will be able to cope at home and to continue in compliance with care, so essential in ophthalmic medical and nursing practice.

PLANNING

The identification of self-care deficits enables us to set goals with and for the patient. These goals are expressed in self-care terms and facilitate the planning of appropriate nursing care.

As we have seen, in her model, Orem identifies five methods which may be used by the nurse in helping the patient with a self-care deficit: acting for, guiding, supporting, providing a development environment and teaching.

The way in which these methods may be utilized, and combined as necessary, will be determined by the patient's needs and degree of dependence, both physical and psychological. The goals which are set must be (1) formulated with and for the patient, (2) realistic and (3) observable in terms of behaviour if nursing care is to be reliably evaluated.

In a speciality such as ophthalmology, where the patient very often receives care on an outpatient basis, or where episodes of hospitalization are short, the care planned should focus on self-care at home.

IMPLEMENTATION

Implementation of care will depend on the patient's personal need, the degree of deficit and independence (dependence). Appropriate nursing action will be determined by accurate assessment and relevant planning of care. Very rarely in the practice of ophthalmic nursing do we encounter patients requiring total support. Exceptions to this, of course, would be during and immediately following general anaesthesia, and particularly in the case of postanaesthetic complications. This may also apply to units where specialities are mixed, such as ophthalmology and neurology, where the neurological state of the patient may necessitate complete compensation for self-care deficits. In such cases the nurse is largely acting for the patient in meeting his self-care needs, with cardiopulmonary support or resuscitation being the priority intervention.

More usually the patient requiring ophthalmic care is identified on assessment as being able to carry out most of his own care, but having certain specific deficits in certain areas, which are met by nursing intervention in terms of acting for, guiding, supporting, providing a developmental environment and teaching. The care is realistic, effective and planned and implemented in order to ensure the feasibility of self-care at home.

Patient education and counselling is of great importance in ophthalmic care, as it forms an essential component of Orem's model. So often the patient is discharged from hospital to continue his care at home. This is particularly true in the case of those patients requiring ophthalmic medication, where the importance of drop compliance in many ophthalmic conditions cannot be overestimated. It is important that the patient understands why the treatment is necessary and that he feels confident in carrying it out.

Donnelly (1987) in her research into eyedrop instillation stresses that: 'in all cases, teaching should be geared to the needs of the individual, and requires knowledge of the patients' background, previous experience and present situation'.

The framework for assessment and planning in Orem's model helps to ensure that effective and appropriate teaching may be carried out. Walsh (1985) states that: 'self-care can only be practised if the individual has the knowledge, material resources and motivation. There is perhaps little that nurses can do about the material resources, but we can impart knowledge and motivation.'

Evaluation

Evaluation provides us with a vehicle for ensuring that nursing intervention in assisting the patient to achieve self-care goals is effective. As previously emphasized, realistic evaluation will only be possible if the patient's goals are expressed behaviourly, in order that we can see that they have been achieved. The criterion for discharge should be that the patient and, where necessary, others concerned with care are able to cope effectively (in terms of self-care at home). Failure to achieve this is failure to provide adequate and sensitive care for those to whom we have a responsibility of care.

In conclusion, Orem's self-care model provides an excellent foundation for ophthalmic nursing practice. Importantly, the Orem model is essentially a model with a nursing core which focuses on needs in terms of health, and emphasizing personal responsibility for health care. It involves, where possible, the patient in the planning of his care and, in so doing, recognizes the autonomy and dignity of the individual.

References

Amos Griffiths, R. (1981) Iatrogenic disease. *Nursing*, **1**, 1103–110.

Blumer, H. (1969) *Symbolic Interactionism: Perspective and Method*, Prentice-Hall, New Jersey.

Donnelly, D. (1987) Instilling eyedrops: difficulties experienced by patients following cataract surgery. *Journal of Advanced Nursing*, **12**, 235–243.

Henderson, V. (1966) *The Nature of Nursing*, Macmillan, New York.

Johnson, D. E. (1980) in *Conceptual Models for Nursing Practice*, Appleton-Century-Crofts, Norwalk, CT.

King, I. M. (1981) *A Theory for Nursing: Systems Concept Process*, John Wiley, New York.

Levin, L., Katz, A. and Holst, E. (1979) *Self-care: Lay Initiatives in Health*, Prodist, New York.

McFarlane, J. (1986) in *Models for Nursing*, (eds B. Kershaw and J. Salvage), John Wiley, Chichester.

Martin, L. and Glasper, A. (1986) Core plans: nursing models and the nursing process in action. *Nursing Practice*, **1**, 268–273.

Orem, D. and Vaughan, B. (1980) *Nursing: Concepts for Practice*, Heinemann, London.

Peplau, H. E. (1952) *Interpersonal Relations in Nursing*, Putnam, New York.

Riehl, J. and Roy, C. (eds) (1980) *Conceptual Models for Nursing Practice*, Appleton-Century-Crofts, Norwalk, CT.

Roper, N., Logan, W. W. and Tierney, A. J. (1990) *The Elements of Nursing*, 3rd edn., Churchill Livingstone, Edinburgh.

Roy, C. (1984) *Introduction to Nursing: an Adaption Model*, Prentice-Hall, Englewood Cliffs, NJ.

Roy, C., Riehl, J. and Roy, C. (1980) in *Conceptual Models for Nursing Practice*, Appleton-Century-Crofts, Norwalk, CT.

Travelbee, J. (1971) *Interpersonal Aspects of Nursing*, F. A. Davis, Philadelphia.

Walsh, M. (1985) in *Models for Nursing*, (eds B. Kershaw and J. Salvage), John Wiley, Chichester.

5

Quality, Standards and Audit

S. Jane Merchant

Chapter Summary

The Concept of Quality

Quality is an often used, but ill-defined, concept. Nevertheless, those involved in health care continue to discuss the quality, or otherwise, of patient care. In most dictionary definitions, the words 'quality' and 'standards' seem to be viewed as interchangeable. Both terms seem to relate to excellence, skill or accomplishment. A recent review of the nursing literature found frequent use of the word 'quality' but no agreed definition, much of the literature being anecdotal or descriptive in nature (Attree, 1993).

In spite of this apparent confusion, nurses and others involved in health care have, especially over the last 30 years, begun to develop numerous methods for 'assuring' the quality of care delivered to patients and clients because intuitively we know this to be important. Much of this work originated in North America, but the concepts and tools applied have been widely adopted in the UK.

This chapter examines some of the reasons why health professionals and organizations should be involved in assuring the quality of service and briefly outlines some of the methods available for doing this.

For clarity, the following terms or definitions will be used:

1. **quality** – a term used to denote excellence or high standards;
2. **assurance** – a method of evaluating and/or ensuring the standard of something;
3. **standard** – a statement against which performance can be measured or evaluated;
4. **audit** – the process of measuring performance against a standard.

Organizational Responsibility and Quality

All organizations have responsibility for evaluating the quality of service delivered to clients. In manufacturing industry strict assurance measures for quality control at every stage in a process have been common for many years. Market forces have ensured that companies providing goods perceived by the general public to be of high quality and backed up by highly publicized customer care programmes have made profits and become brand leaders.

With recent changes in the organization of the Health Service, contracting now takes place between health authorities, GP fundholders and so-called 'provider units'. Contracts cover both quantitative and qualitative aspects of services. Therefore, in the future health services, like other organizations, will be required to demonstrate the operation of effective quality assurance methods in order to ensure the continuation of contracts for patient care. In addition, the Patient's Charter (Department of Health, 1992) has provided a number of standards against which all organizations will be measured.

Professional Accountability and Quality

Health professionals have individual responsibility for the quality of care they give to patients. This is commonly referred to as professional accountability, the nature of which is formulated in guidelines or codes of practice from statutory bodies and, in some cases, from Royal Colleges or other professional organizations (e.g. UKCC, 1992). In addition, educational registration and accreditation schemes that regulate who can practise can be thought of as one method of quality assurance undertaken by the professions themselves.

Although no-one would dispute that individuals and groups of professionals have always been concerned about the quality of care received by patients it is only very recently that national guidelines have ensured that all professionals are involved in quality assurance through the mechanism known as clinical audit (Department of Health, 1993).

An Introduction to Methodologies

There are in fact numerous methods of measuring the quality of clinical care. In the literature these are often divided into retrospective and concurrent methods. Retrospective methods look backwards at what care was given or, more commonly, whether records were adequately completed. Patient surveys conducted after treatment has been concluded also fall into this group, as do post-care case conferences.

Concurrent methods are used at a specific point, or sometimes over a period of time, while the patient is still receiving care. These methods include audit of current patient records, comparing outcomes of care against goals set in care plans or against specially designed care protocols (e.g. management of a patient with cataract), direct observations of care, patient surveys or interviews, and care conferences that include patient, relatives and staff. There are also specific tools designed to measure the competence of the nurse and all disciplines can institute peer review procedures in which a professional discusses and evaluates the handling of a particular patient's care with her peer group.

A number of these methods require that standards are set, or protocols written, to facilitate the observation or audit process. To date, standard setting has largely been undertaken by groups of professionals who have developed standards for their own area of practice. This may be undertaken in-house although some 'off the shelf' packages are available for nursing audit.

CHOOSING METHODS

All methods have advantages and disadvantages and consideration needs to be given to these before choices are made. It should be recognized that, whatever methods are chosen, the time and commitment of staff will be required to ensure successful implementation. There may also be costs in staff time and education input to ensure that staff have the knowledge and skills required. Maxwell (1984) believes that quality of care can never be viewed from one perspective only, and suggests that there are in fact six key areas in a quality service. These are:

1. access (to services);
2. relevance to need;
3. effectiveness for individual patients;
4. equity or fairness;
5. acceptability (to the individual and society);
6. efficiency and economy.

It follows that these very different views of quality will require different methods of measurement. In fact, the outcome of one nursing study has suggested that a variety of methods is the best way to determine quality even when there is only one ward or group of patients involved (Pearson, Durant and Punton, 1989). Since it is the multidisciplinary team that manages care, all members of the team will need to be involved in discussions about the philosophy and aims of the service before methods can be chosen. It is, therefore, likely that in any one ophthalmic service a number of methods will need to be applied, some of which are uni- and some multidisciplinary. Methods for ensuring that patients' views are taken into consideration will also be needed to ensure that a complete picture is achieved.

Methodological Issues

Retrospective Methods

A major concern here is that recollections of patients or staff will not always be accurate some time after events have taken place.

Retrospective audit of nursing records is often viewed as measuring the quality of documentation rather than of care given. It carries the assumption that what is done is what is recorded and there is a risk that staff could learn to make records that produce favourable audit results (Pearson, 1987). An audit of records can, however, be useful if used with a protocol for patient assessment or care; for instance, have all patients undergoing day surgery been assessed as to transport availability? Results from such an audit can be used to inform and influence practice and the audit can be repeated at intervals to see whether standards have been maintained or improved.

Patients' Perceptions

It is important for professionals to understand the patients' perceptions of their treatment and other aspects of the service. Patients tend to be reluctant to offer their views while they are still receiving treatment. The most effective time to obtain opinions is probably at, or immediately after, discharge from inpatient or outpatient treatment. Many hospitals give patients a survey form at this point and provide boxes for collection or provide stamped, addressed envelopes. In spite of this, response rates are often low and it is usually found that patients are reluctant to comment on clinical care even when patient anonymity is assured.

Patient surveys are difficult to construct and professional staff need to ensure that the topics covered are of concern to patients rather than staff (Carr-Hill, Dixon and Thompson, 1989). Some 'expert' patient satisfaction surveys are available but testing will still be required to ensure suitability for particular patient groups. Cang (1989) suggests that, in view of the problems inherent in most questionnaire-based methods, less formal methods should be considered and might in fact lead to a much more accurate picture of user views. In an ophthalmic unit some patients will inevitably find it difficult to read or complete survey forms even if they are in large print. Some patients may be willing to record their comments on a cassette tape or may be happy to be interviewed by someone they see as independent, such as a member of the Community Health Council. Alternatively, 'patient panels' or user groups can be set up to gather the views of patients and relatives.

In spite of the difficulties involved, the potential benefits of involving patients and their representatives need to be recognized; they are, after all, the only people who can comment on some aspects of clinical care such as pain or discomfort (Joule, 1993).

Complaints

All services receive complaints from time to time and these can also be viewed positively in that they provide opportunities to rectify problem areas. Feedback to staff about the subjects of complaints also assist in improving quality as patients often do not complain about the things that staff might expect them to. The majority of complaints tend to be about poor communication and information, and about lack of privacy. Obviously, these are areas where positive action can be taken.

Every health authority and trust must have a complaints policy which is open and easily accessible to members of the public. In addition, complaints should be monitored, action should be taken to rectify faults in the service and complainants should receive an apology and full replies to their complaints or queries (Department of Health and Social Security, 1988). Happily, the majority of comments received from users of health services are positive and can be seen as endorsements of the quality of a service.

Concurrent Methods

Concurrent methods of measuring quality have the advantage of being able to directly affect the outcomes of care for particular patients (e.g. evaluation of the outcomes of care planning, care conferences and peer review meetings) and of being closely related to practice (e.g. Monitor, Qualpacs). The former have the added advantage of involving the staff who are actually caring for patients. They do, however, need to be introduced carefully as nurses and other professionals may be sensitive about opening their practice to the scrutiny of peers. It is important that such new ideas are developed by facilitators who are seen by clinical staff as being objective and clinically competent themselves.

Monitor and Qualpacs are nursing methodologies that depend upon the use of independent observers (although these observers are usually specially trained nurses). Monitor is based on the nursing process and Qualpacs concentrates on psychosocial aspects of care (Harvey, 1988). In both, key criteria are translated into items and scores. These tools have sometimes been criticized in the past as not involving clinical nurses enough or not being relevant to particular clinical areas. Both originate in North America and, although they have been anglicized, this has sometimes raised questions about their relevance to the British health care system. Redfern and Norman (1990) point out that such measures cannot be seen as objective because some kind of judgement on the part of the observer is usually required and they conclude that the reliability and validity of these methods still require extensive testing.

Harvey (1991), however, suggests that the context and method of implementation rather than the tool itself may be the most important factor in success or otherwise. Her study demonstrated that methods implemented by a top-down approach were not accepted well by ward staff who felt that they were not involved, therefore becoming anxious and tending to question the clinical credibility of the observers. She states that a bottom-up approach was more successful because staff felt involved and had some ownership of the process.

Methods That Ensure Staff Involvement

Quality Circles

Ideally, Quality Circles can be viewed as a 'bottom-up' or 'grass roots' approach fuelled by the desire of staff to solve problems and improve services. It is not primarily a system designed for clinical staff only and typically consists of all grades and disciplines of staff, one circle or group representing one ward or department. The leader or facilitator of the group must be someone with enthusiasm who is able to ensure that all members of the group have the opportunity to contribute.

The purpose of the circle is to define problems and, using brainstorming techniques, to find solutions to these. The end product may be a simple change in practice and may require that a policy or standard is agreed. Managers are not necessarily group members, but must give support and be prepared to facilitate exchange of ideas between wards/departments, support policy changes and deal with resource implications where appropriate.

Although Quality Circles will encourage staff participation in developing quality initiatives, they do not provide a method of evaluating or measuring any consequent improvement in quality. They always, therefore, need to be used in conjunction with other methods.

STANDARD SETTING

The best known professional system for standard setting in Great Britain is probably the one developed by the Royal College of Nursing, the Dynamic Standard Setting System for Nursing (RCN, 1989). Here groups of nurses use a structure-process-outcome approach which is based on the work of Donabedian (1969). As in Quality Circles, it is recommended that a group of staff, with a facilitator, choose topics or areas of concern about patient care and use a 'brainstorming' process to define a standard. The process may include investigating current practice, looking for examples of good practice or reviewing the research literature. Because the system was designed by nurses for professional use, it is likely to be more positively viewed by clinical staff than use of BS5750, although work has been done on adopting this for Health Service use (Rooney, 1988) and BS5750 may be very pertinent to some technical areas of practice such as laboratories.

When using the Dynamic Standard Setting System a standard statement, or general statement about the level of care required, is developed first. For example, in order that they can be understood and achieved, all standard statements must be:

1. relevant (to the field of practice);
2. clear and concise;
3. measurable/observable;
4. appropriate and achievable.

Criteria statements are then devised. These can be viewed as the building blocks of the standard. There are three types of criterion:

1. **structure**: the environment; equipment; staff; policies, e.g. the level of knowledge and skill required by the nurse;
2. **process**: the nursing interventions required, i.e. what the nurse must do;
3. **outcome**: the expected changes which will occur as a result of the nurse's actions, e.g. a change in the condition or the knowledge or skill of the patient.

This system can be successfully used by professions other than nurses and by multidisciplinary groups. Once again, although this is a bottom-up approach, the commitment of managers is required. The RCN recommends that there is a formal committee structure through which standards are verified so that all standards are endorsed by a peer group and a relevant senior manager.

It is the responsibility of the group that writes the standard to set a date by which it will be achieved and review dates. Monitoring or audit of standards may be carried out by group members or by selected peers. Either way, information on performance against the standard must be fed back to the staff involved. If the standard is met the group members may be happy to set a further review date some time ahead. If, however, the standard is not met, the group will need to review both the standard itself and the data collected to measure performance. It may be that the standard was not clear enough for the audit information to be collected or that an unrealistic time-scale for achievement was set. On the other hand, the information collected may show that some of the criteria were not met, for instance the correct equipment was not being used or the nurses were unaware of a policy. These issues can then be addressed and another review date can be set. This system, and similar standard setting methods, are now widely used to facilitate the clinical audit process.

Conclusion

This chapter has raised a number of issues about the concept of quality and how it may be measured or audited in a health care setting. It should be remembered that the methods briefly described here are only some of those currently available and that they all have both advantages and disadvantages. The care of ophthalmic patients is a matter of teamwork and, therefore, all team members (including the patient) need to be involved in measuring and assuring its quality. The methods described are merely tools that will assist in this process; the actual quality or otherwise of care will depend on the knowledge and skills of all the team members.

References

Attree, M. (1993) An analysis of the concept 'quality' as it relates to contemporary nursing care. *International Journal of Nursing Studies*, **30**, 350–369.

Cang, S. (1989) Open to criticism. *Health Service Journal*, **99**, 886.

Carr-Hill, R., Dixon, P. and Thompson, A. (1989) Too simple for words. *Health Service Journal*, **99**, 728–729.

Department of Health and Social Security (1988) *Health Service Management: Hospital Complaints Procedure Act 1985, HC(88)37*, DHSS, London.

Department of Health (1992) *The Patient's Charter*, HMSO, London.

Department of Health (1993) *Clinical Audit – Meeting and Improving Standards in Health Care*, Department of Health, London.

Donabedian, A. (1969) Some issues in evaluating the quality of nursing care. *American Journal of Public Health*, **39**, 1833–1836.

Harvey, G. (1988) Raising the standards: the right tools for the job. *Nursing Times*, **84**, 47–48.

Harvey, G. (1991) An evaluation of approaches to assessing the quality of nursing care using (predetermined) quality assurance tools. *Journal of Advanced Nursing*, **16**, 277–286.

Joule, N. (1993) Involving users of health care services: moving beyond lip service (editorial). *Quality in Health Care*, **2**, 211–212.

Maxwell, R. J. (1984) Perspectives in NHS management: quality assessment in health. *British Medical Journal*, **288**, 1470–1472.

Pearson, A. (1987) Nursing and quality, in *Nursing Quality Measurement: Quality Assurance Methods for Peer Review*, (ed. A. Pearson), John Wiley, Chichester.

Pearson, A., Durant, I. and Punton, S. (1989) Determining quality in a unit where nursing is the primary intervention. *Journal of Advanced Nursing*, **14**, 269–273.

Redfern, S. J. and Norman, I. J. (1990) Measuring the quality of nursing care: a consideration of different approaches. *Journal of Advanced Nursing*, **15**, 1260–1271.

Rooney, E. M. (1988) A proposed quality system specification for the National Health Service. *Quality Assurance*, **14**, 45–53.

RCN (Royal College of Nursing) (1989) *A Framework for Quality: Royal College of Nursing Standards of Care Project*, RCN, London.

UKCC (United Kingdom Central Council for Nursing, Midwifery and Health Visiting) (1992) *Code of Professional Conduct*, UKCC, London.

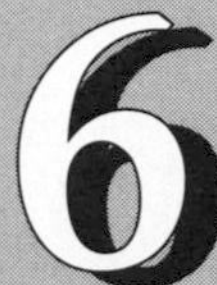

Principles of Emergency Care

Janet Marsden

Chapter Summary

The receiving centre for ophthalmic accidents and emergencies may be a dedicated ophthalmic room in a general Accident and Emergency Department, an ophthalmic ward or a specialist Ophthalmic Accident and Emergency Department. The area may provide a walk-in service or take only referrals from other departments. However the service is organized, the principles of care remain the same.

Design of a Department

All areas within a hospital should take into account the needs of the patient and any area dealing with ophthalmic patients should pay particular attention to the needs of the visually impaired. Signs should be large and clear, the area should be well lit and hazards, such as the edges of corridors and steps, should be well marked. There should be enough space available in the area for accurate estimation of the patient's visual acuity.

The examination area should have black-out facilities, which are essential for effective ophthalmic examination, and should be fully equipped with a slit lamp, direct and indirect ophthalmoscopes, lenses and a tonometer, and a range of diagnostic drops such as stains and local anaesthetics. Hand-washing facilities are essential.

The treatment area should be equipped with ophthalmic chairs (which are easily adjustable, with correct head supports), dressing trolleys and sufficient space for storage of sterile supplies and other equipment. A good light source is essential in order to carry out procedures safely and a suitable one might consist of a ring-shaped fluorescent light with a magnifying lens in the centre. This also proves useful in the examination of the eye. The treatment area should be fully equipped to undertake procedures such as instillation of drops, irrigation, etc.

A dirty utility room should be available and have facilities for urine testing.

A minor operations area should be available for such procedures as suturing of lids and incision and curettage of chalazions. This area should contain oxygen and suction.

An area, with a couch, for patients to recover or be examined on is also necessary in order to provide comprehensive patient care.

Ideally, a supply of drugs and drops should be available for dispensing to patients, to enable total care to be given and any reinforcement of treatment to be undertaken before the patient leaves the department.

Patient Assessment

Patient assessment is like fitting together the pieces of a very important jigsaw. To assess the patient effectively, the nurse needs to put together all the pieces to give a clear picture of the patient's problem. A clear history needs to be ascertained, together with the patient's visual acuity. Observation of the eye should be undertaken. The nurse can then put all these pieces of information together to decide on the priority for care of a particular patient. This process is known as **triage** and is an essential tool in the management of patients in what is often a very busy area.

History Taking

After registration, the patient is greeted by a nurse who will immediately begin to observe the patient's physical and psychological state. To many patients, the hospital is an alien environment and a caring and calm attitude can do much to allay anxiety.

Details of the patient's age are important, as it may lead the nurse to suspect different conditions; for example an elderly patient who presents with gradual visual loss may be suffering from cataracts or senile macular degeneration, conditions that would not come to mind in the assessment of a much younger person. The patient should be asked for details of any allergies, as he may not think these are relevant and so may be given treatment to which he is allergic. The patient's occupation may also give a clue to his condition; for example a welder may not associate his eye problem with his occupation because of the time delay before symptoms of a welding flash appear.

A clear history is an extremely important part of patient assessment. The nurse should allow the patient to say what happened in his own words. Specific questions can then be asked to enlarge on the information given by the patient. Was the visual loss sudden? Was it associated with any pain? These further questions may direct the nurse's thoughts towards various ophthalmic conditions. In the case of an accident, the nurse should find out when the accident happened and under exactly what circumstances. 'Something in my eye' could be anything from a subtarsal foreign body to an intraocular foreign body and details of the circumstances surrounding the injury such as speed of travel of the particle – for example, resulting from the use of a hammer and chisel as opposed to wind-blown – can help to differentiate between major and minor trauma. Any previous history of eye disease, systemic disease such as hypertension or diabetes mellitus, or any drug therapy that the patient may be on may also help the nurse in the assessment.

Visual Acuity Testing

Estimation and recording of visual acuity is an essential part of patient assessment. It can become an important issue in cases of compensation for industrial injury. It is also a baseline for the estimation of progress and further treatment of an eye condition. It is important, therefore, to estimate and record the patient's visual acuity accurately on each visit to the department. The nurse should be acquainted with the various methods of assessing visual acuity (Chapter 10).

For illiterate patients, or those who are unfamiliar with our alphabet, the 'E' test may be used. The chart is set out like a Snellen chart with 'Es' facing different directions instead of different letters. The patient is given an E-shaped card and asked to indicate the direction of the E on the chart. This test can be extremely confusing for patient and nurse alike, and tests such as the Sheridan Gardiner and Kay Picture Test, which are generally used for children, can be much more effective.

Other tests used in the department for testing visual function are the test types for near acuity, the Amsler grid for testing the central visual field and Ishihara charts for testing colour perception.

In cases where the patient's upper lid is swollen or bruised, the nurse can usually raise the lid enough, gently, to allow the letters to be read. A speculum may be used to open the lids enough to obtain the visual acuity or the patient may help by holding his own lid as this may be perceived to be less painful. If the patient's lid swelling is a result of trauma, care should be taken not to press on the globe while opening the lids in case there is an underlying perforating injury. In cases where the patient cannot open the eye due to pain and photophobia, e.g. after welding flash or overwear of contact lenses, a local anaesthetic drop such as benoxinate 0.4% may need to be instilled to facilitate visual acuity recording.

Not only does visual acuity testing aid the nurse in assessing the patient's condition, but a very frightened patient can be reassured when he sees that his condition has not affected his sight.

Observation

The nurse now has a history and visual acuity but needs to examine the eyes to further assess the patient's condition. Before examination, the nurse should explain what is about to happen. This examination may take place, very quickly, by looking at the eye using a pen torch, after recording the visual acuity. The nurse may, however, wish to examine the patient's eyes in more detail while the patient is sitting in a treatment chair or at the slit lamp. The affected eye should be compared with the unaffected eye and any anomalies should be noted. The nurse should examine the structures of the eye in a logical manner in order to ensure that nothing is missed. (For a full account of examination of the eye refer to Chapter 10.)

In cases where the patient is unable to open the eye due to pain, a drop of local anaesthetic can be used to alleviate pain and facilitate examination. When assessing corneal damage, a drop of fluorescein 1%, a staining agent, can be used to outline any disrupted corneal epithelium, for example an abrasion or dendritic ulcer.

Identification of Priorities – Triage

The term 'triage' was first used in a medical context during the First World War, when it was used to describe a system for deciding priorities of treatment for the wounded. In the Vietnam War, effective triage was credited with ensuring a high level of medical care. The development of triage in the accident and emergency setting means that patients receive treatment according to the severity of their condition, not on a first-come, first-served basis. It ensures that those needing urgent treatment receive it, and those with less immediate problems may need to wait longer. Information about such a system should be given to all patients so that those that have to wait longer do not feel abandoned and unfairly treated.

The priorities and grading system will vary according to local conditions but are designated in the ophthalmic setting as follows.

1. **Category 1**: where a delay in treatment could lead to ocular damage, facial disfiguration or systemic complications; or patients with physical, mental or social problems which make rapid treatment advisable. This may include conditions such as:
   (a) chemical injuries;
   (b) open injuries of the eye, face or lid;
   (c) hyphaema;
   (d) hypopyon or corneal abscess;
   (e) acute glaucoma;
   (f) very recent, sudden loss of vision;
   (g) suspected retinal detachment;
   (h) patients in acute pain;
   (i) tiny babies.
2. **Category 2**: where a short delay in treatment would not lead to permanent damage but could cause severe anxiety or discomfort to the patient; or patients with physical, mental or social problems where fairly rapid treatment is advisable. This may include situations such as:
   (a) babies and young children;
   (b) inpatients from other hospitals;
   (c) recent ophthalmic inpatients with problems;
   (d) recent loss of vision (detachment not suspected, longer history);
   (e) acute infection (e.g. orbital cellulitis) or inflammation (e.g. uveitis).
3. **Category 3**: where a delay in treatment would not lead to permanent damage or cause severe anxiety or discomfort to the patient. This may include problems such as:
   (a) corneal foreign body;
   (b) abrasion;
   (c) conjunctivitis;
   (d) dry eye;
   (e) patients referred with suspected chronic, open-angle glaucoma;
   (f) patients referred with suspected cataracts.

Each patient should be assessed holistically and the history, visual acuity and eye examination should be brought together to assign a triage category. This assessment should be carried out by a trained and experienced nurse and should be comprehensively documented in order to facilitate communication with other nursing and medical staff. A list of conditions and situations can only be used as a guideline and is no substitute for the clinical knowledge and skills of experienced staff.

PROCEDURES

After initial assessment, the nurse may need to carry out various specialized procedures such as irrigation of the eye or removal of subtarsal or corneal foreign body to minimize the damage to the eye before the patient is seen by a doctor. Adequate and full explanation of any procedure, prior to it being undertaken, will enhance the patient's compliance and go some way to allaying any fears or apprehensions he may have.

IRRIGATION

A prompt and effective response to a chemical injury is vital to minimize tissue damage. Copious irrigation is needed initially, to dilute the chemical and remove particulate matter. Buffer solutions may be used to irrigate the eye but the most common (and cheapest!) irrigation solution is 0.9% (normal) saline. Any delay caused by attempting to identify the nature of the chemical or the appropriate neutralizing solution extends the contact time and increases the risk of more severe injury. Beare (1989) points out that neutralizing solutions are probably no more effective than neutral ones. The eye is irrigated using an irrigation set or intravenous infusion and a bottle or bag of normal saline. This provides a directable and controllable stream of fluid. An undine may be used, but the volume held makes it a very repetitive, fiddly and inefficient procedure.

The patient should be positioned comfortably, either lying or sitting with the head well supported and inclined to the side to be irrigated. The eye should be anaesthetized using preferred local anaesthetic drops to prevent blepharospasm and aid examination and irrigation. The patient's clothes should be protected with a waterproof cape and a receiver held to the cheek to catch the irrigation fluid.

The flow of lotion is started on the cheek to accustom the patient to it before it is directed on to the conjunctiva. All aspects of the conjunctiva and cornea must be irrigated and the upper lid doubly everted if necessary. The patient needs to be encouraged to look in all aspects of gaze to expose different parts of the conjunctiva. A swab on a stick may be used to assist in the removal of solid matter from the fornices. Immediately after irrigation, which may use 2–3 litres of fluid, the patient should be examined by the doctor to assess damage and start treatment and thereby minimize any long term effects.

Removal of Subtarsal and Corneal Foreign Body

Subtarsal foreign bodies are a common cause of irritation and pain – a small foreign body becomes trapped between the upper lid and the eye, and each time the patient blinks the foreign body is rubbed over the cornea, causing a distinct pattern of linear abrasions that are easily seen after staining with fluorescein.

A patient complaining of a foreign body sensation should have his lids everted to ensure that there is no subtarsal foreign body present. The procedure should be explained to the patient and he should be reassured that, while the procedure may feel a little strange, it is not painful.

The patient should be encouraged to look down while the nurse grasps the upper eyelashes and everts the lid. The lid should be wiped with a swab to remove any foreign material and its presence or absence should be recorded on the patient's notes. The patient should then be examined for assessment and treatment of any corneal abrasions. Local anaesthesia is not usually necessary for lid eversion.

Corneal foreign bodies are a major source of self-referrals to any area dealing with ophthalmic patients. Many happen at work – particles flying at relatively high speed into the eye during drilling or grinding with insufficient eye protection. Others are caused by particles hitting the eye at fairly low speeds, being blown in by the wind, for example. Corneal foreign bodies cause irritation and a variable degree of pain which may be accompanied by lacrimation and blepharospasm.

The history of the injury should be taken into account as this may indicate whether the foreign body is likely to be superficial or more deeply embedded. Before any attempt is made to remove the foreign body, the eye should be anaesthetized with the topical anaesthetic of choice. The patient should be positioned either sitting or lying down with his head well supported and should be asked to fix his direction of gaze so as to maximize the view of the foreign body. Removal should be attempted using a moistened, cotton-tipped swab. A more deeply embedded foreign body may be removed by 'picking' it off the cornea with a hypodermic needle, usually a 'green' or 21 G. In a department with access to a slit lamp, it is not appropriate that an embedded corneal foreign body be removed by any other method than at the slit lamp, as this is by far the safest method.

After removal of the foreign body, the patient should be examined by the doctor to assess corneal damage and prescribe treatment. It is likely that antibiotic ointment will then be instilled and eye pads applied. Iron and steel foreign bodies often leave a rust ring, which needs to be removed at a follow-up appointment, in 24–48 hours.

CONSULTATIONS

After the triage procedure has been carried out and any immediate care has been given, the patient will be examined by a doctor. The nurse's role during the consultation is to facilitate smooth progress by explaining techniques, reassuring the patient to ensure that he does not become agitated or upset and reinforcing explanations given by the doctor. The nurse may need to fill in details that the patient has forgotten to tell the doctor. Sometimes, two totally different histories may be heard – one by the nurse making the initial assessment and one by the doctor. Before the beginning of each session, the nurse should ensure that the room is set up correctly, that all equipment is working and that there are adequate supplies of drops, tissues, stationery, etc.

CORNEAL STAINING

The technique of corneal staining is used to assess corneal damage. The two main staining agents used are fluorescein 2%, which is orange and is used to demonstrate epithelial defects, and rose Bengal 1%, which is red and stains dead tissue.

The patient should be warned that when he wipes his eye, the colour seen is just a stain which has been instilled (and not, in the case of rose Bengal, blood!), and that he may find the stain on his handkerchief after he has blown his nose because of the connection between the lacrimal system and the nose. (Corneal staining is discussed more fully in Chapter 16.)

DILATION OF THE PUPIL

Mydriatics dilate the pupil and usually have a cycloplegic effect, i.e. they paralyse the ciliary muscle and therefore prevent accommodation. They are used in the Accident and Emergency Department for a variety of reasons:

1. to assist in the detailed examination of the posterior segment;

2. to prevent or break down posterior synechiae (adhesions between the iris and the lens) in uveitis, and anterior synechiae (between the iris and the cornea) in perforating injury.
3. to overcome ciliary spasm and thus reduce pain, e.g. after a corneal abrasion or in uveitis.

Before dilating drops are instilled, it should be explained to the patient that they paralyse accommodation and therefore he will have blurred near vision for some hours after the examination. It is for this reason that phenylephrine may sometimes be used on its own as it has no cycloplegic effect and therefore does not interfere with accommodation. The patient may also experience some photophobia due to the increased amount of light entering the eye.

The patient may wish to make arrangements for transport home if he experiences particular difficulties with his vision while dilated. Most patients, however, have no problems with their distance vision and feel quite happy and safe using their usual form of transport. It should be left entirely up to the patient whether he drives or not as distance visual acuity is unchanged and accommodation is not generally used while driving. Patients often find it much easier to adjust if both pupils are dilated, rather than just one.

Before instillation, as with all drugs, the nurse should check that she is dealing with the correct patient, the correct eye and the correct medication and strength; and the expiry date.

The instillation may be repeated as instructed by the doctor or by local policy until dilation is complete. The nurse should have a good knowledge of the drug used and be able to advise on its duration and any side effects if necessary.

After the examination, the doctor will have made a diagnosis and may, if necessary, have prescribed treatment. The nurse may have to initiate treatment by carrying out procedures such as heat treatments, subconjunctival injections, instillation of medication and application of dressings.

All information given by the doctor should be reinforced by the nurse both verbally and by the use of written information if necessary. The nurse should ensure that the patient understands his diagnosis and treatment, the likely course of his condition, any follow-up appointments that may be needed, where to get any medication and what to do if his condition deteriorates, before leaving the department. This may take some time, but is essential to ensure compliance with treatment and to minimize preventable complications.

SUBCONJUNCTIVAL INJECTION

In some conditions, such as acute anterior uveitis and intraocular infections, a high concentration of a drug is needed quickly for optimum effect. This can be achieved by subconjunctival injection – the aim of which is to inject drugs into the potential space between the conjunctiva and the sclera. A maximum of 1.5 ml of fluid can be injected at a given site. If there is more than this amount, or if drug incompatibilities are likely, more than one injection site will be required. The first should be in the upper bulbar conjunctiva if possible. Either a doctor or an ophthalmic trained nurse may carry out the procedure, depending on hospital policy.

Subconjunctival injection may be uncomfortable or frightening for the patient and, therefore, correct and adequate explanations should be given at all stages of the procedure (which may involve a small subconjunctival injection of lignocaine).

Briefly, the procedure is as follows.

1. The eye is anaesthetized with a topical local anaesthetic. Anaesthesia should be checked before injection, by gently touching the bulbar conjunctiva with a pair of conjunctival forceps.
2. A speculum may be inserted to keep the lids apart if required.
3. The patient should be asked to hold a fixed direction of gaze to present the best view of the chosen site for the injection (for example, if the upper bulbar conjunctiva is chosen as the site for injection, the patient should be asked to look down to expose as much of it as possible).
4. The tip of the needle should be gently inserted, bore uppermost, into the conjunctiva and the medication released slowly. Conjunctival forceps may be used to grasp the conjunctiva if necessary.
5. The eye should be padded with a folded pad, followed by a single pad – a bandage may be applied if requested.
6. The patient should be given instructions about the length of time to leave the pad on and should be advised to take analgesia if necessary.

HEAT TREATMENT

Heat can be applied to the eye and lids to relieve pain, aid absorption of drugs and promote the circulation of blood in cases of local infection such as stye and chalazion.

Both dry and moist applications of heat may be used, although moist heat treatments may be considered more useful as they can be continued by the patient at home.

Dry Heat Application

The electric heater consists of an element, contained in a flat pad (Maddox pad), which is placed in the middle of an eye-pad and bandaged over the patient's closed lids. The supply of current and therefore the amount of heat produced is controlled by a rheostat in the form of a control box. The warmer should be adjusted until the patient feels the pad to be comfortably warm. The pad may be used for 20–30 minutes at a time.

Mains electricity is potentially dangerous, as is excess heat, and the pad should only be loosely strapped or tied to the head so that if it should overheat it can be removed quickly.

Attention should be paid to the hazard warning given by the Department of Health and Social Security on this subject (HN(HAZARD)(*81)5), dated 21 April 1981. This discusses the problem of control boxes overheating, suggests that all heaters should be regularly examined by suitably qualified personnel to assess their electrical safety and recommends that all heaters without a green pilot light should be withdrawn from use.

Moist Heat Application

Hot spoon bathing is used to apply moist heat to the eye, steaming it rather than bathing it with water. A wooden spoon is padded with absorbent material.

The patient must sit comfortably with a bowl of freshly boiled water in front of him resting on a firm surface such as a table. A waterproof cape may be used to protect the patient's clothing. He should be instructed to keep his eye closed and his head over the bowl, and then to repeatedly lift the spoon towards his eye until he can feel the heat, but not to touch his lids with the spoon as this would cause a scald.

This may be continued for 5–10 minutes, or longer, changing the water as it becomes cool. Most patients should have little difficulty in carrying out this treatment at home if full explanations and a demonstration are given before they leave the hospital. Alternatives to hot spoon bathing may include the following.

1. The patient is instructed to fill a jug or bowl with boiling water and to lean over it, holding the face in the steam and keeping the eye closed.
2. The patient puts some boiling water into a jug or bowl and stands a tablespoon in it. Once the bowl of the spoon is hot, he quickly removes the spoon from the water and dries it. He then holds the bowl of the spoon close to his closed lids until he can feel the heat from it (being careful not to touch his lids with the spoon). This is repeated as necessary.

   Both these methods are less complicated both in terms of method and equipment and are less likely to contaminate household equipment with infected secretions.

3. Another simple and effective way of using heat is by asking the patient to wring out squares of lint or other absorbent material in hot water and place them over the closed lids, changing them as they cool. This is particularly suitable for children and the temperature of the pads may be increased as the child gets used to it. The lids may be protected with a light application of petroleum jelly if required.

Instillation of Medication and Application of Dressings

In many cases, treatment is started in the department by the instillation of medication, both before the application of various dressings such as eyepads and bandages and in order to teach the patient how to instil his medication at home.

Prior to the instillation of medication, the patient should be seated comfortably in a treatment chair with his head well supported. A child may sit on his parent's knee, both so that the parent can assist the nurse and to give the child more security. Adequate light is necessary and an anglepoise type of lamp is very useful.

Before instilling any medication, the nurse should check the patient, the correct eye, the correct medication and strength and the expiry date. In order to adhere to the principles of asepsis, procedures must be preceded by thorough hand-washing.

Instillation of Drops

The nurse holds a swab to the lower lid, everts it slightly and asks the patient to look up. The dropper or bottle is held in the other hand and a drop is instilled into the lower fornix. The lids are dried with a swab. Various devices are available to assist patients who have difficulties with the instillation of eye drops at home. Most are readily available at pharmacies, at a low cost, and may help patients to be independent of neighbours or of overstretched community services.

Application of Ointment

Ointment may be applied either to the lid margins or instilled to have an effect on the eye.

1. To apply to the lid margins, for example in blepharitis, a small stream of ointment is squeezed along the margins of the closed lids and spread with a swab from the medial to the lateral aspect. To carry out this procedure at home, the patient may be instructed to first wash his hands, then to apply a little ointment to the tip of his little finger and then rub the ointment on to the lid margins where the lashes grow, both on the top and bottom lids. If both eyes are to be treated, he should be instructed to wash his hands in between the treatment of each eye and again at the end of the procedure.
2. To insert ointment into the eye, the lower lid should be held with a swab and the patient should be asked to look up. A small stream of ointment is squeezed in to the lower fornix, from the medial to the lateral aspect. The patient then closes his eyes and any excess ointment is wiped off his lids.

Parents may be advised to instil drops or ointment when babies or small children are asleep as this is often much easier and less distressing for all concerned.

Eyepads and Bandages

If the patient has a corneal abrasion, an eyepad is normally applied to keep the lid closed and to keep the patient comfortable. There does not appear to be any empirical evidence that padding aids corneal healing, but most patients appear to be far more comfortable and suffer less pain when the eye is padded and, for this reason alone, the procedure is worth carrying out.

A double pad should be applied, the first folded in half and placed over the closed lids (in order to keep them closed and prevent any further abrasion of the eye on the inside of the pad) and the second open over the top, the whole taped down with two or three pieces of skin-safe tape. A bandage may be applied over the pad to provide more pressure and support.

The nurse must make sure, after the application of a bandage, that the patient can still hear – the bandage should not cover his ears – and that he can still see through the other eye – again, it should not be covered by the bandage! The patient should be told how long to keep the pads on for and whether any follow-up appointment is required, before he leaves the department.

Patients should always be asked if they are driving home before eyepads are applied. Driving with an eyepad on is extremely dangerous as the whole of one field of vision is lost and, as the patient is not used to this, he will not be able to compensate for the loss of visual field as would a driver who has had only one eye for some time. (All changes in circumstance such as the loss of an eye must be reported to the Driver and Vehicle Licensing Authority and a period of adjustment undertaken before driving again.) Driving with an eyepad on is likely to invalidate insurance and to be regarded with disfavour by the police.

There is little point in telling someone that they must not drive after putting an eyepad on. They are likely either to drive anyway or to take off the pad to enable them to drive, and thus not receive the correct treatment. If the patient needs to drive home, it is more effective to instruct him how to pad his eye at home, give him the pads and any medication and let him get home before commencing treatment.

Patients should never have pads applied to both eyes at once. This is very disorientating and can be quite dangerous as the patient's companion is not likely to be experienced in leading and helping a totally blind person. It is safer to pad the worst affected eye and give extra pads to enable the patient to pad the eyes alternately, or to pad the second eye when he goes to bed.

Minor Operative Procedures

Minor operative procedures such as the suturing of lid lacerations and the incision and curettage of chalazion may be carried out within the area. The nurse must be able to prepare the patient for these procedures, both physically and psychologically. Knowledge of surgical techniques and the ability to assist is also necessary. Nurses who carry out procedures such as incision and curettage of chalazion should ensure that a fully informed consent is obtained prior to surgery. The patient, following surgery, usually waits for a short period in the department and has the dressing changed before going home. It must be recognized that the covering of one eye produces a visual disablement and patients must be given instructions to enable the safe adaptation to this temporary situation.

ON LEAVING THE DEPARTMENT

Successful treatment depends on patients' compliance with their treatment regime at home and their understanding of their situation. Each patient therefore needs to fully understand his condition and treatment before leaving the department.

If a patient has never instilled drops or ointment before, a demonstration might be given and reinforcement can be given to all patients with the use of simple, comprehensive instructions, which should include line drawings.

The patient should be given time to ask questions about the diagnosis and treatment and the nurse should ensure that he gets adequate answers before he leaves. Again, written information is useful. It should be comprehensive but straightforward and designed not to overwhelm the patient with information. A patient who is given too much to assimilate will probably not bother to read the information at all or will stop halfway through.

The patient may be given the telephone number of the unit in case he has any problems at home. The Patient's Charter introduced the concept of the Named Nurse and this is also a very useful tool, giving the patient the name of a nurse who has cared for him in the department and whom he can contact should any problems or queries arise. Reassurance or further explanation given over the telephone may be all that is needed if he becomes worried, rather than a repeat visit.

HEALTH EDUCATION

A significant part of the nurse's role when dealing with ophthalmic patients is health education, both with reference to the patient's present condition and generally. For example, the nurse should be able to advise on contact lens care (Chapter 20), types of safety glasses and the employer's and employee's roles in eye protection. Other information given might include how to prevent welding flash injuries, how to remove foreign bodies or how to irrigate the eye effectively after chemical injury.

There should be a good selection of health education booklets and posters in waiting areas. Patients will read booklets while they are waiting and may then take them home if they are interested. Topics might include smoking, drinking, HIV and AIDS and other current topics. A wide selection of material is available from the Health Education Authority and local health education departments.

Role of the Specialist Nurse in the Emergency Service

It can be seen that the ophthalmic trained nurse has an extensive role to play in the accident and emergency treatment of patients with ophthalmic problems. The role of the nurse in the receiving centre for ophthalmic accidents and emergencies is complex. As a triage nurse, she is involved in identifying priorities and ensuring that those patients in most need get medical aid first. As an educator, communicator and clinical nurse, she initiates first aid and treatments, promoting compliance by enhancing motivation and skills and helping to prevent further episodes by health education.

Jones *et al.* (1986) point out that an ophthalmic 'accident and emergency department' is really a primary care centre, many patients presenting with conditions such as conjunctivitis that could adequately be treated by their general practitioner. They suggest that many of these patients could be diagnosed and treated initially by an ophthalmic nurse practitioner. This might lead eventually to a wholly nurse practitioner-led service, treating a proportion of the patients that present and referring others to ophthalmologists. This scenario presents many problems of training, skill and accountability. These may be overcome, however, by protocols and guidelines on treatment and care, by programmes of training and assessment of suitability for the role and by the recognition of the role by health authorities who accept vicarious liability for the practice of the nurse practitioner.

This is a very exciting development in the role of the ophthalmic nurse and one which may be very rewarding. Indeed, this scenario has become a reality at Manchester's Royal Eye Hospital where the Emergency Eye Centre operates daily between 8 am and 9 pm, undertakes the initial care for all walk-in patients and the total ophthalmic care for a high proportion and is entirely nurse practitioner-led. A separate Acute Referral Centre accepts secondary referrals from health care professionals such as general practitioners, optometrists and nurse practitioners. There are many possible pitfalls in the development of such a role, however, and adequate time must be given to identify potential problems and to decide on strategies to deal with them should they occur so that the eventual implementation of such a scheme is to the best possible advantage of all concerned.

References

Beare, J. (1989) Management of chemical burns of the eye, in *Major Chemical Disasters – Medical Aspects of Management*, (ed. V. Murray), Royal Society of Medicine Services International Congress and Symposium Series No. 155, Royal Society of Medicine, London.

Jones, N. P., Hayward, J. M., Khaw, P. T. *et al.* (1986) Function of an ophthalmic 'Accident and Emergency' Department: results of a six month survey. *British Medical Journal*, **292**, 188–190.

Further reading

Proctor, T. (1989) Protection of the eye during welding. *Occupational Health*, 41 (10), 279–288.

Eagling, E. M. (1974) Ocular damage after blunt trauma to the eye: its relationships to the nature of injury. *British Journal of Ophthalmology*, **58**, 126–139.

Tannen, M. and Marsden, J. (1991) Chemical burns of the eye. *Nursing Standard*, 6(6).

7 PRINCIPLES OF INPATIENT CARE

Linda Whittaker

CHAPTER SUMMARY

GENERAL PRINCIPLES

The skills required to nurse the ophthalmic patient range from the manual dexterity necessary to carry out procedures on the eye to the social skills required to allay fears and apprehensions. The surgeon performs delicate microsurgery and relies on the nurse to use her skills in the postoperative period to facilitate recovery. Observational skills are also important so that complications can be noted quickly and appropriate action taken. For this to be possible, it is necessary to have a detailed knowledge of the structure and function of the eye, and of complications that may occur. In addition, systemic diseases may have ocular sequelae and, in some instances, these may be the first manifestation of the disease process. A good ophthalmic nurse should be able to recognize these and take appropriate action, ensuring her patient receives the attention required.

Many manifestations of behaviour may be apparent in a patient with visual problems. These include fear, withdrawal, demands and hostility. These reactions are normal when an individual is faced with the prospect of losing his sight. The ophthalmic nurse must meet these expressions with confidence, sensitivity, gentleness and efficiency and take appropriate nursing action to help the patient reach acceptance of the situation so that rehabilitation can be commenced. These reactions can apply as much to those patients with a temporary visual impairment as to those with a permanent loss of vision. With a visual impairment, everyday tasks that we all take for granted may prove difficult. The patient may not want to perform them for fear of making errors and, unless the nurse uses her skills to reeducate the patient, he may become apathetic and even depressed.

Until the patient comes to terms with his handicap it is difficult to attempt rehabilitation. If the nurse is aware of aspects related to the rehabilitation of visually handicapped people, she can give accurate and relevant information to aid this. A knowledge of registration details, financial benefits, mobility training, services available from statutory and voluntary agencies, aids and adaptations to carrying out daily activities, low vision aids, the importance of good lighting, employment, hobby and leisure pursuits and education can enable the nurse to give practical information both to the patient and his relatives (Chapter 3).

An integral part of the role therefore involves the patient being encouraged to be as independent as is 'safely' possible. The aspect of 'safe' independence is important because a visually impaired person may be independent in his own environment but, when placed in an unfamiliar environment and being unable to use mobility aids such as guide dogs and long canes, he may endeavour to maintain the amount of independence that is normal to him. In a hospital ward, the potential hazards to safety can include wet floors, trolleys, chairs, equipment not readily seen, etc. It is therefore essential that education of the patient in safety aspects is instigated and the balance achieved between promoting independence and maintaining safety. When guiding a visually impaired person it is preferable for them to take the arm of the person who is guiding them. This places them slightly behind the sighted guide, who will stop before an obstacle is reached; being pushed or pulled along only serves to heighten anxiety. Also, by holding the guide's arm, the guided person can feel any change of direction without having to be told.

Facial expressions and the use of hand gestures are meaningless to a visually impaired person. It is essential to communicate your presence to a visually impaired person so that he is not startled by a sudden touch. Similarly, it is of vital importance to announce your departure as it can be very embarrassing to find the conversation he is having is with himself. Visually impaired people often find difficulty in coming into a conversation, as they are denied the usual non-verbal cues that indicate that interaction from them is now appropriate. Their concentration span is lessened and so any information given must be concise. Additionally, it is difficult for them to know when they are being addressed unless their name is used. Their preferred name should be elicited from them as soon as possible.

Overall, it is important for the nurse to act as the patient's 'eyes'. Whatever she sees that is relevant should be transmitted to the patient so that he is aware of what is occurring and so can feel a part of it. This often requires a conscious effort on the part of the nurse because we often register information such as changes in floor levels or surfaces subconsciously. An accident can result in a loss of confidence. Trust, therefore, is an integral part of the relationship between ophthalmic nurses and visually impaired patients and has to be earned.

Patient Assessment

An assessment is used to identify specific patient problems and so forms the basis for prescribing nursing care. If this part of the nursing process is not carried out adequately, it will be reflected in the other stages. Crow (1981) recognizes this, and states 'a nursing care plan, and nursing care generally, can only be as good as the information on which it is based.' The assessment is usually carried out by taking a nursing history, and this can incorporate information gained from the patient, his relatives, and friends so that all aspects of the patient can be assessed, e.g. 'aspects of him as an individual, as a patient, as a member of a family, and as a member of a community' (Crow, 1981).

Models of nursing may be used as a framework for the basis of care. These comprise systems, adaption, interaction and behavioural models (Chapter 4). The assessment of an ophthalmic patient is often made using Roper's Activities of Living as the criteria, because visual impairment may have a marked effect on the patient's ability to carry out the majority of these activities. Other models of nursing, however, may need to be applied to certain problems, e.g. the educational needs of the patient.

Assessment of any patient should include physiological, psychological, social and spiritual needs. An accurate record should be made so that the patient is not repeatedly asked the same questions by different members of staff. It is important, however, to remember the assessment should be continuous and not a 'one-off' so that relevant information offered by the patient is not overlooked. Time is required to build up a relationship with a patient and if he has a personal problem, he might not at first be inclined to disclose this to what is really a complete stranger. Only by building up relationships with patients will they be given confidence to discuss their problems. As some ophthalmic patients may only be in hospital for a relatively short time, it is essential for the ophthalmic nurse to be efficient in facilitating this interaction. This has been assisted by part of the Patient's Charter (1991) which lays down that 'a named qualified nurse will be responsible for nursing care'.

Actual assessment forms will vary from hospital to hospital, and this should be borne in mind when considering the following information: patient's name and address, name and address of the general practitioner and medical diagnosis can be obtained from the patient's medical records, so that they are not repeatedly asked for this information. Relevant additional information can then be obtained from the patient to establish previous routines, what he is able or not able to do for himself (previous coping mechanisms in order to interpret the information) and to identify any actual or potential problems.

It is essential to establish what the patient understands about his condition and the reasons for his admission to hospital. This should be obtained by asking open-ended questions and recording the information given in the patient's own words because this could indicate his level of knowledge. The majority of patients are aware of the term 'cataract' but on further questioning have little knowledge of what it means. This lack of knowledge can be rectified by the nurse.

A record should also be made of the patient's recreational activities and of previous or present work. This information can be useful to the nurse to develop her interpersonal relationships with her patients, as it gives her topics to discuss. A patient with a visual impairment may become bored easily, as with the majority of ophthalmic conditions patients don't feel 'ill'. If a note has been made of hobbies that the patient enjoys, it may be possible for him to carry on with these and so alleviate his boredom.

Past medical, surgical and ophthalmic history should also be recorded if relevant. Systemic disorders often have ocular sequelae and may be relevant to the care needed by the patient. Examples of this include diabetes mellitus, thyroid gland dysfunction, multiple sclerosis and rheumatoid arthritis. Previous surgical treatment may assist in indicating the amount of information the patient needs regarding anaesthesia and whether it will be possible to build on existing knowledge. This is obviously true of previous ophthalmic history.

An assessment should also be made of the patient's general condition. This should include aspects of mobility, diet, sleep pattern, breathing, elimination, personal hygiene, dentition, hearing, speech and any known allergies. In addition to this, assessment of the patient's sight should be made and whether any spectacles are used. The visual acuity on admission should be determined if this information is not available in the medical records and should be transferred to the nursing record to give an indication to other nurses carrying on with the patient's care the amount of vision they have. With some ophthalmic patients, for example those with glaucoma, it should be remembered that they may have a defect in their field of vision and that although the visual acuity may be good there may be a gross field defect and problems of navigation.

Any medication that the patient is taking should be recorded. Systemic medications are usually continued unless there are ocular complications associated with them. Anticoagulants may be stopped prior to surgery. Topical ophthalmic medications may also be continued; for example, a patient who has been admitted for cataract surgery may already be receiving treatment for glaucoma.

Measurement of blood pressure, pulse and urinalysis should also be made and any abnormalities reported to the medical staff. Any evidence of hypertension could have a direct influence on any ophthalmic surgery undertaken as it can lead to complications occurring at the time of surgery. Any irregularities of the pulse could determine whether the patient for surgery is given a local or general anaesthetic. Urinalysis is also necessary to determine any underlying medical complications such as undiagnosed diabetes.

Any investigations the patient is expecting or that have been arranged should also be recorded on the nursing record. As the majority of patients for surgery are elderly, these may include chest X-rays, electrocardiography, a full blood count, and urea and electrolyte balance. If the patient is diabetic, blood sugar levels will be necessary. For dacryocystorhinostomy, where there may be appreciable bleeding, the blood group may be requested prior to surgery. If the patient takes anticoagulants a clotting test may be requested. If a patient has been admitted with uveitis, it will be necessary to investigate any underlying systemic condition by X-rays of spine and chest and blood investigations for a variety of disorders. In patients having an intraocular lens implant at the time of cataract surgery, biometry may be carried out to determine the power of the implant required. Fluorescein angiography and ultrasonography investigations may be required by other patients. Recording these investigations will give an indication of the need for explanations to these patients.

Psychological assessment of the patient should also be made and recorded to enable the nurse to give practical advice and support to assist in alleviating any worries the patient may have. Individual patients may need more psychological support than others. If the patient has had a previous admission he may not be unduly anxious about his stay in hospital. Similarly, a patient who has had notification of admission from the waiting list will usually exhibit lower anxiety levels than a patient admitted as an emergency. The nature of any operation may also have a bearing on the patient's reactions. A patient admitted for removal of an eye may require a great deal of psychological care. With this type of problem, it may be very helpful for the ocular prosthetist to visit the patient to discuss his fears and to give him practical information regarding how soon the artificial eye will be fitted and the cosmetically acceptable results that are possible (Chapter 21).

Assessment of the patient's social needs is of crucial importance while in hospital and in preparation for discharge. Most assessment forms will have space available to record any support the patient is receiving from the community prior to admission, and also from relatives or friends. It is necessary to determine who will be available to care for him on discharge. If the patient lives alone, it will be difficult for him to carry out household duties, shopping and washing his hair. It may therefore be necessary to arrange interim support services such as district nurse, home help and meals-on-wheels. In addition, most ophthalmic patients are discharged home on topical medications and it is necessary to determine who will instil the prescribed treatment so that the education of the patient, relatives or friends in this technique can be fulfilled prior to discharge. This information is required early during a short stay, in order to arrange services and teach effectively.

Nursing Care

Once the initial assessment has been completed, it should be possible to determine the patient's actual and potential problems. These identified problems should be listed in order of priority. Bower (1977) states: 'priority setting does not negate the importance of the lower-priority needs or problems; it simply puts them into a realistic framework for consideration and solution'. Patients' problems should be stated in clear and precise terms, and include how the problem is affecting the patient, what is causing the problem and if it is amenable to nursing intervention. Therefore, a medical diagnosis alone is not sufficient. It may be, however, that the medical condition has an obvious consequence. For example, a patient admitted with acute glaucoma may have considerable pain due to raised intraocular pressure, and nursing interventions can assist in alleviating this problem for the patient.

Following problem identification, the goals can be stated and the nursing care plan compiled. Bower (1977) states:

> the nursing care plan is the tool to implement the nursing process and the key to quality nursing care lies in the nurse's desire, interest, and ability to systematically plan care. A process that includes comprehensive assessment, accurate problem identification, plans for action, and an evaluation based on the desired outcome is the most efficient and practical way to plan nursing care.

These points are just as applicable in an ophthalmic nursing setting as in any other. Indeed, because a patient with a visual impairment is physically 'well' it can be easier to include the patient in the care plan discussion. This will also pave the way for promotional and rehabilitative aspects of care with education and practical instructions necessary for continuance of care following discharge to be included, and the patient to understand why they are necessary.

The following section will cover most aspects of admission, pre- and postoperative periods and preparation for discharge. It should be remembered, however, that specific problems may arise with different conditions, and it will be necessary to refer to the appropriate chapters.

Patients are usually anxious when admitted to hospital. This quite often results from insufficient knowledge of their condition and treatment, of anaesthetics, and a general fear of the unknown. Numerous studies have been carried out relating to stress and anxiety levels among patients in hospital. Wilson-Barnett (1979) suggested that the first 24 hours following admission were when the patient had the highest stress levels and that a proper nursing assessment can directly affect the length of time it takes to help the patients adapt to their new environment. The giving of information preoperatively has been found to have an effect on patients' postoperative recovery. Hayward (1975) found that informed patients recovered more quickly and required less analgesia than patients who lacked information. Similarly, Boore (1978) found that 'the preoperative giving of information about prospective treatment and care, and the teaching of exercises to be performed postoperatively, will minimize the rise in biochemical indication of stress.'

Problem	Goal	Nursing intervenion
Anxiety due to insufficient knowledge regarding: 1. condition and treatment; 2. anaesthesia; 3. fear of the unknown.	Anxiety levels reduced to a level acceptable to the patient within 24 hours following admission.	1. Establish patient's knowledge base. 2. Elicit patient's specific worries. 3. Briefly explain the condition and the reasons for operation. 4. Explain length of anaesthesia and briefly outline what the patient can expect to happen in the theatre. 5. Outline the expected visual prognosis. 6. Instruct on postoperative restrictions and why they are necessary. 7. Make sure the patient understands the information given. 8. Observe for reduction in anxiety levels at each interaction.

The patient with a visual handicap may fail to 'notice' things going on around him. He will be unsure of the ward layout and will need to be informed of the ward routines. It is necessary to introduce such a person to his fellow patients and members of staff to avoid him becoming isolated. It is essential also to escort the patient around the ward environment so that he becomes familiar with it. Franklin (1974), in her study on patient anxiety on admission to hospital, found that only 38% reported noticing such information as location of areas, or reading signs about, for example, visiting times. A patient with poor vision is even less likely to absorb such helpful information. This is the rationale for explaining and showing the patients around the ward environment, explaining routines and introducing them to staff and patients. In addition to helping patients become familiar with the environment, taking them around the ward can assist in assessing the level of visual handicap and give an indication to the nurse of the amount of support and assistance the patient may require.

Problem	Goal	Nursing intervention
Unsure of ward layout, ward routine and other people due to visual handicap.	Knows ward layout and routine, can move safely around the ward within 24 hours and is able to summon help if needed.	1. Introduce patient to other patients and staff. 2. Show the patient around the ward; explain its layout. 3. Observe the effect the patient's visual handicap has on moving safely around the ward. 4. Explain the ward routines. 5. Explain the call bell system. 6. Make sure the patient understands the information given. 7. Provide opportunities for patient to ask questions and answer them promptly.

Another aspect of the effect of a visual impairment is that of being unable to mobilize safely due to their low vision. Ward areas can provide potential hazards to the patient's well-being, for instance wet and slippery floors, trolleys and equipment lying in the patient's path. Similarly, a patient who may be fully mobile in his own environment using mobility aids such as long canes and guide dogs will not be able to use them in the ward areas because of restrictions on space, possible injuries to other patients and hygiene regulations. Therefore, it may be necessary to restrict full mobility to ensure the patient's safety needs are met. This should be done on an individual basis for each patient because, while adequate safety is desirable, it is not desirable for the patient to be totally dependent on the nurse, as this may create problems on the patient's discharge home if he is not able to cope for himself.

Problem	Goal	Nursing intervention
Unable to mobilize safely due to visual handicap.	To be as independent as is safely possible during stay in hospital.	1. Establish patient's normal level of mobility. 2. Make sure obstacles are not left in the patient's path. 3. Warn the patient of any change in floor surface levels. 4. Warn the patient when the floors are wet. 5. Observe the patient while he is mobilizing and give assistance when necessary. 6. Explain to the patient why full independent mobility is not feasible and make sure he understands.

Another problem facing the patient is that of being unable to sleep due to the change in environment. Sleeplessness may cause further safety problems for the patient when he is mobilizing. Hospitals are notoriously noisy places, and because background noise can be more intense to a visually handicapped person, it is essential to ensure that noise levels are kept to a minimum. In order to cater for the individual patient, normal routines should be adhered to as closely as possible.

Problem	Goal	Nursing intervention
Potential problem of being unable to sleep due to the change in environment.	To feel adequately rested throughout his stay in hospital.	1. Establish patient's normal sleep pattern. 2. Allow patient to follow normal pre-sleep routine. 3. Ensure noise levels are kept to a minimum. 4. Provide hot drink if patient wishes if he wakes during the night. 5. Escort to the toilet if required. 6. Observe amount of sleep patient has and if he feels this is acceptable. 7. Provide night sedation if required.

Some surgeons request a conjunctival swab in order to identify any pathogenic bacteria present. The eyelashes are very rarely cut before intraocular surgery. These procedures should be explained fully to the patient prior to them being carried out (see also page 99).

If the patient is to have a general anaesthetic, routine preparation is carried out, such as starvation for six hours preoperatively, removing jewellery and prostheses, etc. However, if the patient is having a local anaesthetic it is not necessary for him to starve, but to have a light meal only before surgery. A 'bonus' for the patient undergoing local anaesthetic is that he is allowed to keep his dentures in.

Specific preparation for the ophthalmic patient includes checking that the correct eye is marked for surgery and that any prescribed preoperative drops are instilled. Dilation of the pupil in cataract surgery is essential to the success of the operation.

Once the patient is prepared, including premedication if required, the patient's call bell should be placed within his reach so that he is able to summon assistance if necessary. Immediately prior to theatre a bedpan or urinal should be offered to the patient and when the patient is transferred to theatre a careful check should be made that the correct patient is being transferred and that all relevant documentation is transferred with him. This is all part of ensuring that the correct operation is performed on the correct patient. It is particularly desirable for a nurse with whom the patient is familiar to accompany him to theatre to help keep anxiety levels to a minimum.

Problem	**Goal**	**Nursing intervention**
Potential of post-operative complications due to being physically unprepared for surgery.	Safely and efficiently prepared for surgery prior to transfer to theatre.	1. Ensure patient understands the reasons for any preoperative investigations necessary, e.g. chest X-ray, electrocardiograph, blood investigations, conjunctival swabs for culture and sensitivity, urinalysis and blood pressure check. 2. If required, cut eyelashes on the eye for surgery and explain the reasons for this. 3. If for general anaesthesia, ensure the patient remains 'nil orally' for six hours preoperatively. 4. Prepare in gown and cap before giving premedication. 5. Check consent form is signed. 6. Administer premedication at prescribed time. 7. Remove dentures, jewellery, and any prostheses. 8. Check correct eye is marked for surgery. 9. Instil prescribed preoperative drops. 10. Place call bell within patient's reach. 11. Provide opportunities for any questions the patient may have and answer them promptly. 12. Provide bedpan/urinal for patient to empty bladder immediately prior to transferral to theatre. 13. Ensure all relevant documents are transferred to theatre with the patient.

Following surgery, it is necessary to ensure that the patient has a safe recovery from the anaesthetic and that any complications that do occur are detected early. For this reason the patient should be nursed in the semi-prone position, making sure a clear airway is maintained. Ophthalmic patients are placed on their sides to avoid pressure on the operated eye. An exception to this is when a patient has had an enucleation. The main complication is haemorrhage and, by placing the patient lying on the affected side, pressure is applied to the socket and the risk of haemorrhage is reduced. Similarly, patients undergoing vitreoretinal surgery may require specific positioning postoperatively and in this case the patient will be positioned according to the surgeon's directions. Regular observations of pulse, blood pressure and skin colour should be made and any abnormalities should be reported. Once the patient has fully recovered from the anaesthetic, he can be nursed sitting, with the bed head at an angle of 45° unless contraindicated by the surgery. As the majority of ophthalmic patients are elderly the complications of bedrest such as pneumonia and deep vein thrombosis are real. Gentle leg exercises and deep breathing should, therefore, be encouraged when the patient has recovered from the anaesthetic and is back on the ward, and early mobilization is encouraged wherever possible.

Problem	Goal	Nursing intervention
Potential problem of shock and asphyxiation due to surgery and anaesthesia.	Safe recovery from anaesthesia; early detection of any complications within 24 hours postoperatively.	1. Maintain clear airway. 2. Nurse in semi-prone position till awake. 3. Ensure suction working and to hand. 4. Measure and record half-hourly pulse and blood pressure readings until stable, then reduce to 4 hourly for 24 hours. 5. Report to nurse in charge if any deviations from patient's baseline observations. 6. When awake from anaesthetic, position according to surgeon's wishes or at an angle of 45°. 7. Observe for physical signs of shock and report immediately if present. 8. Encourage deep breathing and leg exercises when recovered from anaesthesia, or early mobilization.

The majority of ophthalmic patients do not experience significant pain postoperatively. It is most likely following surgery for retinal detachment, dacryocystorhinostomy and injury. Pain results in restlessness, and if a patient moves around the bed a great deal or rubs his eyes complications such as haemorrhage or prolapsed iris can occur. The patient should be allowed to verbalize the amount of pain he feels and the nurse should be willing to listen and observe for non-verbal signs of the presence of pain such as tenseness, restlessness and facial grimaces. Analgesia should then be given as appropriate and its effect monitored.

Problem	Goal	Nursing intervention
Potential problem of pain due to surgical wound/ ET tube.	Patient pain free or pain at a level acceptable to patient at all times following surgery.	1. Assess levels of pain 3–4 hourly. 2. Administer postoperative analgesia as prescribed. 3. Observe and report on its effect. 4. Ensure the comfort of the patient.

Retention of urine following general anaesthesia should be anticipated, especially in the elderly male. The patient should be encouraged to pass urine and offered at least 2-hourly toileting facilities.

Problem	Goal	Nursing intervention
Potential problem of retention of urine due to anaesthesia.	No anxiety, bladder distension or discomfort reported by patient during postoperative recovery period.	1. Offer 2-hourly toileting facilities. 2. If patient has not passed urine within 12 hours of surgery, report to nurse in charge.

Enforced bedrest because of the surgery has two important consequences. As the majority of ophthalmic patients are elderly it is important to monitor pressure areas and encourage a change in position at least 2-hourly. Hygiene and dietary needs during this period should be attended to by the nurse and independence encouraged as much as possible, for example, by using the clock face to describe the location of food on the patient's plate so that he can then feed himself. During this period the patient is usually anxious regarding the visual prognosis, and time should be taken to talk to the patient, allowing him to verbalize any worries he may have and letting him know how the operation went.

Problem	Goal	Nursing intervention
Unable to carry out activities of living due to enforced bedrest following surgery.	Will return to normal pattern of self-care within 48 hours.	1. Explain reasons for bedrest and make sure patient understands. 2. Place call bell within patient's reach. 3. Change patient's position in bed 2-hourly and observe for pressure area breakdown. 4. Assist with dietary needs as necessary. 5. Place fluids within patient's reach. 6. Provide postoperative wash and change into night attire when recovered from anaesthesia. 7. Take time to talk to the patient and allow him to ask any questions or verbalize any worries he may have. Answer questions promptly.

Patients may wear a pad or shield over the operated eye. The extent to which this affects the patient can be directly related to the amount of vision the patient has in the unoperated eye. This can vary enormously and so attention should be paid to each individual patient. This problem can be reduced to some extent by placing the patient's bedside locker on his unaffected side and ensuring all articles the patient requires are within reach. It is important to approach such patients from the unoperated side so as not to startle them.

Problem	Goal	Nursing intervention
Patient has blind area due to operated eye being occluded by a pad.	Will be safely independent until pad is removed and usual field of vision is restored.	1. Place locker on patient's unaffected side. 2. Ensure all articles are within reach. 3. When attending to patient, approach from unoperated side.

In order to help avoid complications of pain, infection and haemorrhage it is necessary to ensure the patient receives his topical medication as prescribed. Strict asepsis is maintained at all times, observations of the eye are made at each dressing and adequate analgesia is given. Although the vision of the patient is not tested at every dressing, it is important to note any comments the patient may make about improvement or deterioration in vision in order to instigate action in the event of possible complications occurring.

Problem	Goal	Nursing intervention
Potential ophthalmic complications of pain, infection, inflammation and haemorrhage due to intraocular surgery.	No discomfort or reduction in vision reported by the patient up to his discharge home.	1. Instil prescribed eye medication using aseptic technique. 2. Observe ophthalmic condition at each dressing and report observations to nurse in charge. 3. Discourage patient from touching the eye or pad, explaining why this is necessary and ensuring understanding. 4. Note any comments made by the patient regarding vision or discomfort. 5. Reinforce activity restrictions and explanations. 6. Give prescribed analgesia as required and monitor its effect.

While busy at times, most ophthalmic wards are quiet compared to the 'hurly burly' of an acute surgical ward, so there can be a potential problem of boredom for the ophthalmic patient. The pace of nursing in an ophthalmic ward is slower in order to give visually impaired patients time to carry out activities as independently as possible.

It is, therefore, important to allow the patient to have an appropriate amount of activity and rest. In order to prevent boredom, the nurse should ascertain the patient's interests on admission and, where possible both from a practical and visual aspect, allow him to carry on with these. Time should also be taken to engage the patient in conversation on topics that are of interest to him and in such a way that the patient does not feel he is preventing the nurse from carrying out her work or using up her 'valuable' time. Friends and relatives should be encouraged to visit, with possibly extra care being taken with young babies, who seem to have a knack of poking their fingers into eyes! Opportunities should also be provided for the patient to listen to the radio, watch television, listen to cassette tapes or talking books, read large print books and play card or board games if he wishes. Many games are available from the Royal National Institute for the Blind and a catalogue and price list is available both in normal and large print.

Problem	Goal	Nursing intervention
Potential problem of boredom due to inactivity.	Patient will have appropriate amount of activity and rest acceptable to him during his stay in hospital.	1. Ascertain patient's interests. 2. Take time to converse with the patient on topics that interest him. 3. Encourage normal interests if visual handicap and surgical considerations allow. 4. Encourage friends and relatives to visit. 5. Provide radio, television, cassette tapes and large print books as patient wishes.

Preparation for Discharge

A common problem on discharge is the instillation of eye drops. This may apply equally to patients who have instilled drops previously and those with no previous experience. Donnelly (1987) suggested that the patients appeared to be unable to determine their own learning needs at this time. The ophthalmic nurse should explain the importance of a need for compliance with treatment, emphasizing that some drops such as cyclopentolate may themselves cause blurring of vision. The actual procedure for instilling the drops and the importance of handwashing before and after treatment should be explained to the patient. In addition, emphasis should be placed on avoiding contamination of the drop bottle from the skin, conjunctiva or lashes. The patient should be observed instilling his own drops each time they are prescribed. Encouragement should be given and alternate methods discussed with him so that he adopts the one that suits him most. This may vary from instilling the drops while sitting in a chair, in front of a mirror or lying on his bed. Throughout the teaching of the patient in this technique, the nurse should always make sure he understands the information he has been given. The patient should also be advised that, if the eye gets sticky, he should boil some water, allow it to cool and gently bathe the eye from the nasal to the temporal side using cotton wool moistened in the solution.

Problem	Goal	Nuring intervention
Unable to instil own drops due to lack of knowledge and practice.	Patient to be confident of his ability to carry on treatment following his discharge home.	1. Explain need for compliance with treatment and ensure patient understands. 2. Explain the procedure for instilling drops, using appropriate terminology. 3. Observe the patient instilling his own drops each time they are prescribed, giving encouragement. 4. Monitor and report on patient's progress. 5. Explain the effect of treatment, including visual effects, and make sure patient understands.

The final problem considered is that of the patient being inadequately prepared for discharge home through lack of knowledge. It is important that the patient is given the necessary information in order to carry out self-care at a safe level independently on return home. It may be necessary in some instances for community resources to be arranged (e.g. district nurse, home help, meals-on-wheels), to enable the patient to go to his own home following discharge and this should be considered and organized on an individual basis. All previous information given on cleaning the eye, instilling drops and postoperative restrictions should be reinforced to both patient and relatives. Written instructions can also be given to enhance the verbal instructions. It should be remembered, however, that written instructions alone are not of benefit to the patient. An outpatient appointment is usually issued for up to 2 weeks following discharge and the nurse should make sure the patient has transport to attend and, if not, arrange for an ambulance. Both the patient and the relatives should be advised on how to contact the hospital if any problems occur, such as deterioration of vision and worsening pain. Advice should also be given, if necessary, on rehabilitation services, aids available for use in the home such as timers, auditory gadgets to make daily living easier and any ways in which the patient's eyesight can be used to his full advantage. This may include increasing the size of objects, using suitable lighting and decorations and incorporating the use of contrast to make objects more visible.

Problem	Goal	Nursing interverntion
Inadequately prepared for discharge home due to lack of knowledge.	Understands necessary information in order to carry out self-care on return home, by time of discharge.	1. Reinforce instructions given on cleaning the eye and instilling drops. 2. Reinforce postoperative restrictions. 3. Issue drops and explain times to be instilled and visual side effects. 4. Issue follow-up outpatients appointment. 5. Give written instructions in addition to verbal ones. 6. Arrange any necessary community services. 7. Advise the patient and relatives to contact the hospital if any problems occur. 8. Ensure both patients and relatives understand the information given. 9. Allow both patients and relatives to ask any questions and answer them promptly. 10. Advise on rehabilitation services, both statutory and voluntary, aids available for use in the home and ways in which the patient's eyesight can be used to his full advantage.

Finally, it should reiterated that the patient must always be treated as an individual, and his care planned according to needs. The problems identified in this chapter are intended to give a broad aspect of general problems relating to the ophthalmic patient.

Procedures

The following section covers some of the common ophthalmic nursing procedures that may be required for the ophthalmic inpatient.

Taking Conjunctival Swabs

This investigation is still used by some surgeons to determine the presence of any pathogenic micro-organisms in the conjunctival sac. This is most commonly done as a routine preoperative investigation before any drops are given. If any discharge is present following surgery, it may be done postoperatively. A sterile swab on a stick is used and placed in the appropriate transport medium for bacterial or viral culture. Before taking the swab, the procedure must be explained to the patient so that he understands and is able to co-operate fully. For patient safety, he should be seated in a chair with his head well supported, and adequate illumination should be available. The nurse must ensure that the skin is not touched in order that the swab is taken from the correct surface and that the highly sensitive cornea is not touched or damaged. The bottom lid should be gently everted and the patient should be instructed to look up so that the conjunctival surface is exposed. The swab is passed gently along the exposed surface from the inner to the outer canthus. This should only take a couple of seconds and any secretions will be absorbed on to the swab. The swab is then placed in the transport medium and despatched to the laboratory with the appropriate investigation form, correctly completed.

Cutting Lashes

This procedure may very occasionally be carried out on ophthalmic patients. It is necessary to ensure that no lashes or parts of lashes remain in the conjunctival sac following the procedure, as they may enter the eye during surgery. Although it is necessary to trim the lashes as close to the lid margin as possible, it is essential that care is taken not to cut the skin surface, as any break in skin integrity provides an entry site for infection. It is necessary therefore to gain the full co-operation of the patient and for this reason it is recommended that confused, anxious or agitated patients, or children requiring their lashes trimmed should have this done under anaesthesia, if at all. The patient should be informed that the lashes will re-grow within six weeks to their previous length.

Aseptic Dressings

Once a patient has undergone surgery, it is necessary to incorporate strict asepsis when carrying out dressings to minimize the risk of postoperative infection. The principles for ophthalmic dressings are modified from those used for general dressings, but the same rules apply regarding avoidance of contamination from the air. The actual contents of dressing packs vary from hospital to hospital, but should contain some form of sterile swab and gallipot for holding normal saline. Supplementary sterile swabs and eye pads should be taken and used as necessary. Scissors and a pen torch cleaned with an alcohol-impregnated swab should also be available for opening supplementary packs, cutting tape and examining the eye respectively. The patient should be seated or lying down with his head supported and adequate illumination is necessary. Forceps should not be used as the risks of damaging the eye are increased. It is desirable to use one hand for picking up clean items from the trolley and the other hand for cleaning the eye.

The sterile swabs should be moistened in the normal saline, transferred to the other hand, and the eye cleaned from the inner to outer aspect. (By cleaning the eye in this way, it moves any infected material away from instead of towards the eye.) The swab should be passed along the lid margins once only in one smooth motion. To clean the lower lid effectively, the patient should be asked to look up so as to expose the area more fully and then to clean the top lid the patient should be asked to gently close his eyes. A firm but gentle pressure is necessary in order that the patient is not caused undue discomfort due to clumsiness on the nurse's part. The eye lids are swabbed as many times as necessary until they are clean.

A dry swab is then used to draw back the lids while shining a light on to the eye, to observe for any signs of complications and to monitor the progress towards healing. The specific observations necessary often relate to the type of surgery the patient has had, and so reference should be made to the appropriate chapters dealing with the specific disorders. It is important to observe the eye at each dressing, otherwise complications may be missed and a delay in taking appropriate action may result. If an eye pad is required, it should be applied to the eye without actually touching the surface that will lie against the patient's lids. It is possible to do this by placing a piece of tape over the pad and using that to lift the pad from the sterile surface, sticking it to the patient's forehead and cheek above and below the eye that is being covered. It is important to instruct the patient to gently close his eyes when applying a pad, and to make sure the eye is closed underneath the pad. As with any dressing where asepsis is required, it is essential that the nurse pays attention to her own hygiene, that hands are thoroughly washed and dried prior to and following this procedure and that all used equipment is disposed of adequately.

INSTILLATION OF MEDICATION

Topical medications are used in the prevention and treatment of ophthalmic disorders. It should be remembered that ophthalmic medications are drugs and that checks are made before giving an ophthalmic drug as you would with a systemic drug. The following checks should be made prior to instilling ophthalmic medication:

1. it is the correct patient;
2. it is the correct eye;
3. it is the correct medication;
4. it is the correct strength of medication;
5. the expiry date on the medication has not been reached;
6. the time and date of instillation are correct;
7. the date of commencement of the medication;
8. the medical staff have signed for the prescription.

These checks are necessary for safety considerations and are doubly important when different medication is instilled into each eye of the same patient. For instance, a patient may be on a long-term treatment for glaucoma and may require a cataract extraction for the other eye. He may, therefore, be on a miotic drop to one eye and a mydriatic drop to the other. It cannot be emphasized enough, therefore, how important these safety checks are.

When instilling a drop, a dry sterile swab should be held to the lower lid, slightly everting it. The patient should be asked to look up, so that the drop is instilled into the lower fornix and not directly on to the highly sensitive cornea. The drop container should be held inverted with the tip at least 13 mm from the eye to avoid contamination of the container. One drop is instilled into the lower fornix between the middle and outer third of the eye. The patient is then asked to gently close his eyes, and the eyelids and cheek are gently dried.

Eye ointment may be either inserted to have an effect on the eye or applied as treatment to the lid margins. To insert ointment into an eye, the lower lid is held with a swab and the patient is asked to look up. A small stream of ointment is squeezed into the lower fornix from the inner to the outer aspect, the patient is asked to close his eyes gently and the excess ointment is wiped from the lashes. The patient who has had ointment inserted should be advised that his vision will be blurred for at least a couple of hours, due to the oily base of the ointment, and that this is normal. To apply ointment to the lid margins, a small amount of ointment should be squeezed along the margins of the closed lids and spread evenly with a sterile swab from the inner to the outer aspect.

In order to adhere to the principles of asepsis all of the procedures described must be preceded by the scrupulous washing of the hands.

Standard Care Plans

This chapter will conclude with a brief mention of the use of standard care plans in ophthalmic nursing. I feel that they are of benefit in this nursing field for a number of reasons. First, the length of time the ophthalmic patient is in hospital has considerably reduced over the past 10 years. In addition, certain problems are common for any patient undergoing certain types of surgery and to have those problems identified on standard care plans allows for time to be given to problems affecting the individual patient, e.g. physically preparing the patient for surgery and alleviating anxiety. These plans could then be expanded to create an individual care plan to provide individualized care for each patient. Standard care plans can be used to give care that is common to all patients admitted with the same diagnosis. Mayers, citing Kershaw (1979), advocated this concept and stated 'the nurse would then build the individual problems from the nursing history'. Kershaw (1979) incorporated the use of standard care plans in the care of ophthalmic trauma patients and it could be suggested that this be tried with other conditions, especially where the length of stay in hospital is short.

Kershaw (1979) identified nine problems that were routine and normally experienced by patients with eye injuries:

1. anxiety about family and admission;
2. anxiety about sudden loss of sight and its implications;
3. anxiety about anaesthesia and surgery;
4. not understanding condition and urgency;
5. possible chest infection due to general anaesthetic and bed rest, as well as inadequate preoperative preparation;
6. possible infection due to wound contamination at time of accident;
7. anxiety about visual progress;
8. lack of understanding of surgery and of nursing and medical care;
9. anxiety about family, job and money.

By implementing and evaluating the use of standard care plans, their use should become apparent. However, it is essential to emphasize that standard care plans should never be used in isolation, otherwise individual nursing care will not be provided.

References

Boore, J. R. P. (1978) *Prescription for Recovery – The Effect of Pre-Operative Preparation of Surgical Patients on Post-Operative Stress, Recovery and Infection*, Royal College of Nursing, London.

Bower, F. L. (1977) *The Process of Planning Nursing Care – A Model for Practice,* 2nd edn, C. V. Mosby, St Louis, MD.

Crow, J. (1981) *The Nursing Process,* (ed. C. R. Kratz), Baillière Tindall, London

Department of Health (1991) *The Patient's Charter*, HMSO, London.

Donnelly, D. (1987) Instilling eye drops: difficulties experienced by patients following cataract surgery. *Journal of Advanced Nursing*, **12**, 235–243.

Franklin, B. L. (1974) *Patient Anxiety on Admission to Hospital,* Royal College of Nursing, London.

Hayward, J. (1975) *Information – A Prescription Against Pain*, Royal College of Nursing, London

Kershaw, J. E. M. (1979) Teaching the nursing process – standard care plans. *Nursing Times,* **16 Aug,** 1413–1416.

Wilson-Barnett, J. (1979) *Stress in Hospital – Patients' Psychological Reactions to Illness and Health Care,* Churchill Livingstone, Edinburgh.

Further Reading

Allen, M., Knight, C., Falk, C. and Strong V. (1992) Effectiveness of a preoperative teaching programme for cataract patients. *Journal of Advanced Nursing*, **17**, 303–309.

Beed, P. (1991) Losing her eyes. *Nursing Times*, **87** (47), 26–28.

Bickford, M. E. (1988) Patient teaching tools in the ophthalmic unit. *Journal of Advanced Nursing and Technology*, **17**, 50–55.

Department of Health and Social Security (1988) *Causes of Blindness and Partial Sight Among Adults in 1980/81 in England – New Registrations,* HMSO, London.

Dobree, J. H. and Boulter, E. (1982) *Blindness and the Visually Handicapped: The Facts*, Oxford University Press, Oxford.

Field, D. (1992) Managing chronic simple glaucoma. *Nursing Standard,* **16** (18), 28–30.

Ford, M and Heshek, T. (1992) *In Touch – Aids and Services for Blind and Partially Sighted People,* British Broadcasting Corporation, London.

Klemz, A. (1977) *Blindness and Partial Sight*, Woodhead-Faulkner, Cambridge.

Guiding a Blind or a Partially Sighted Person; Information for People Losing Their Sight; Helping People Who are Deaf as Well as Blind; Leaflets available from the Royal National Institute for the Blind.

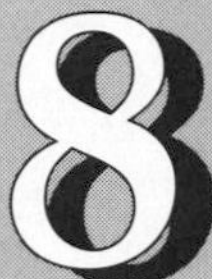

Principles of Outpatient Care

Deirdre Donnelly and Meg Johnson

Chapter Summary

Advances in ophthalmic medicine and in the application of technology to eye disease have resulted in marked changes in management in recent years. Many conditions can now be treated on an outpatient basis, including major ocular surgery. The following chapter considers the care required by patients who are attending for consultation and/or investigations and those who are attending for surgical procedures.

Outpatient care means that there is only minimal contact between the patient and the doctor or nurse initiating care. A vitally important part of the nurse's role in this area is to ensure that the best possible use is made of the time when patient and carer come together. Ensuring that the patient has understood the information given to him while in the outpatient department, giving further information and assessing the patient's practical ability to carry out his treatment safely and with confidence have become the primary objectives of the ophthalmic trained nurse in the outpatient setting.

Outpatient Consultation/Investigation

Reception of Patients

In order to avoid congestion and confusion it is essential to make it as easy as possible for each individual to find out where he wants to get to in the department.

Signposting

Where a large number of the patients attending have some visual impairment it is obvious that any signs intended to give information to patients are large, clear and easy to read. Good signposting covers a wider area than simply written notices, however. Doors and doorways should be painted in colours which contrast sharply with surrounding walls so that visually impaired patients can readily distinguish between them. (Black on yellow, as in car number plates, provides good contrast.) Floor coverings should be plain – some patterns can look like potential obstacles in the path of a patient with poor vision. Large symbols on the walls can also help people to find their way around the department – large eyes looking in a particular direction might be an appropriate symbol to use in an ophthalmic department!

However much care is taken with signposting, there will always be some patients who simply cannot find their way around without help. They may be unable to see or they may be simply overwhelmed by all the hustle and bustle of the department. When dealing with such a patient, the nurse should be able to provide the guidance and individual attention of which these patients are particularly in need.

Layout of the Department

The most suitable layout for any outpatient department is probably what is known as the 'racetrack' design. This means that the areas which the patient is likely to visit are arranged in logical progression – reception is followed by the visual acuity room, then the clinic areas, nursing treatment rooms, testing department, dispensing opticians, appointments and pharmacy, etc., finally leading the patient back to the main reception/waiting area. Arranging the department as far as possible in this sequence means that patients are able to proceed from one area to another with the minimum of upheaval and risk of anyone 'getting lost'.

Needs of the Patient

Poor vision may not be the only problem affecting patients attending the ophthalmic outpatient department. Many of the patients will be elderly and may have a hearing impairment or limited mobility. Other groups of patients may have general medical problems such as diabetes, which frequently has ophthalmic complications.

The nurse in the outpatient department should be aware of these additional problems with which ophthalmic patients may be burdened, as it is important to take these into consideration when planning and giving nursing care.

Some of the commonest of these problems and possible ways of dealing with them are listed below.

Problem	Goal	Nursing intervention
Patient is slightly/very deaf. Unsure of what is being said to him. He is worried about not hearing his name being called.	To relieve patient anxiety. To ensure patient understands what is being said to him.	1. Establish which patients in your area have a hearing problem and find out their names. 2. Reassure each patient by telling him that you are aware of his disability and will ensure that he does not miss his turn. 3. Inform other staff of patient's problem and of the need to speak clearly to him. 4. Listen to what is said to the patient by, e.g., medical staff. Determine how much patient has heard before repeating information and ensuring that it has all been understood.
Patient frail and elderly. Unable to walk far without assistance. Has difficulty getting from one department to another.	To help patient to move from one department to another without overexerting himself.	1. Assess patient's level of mobility by asking him how far he can walk. 2. Supply patient with a mobility aid if appropriate. Ensure that he knows where he is going and, if necessary, accompany him. 3. Make sure there is adequate room for the patient to use his frame, wheelchair, etc., by clearing corridors of any clutter or items which he may bump into or fall over. 4. Check that he reaches his destination without unnecessary exertion or anxiety. 5. Inform other staff who will be dealing with the patient of his mobility problem and how to deal with it.
Patient is a known diabetic and has been in the department for some time.Potential risk of hypoglycaemic episode.	To prevent hypoglycaemic attack from occurring while in the department.	1. Discover whether any of the patients in your area are diabetic either by consulting the notes or by asking them. 2. Ask the diabetic patient how his diabetes is controlled (whether by insulin, tablets or diet), when he last had his medication (if any) and when he last had something to eat. 3. Ask patient what his normal eating pattern is and at what time he would normally have his next meal or snack. 4. Ensure that the patient knows where he can obtain food or drink should he need it. If unable to obtain it himself, arrange for it to be brought to him. 5. Observe known diabetic patients for any signs of hypoglycaemia – pallor, sweating, disorientation, faintness, etc.

ORGANIZATION OF THE DEPARTMENT

ADULTS

The majority of adults attending the outpatient department have two main concerns: 'What will they say about my eyes?' and 'How long will I have to wait?'

The department should be organized in such a way that:

1. the patient leaves the department with a clear understanding of what his eye condition and/or its treatment involves;
2. the waiting time is kept to a minimum.

While in the department the patient may see several specialists – ophthalmologists, optometrists, etc. All these people will give him information to remember and instructions to follow. This amount of information may be difficult to assimilate. The effect of anxiety about his eye condition, the short space of time given to each patient to absorb the information and the further anxiety caused by wanting to remember everything exactly mean that his chances of recalling even half of what he has been told are slight.

The nurse can play an important role here by assimilating the information given to the patient by various people and interpreting what has been written in the medical casenotes for him. She can also suggest to other members of staff ways in which they could improve patient recall of and compliance with their advice.

Problem	Goal	Nursing intervention
Patient is unable to recall all the advice given to him, due to anxiety about his eye condition and to the speed at which this information was given.	To improve patient recall of advice and thereby improve compliance with treatment and care.	1. Ask the patient what he has been told by doctor, optometrist, etc. Assess his level of anxiety and ability to remember what has been said. 2. If a relative or friend is accompanying the patient, ensure that they also are listening to what you are telling the patient. 3. Ask patient if there are any points about which he is unclear and try to clarify these. If necessary, go back to the source of the information, e.g. casenotes or doctor, to check. 4. Repeat information to patient. Emphasize the important points verbally and also write them down for the patient to keep. Ensure that your explanation is clear and easy to understand.

Problem	Goal	Nursing intervention
		5. Suggest to other members of staff means by which they could improve patient recall and compliance – repetition, written information, diagrams, etc. 6. Try to relieve patient anxiety by assuring him that he is now aware of the important information he has been given and need not worry about having forgotten anything vitally important.

The other main concern is the length of waiting time. Some consultations are inevitably long and the patient should be made aware of this prior to his first appointment. Waiting time targets to see the doctor are now stated in the Patient's Charter.

The nurse can help to minimize delays by preparing the department prior to the arrival of patients.

The treatment room should have adequate supplies of equipment and packs for the procedures which may be performed during the session. The medical consulting rooms should also be prepared with adequate supplies of topical medication and stationery. Routinely used equipment, such as a slit lamp, should be prepared ready for use and checked to ensure that it is in good working order. Less frequently used equipment that may be shared between consulting rooms should be conveniently stored and also checked daily to ensure that it is in good working order.

In the long term, the head of the nursing team may be responsible for ensuring that major pieces of equipment are regularly serviced and that old equipment is replaced to ensure continuity. It is usually the nurse who is responsible for arranging urgent repairs and informing the medical staff when equipment is not available.

Children

Children require a different set up to adults for outpatient care. The outpatient department, like the hospital ward, is an alien environment and one to which the child should be exposed for as short a time as possible. It is, therefore, necessary to organize an area of the department to cater specifically for their needs. Many of the children attending the outpatient department will previously have been inpatients, e.g. following squint surgery. Children, even more than adults, welcome the sight of a familiar face. If it can be arranged, nurses from the paediatric ward area should help to run special paediatric clinics. This is valuable not only to those who have already been in hospital but also to those children who are soon to be admitted, as it gives them the opportunity to get to know at least one or two of the ward staff.

Problem	Goal	Nursing intervention
Children in the outpatient department are potentially restless and upset. Need to minimize the trauma experienced by children attending outpatient department.	To occupy children happily while in outpatient department.	1. Section off an area of the department exclusive for a children's play area. 2. Decorate this area to suit a child's taste and ensure there are plenty of safe toys for them to play with. 3. Ensure children attend special paediatric clinics as far as possible. 4. Staff these clinics with nurses from the paediatric ward(s), to provide continuity of care between the outpatient department and the ward areas, and also to reassure children through seeing familiar faces. 5. Keep children's waiting time to a minimum to avoid restlessness. 6. Involve parents as far as possible in care, e.g. get mother to hold her child while the doctor is examining him. Ensure parents understand care and treatment. 7. Introduce the children who are going to be admitted to hospital to some of the nurses they will meet on the ward.

Communication and Liaison with other Departments

Co-ordinating the care each patient receives is a nursing responsibility. Ensuring that there is a good system of communication and liaison between departments is an essential part of this and is vital if a high standard of patient care is to be achieved.

It is generally the nurse who oversees the passage of the patient through the outpatient department and who is mainly responsible for communicating with the various departments through which the patient passes. The nurse can communicate useful pieces of information about an individual patient to the people the patient will come into contact with in each department. Information given to others about, for example, the patient's hearing problem or high level of anxiety, can give them valuable clues about how to deal with a particular patient. In return, the nurse can receive information about the future care and treatment needed which she can then pass on to the patient or to the next person dealing with him. This kind of communication extends beyond the boundaries of the outpatient department to the wards and to the community as well.

Effective communication can save time and improve patient care. Responsibility for communication of patient care is best undertaken by the Named Nurse who is responsible for that care.

Procedures in the Department

The nurse or other healthcare professional in the outpatient department may be required to carry out a variety of procedures. The equipment used may vary slightly between hospitals; however, the same basic principles of nursing care apply.

An outline of the care of patients undergoing five procedures commonly carried out in the outpatient department – field analysis, lacrimal sac washout, Schirmer's tear test, epilation of lashes and strapping of entropion – are given below. (Applanation tonometry is described in Chapter 18.)

Visual Fields Testing

This test is generally indicated for two main reasons: 1) glaucoma and 2) neurological defects. It may be carried out periodically to assess the progress of the condition. Although painless and non-invasive, patient co-operation is essential for this test. Good concentration is also important as the test may take up to half an hour for each eye. The Goldmann Perimeter is rapidly being replaced by semi-automated methods, e.g. Humphrey visual field analysis.

Problem	Goal	Nursing intervention
Patient requires field test. Unable to co-operate as he does not know what this involves.	To obtain patient co-operation with test by explaining what it involves.	1. Explain test to patient and what he will be expected to do during it – that he will have one eye covered and will be asked to place his head against a headrest and fix the uncovered eye on a central target on the machine. Explain how long the test will take and that he will be asked to fix on the target for this time. 2. Have several practice runs until the patient feels happy to proceed with the test. 3. If the patient has difficulty concentrating for the duration of the test, suggest a few minutes break before continuing. 4. Explain to the patient the results of the test and what they mean.

Lacrimal Sac Washout

This is an uncomfortable procedure carried out primarily on patients complaining of a watering eye. Its aim is either to clear or to locate any blockage in the lacrimal drainage system. Some fluid may run down the patient's cheek during the test so it is advisable to place a towel or cover around the patient's shoulders prior to carrying it out.

Problem	Goal	Nursing intervention
Patient apprehensive about having sac washout test as unaware of what it involves or why it is being done.	To prepare patient mentally and physically for test. To carry out test safely and successfully.	1. Tell patient what you are about to do and what he will be expected to do during the test. Ask him to sit well back in the chair and ensure that his head is well supported. Explain that you are going to instil some anaesthetic drops in his eye and will then syringe his tear duct in the hope of clearing the blockage. 2. Point out that the test will be uncomfortable but not painful. Emphasize the importance of keeping his head still during the test to prevent him from hurting himself. Explain that he will feel a sensation of pressure or filling in the tear duct. Ask him to let you know if he feels any water running into his throat. 3. Wash hands and prepare equipment for test. Fill syringe with 1–2 ml of sterile saline. Instil anaesthetic drops in eye and wait 30 seconds until effective. Ask patient to look up and approach him from the side. Dilate punctum by gently rotating Nettleship's dilator downwards through punctum for about 2 mm before twisting it gently horizontally for about 1 mm. Introduce lacrimal cannula into dilated punctum and inject fluid at the back of his throat as this indicates that the system is patent. 4. If the patient does not feel water in his throat, observe upper and lower puncta for reflux and whether this is clear or purulent. If unable to clear blockage, refer patient back to doctor. 5. Explain result of test to patient and what it will mean to him in terms of aftercare. 6. Ensure patient feels alright following test. If shocked afterwards advise him to stay seated for a little while until he feels well enough to leave.

Schirmer's Tear Test

This test is a quick and practical, though relatively crude, way of assessing the adequacy of tear production. One end of a strip of absorbent paper is placed inside the lower lid for a set period and the length of the paper that has been wetted by the tear film is then measured. This is the commonly preferred basic test, referred to as Schirmer's I.

It is possible to gain additional information by modifying the test. Irritation of the eye, including that caused by the pressure of the paper strip, can cause reflex lacrimation. If, however, local anaesthetic drops are first applied this response is obliterated and the tear strip measured indicates the basal secretion (Schirmer's II).

Problem	Goal	Nursing intervention
Patient has poor tear production and is complaining of his eyes feeling dry. Need to assess this.	To provide a measurement of the amount of tears produced by the eye.	1. Explain test to patient by saying that it measures tear production by the eye. Say that you will be placing a small strip of blotting-type paper inside the middle of each lower lid, which will feel like grit or an eyelash in the eye for a while. 2. Instil local anaesthetic drops at this stage if test II is being carried out. 3. After the strips are in place, ask the patient to sit back in chair with his eyes closed for about 5 minutes, and to try and tolerate the strips for this length of time. 4. Give patient regular time checks while his eyes are closed, so that he knows how long is left. 5. After 5 minutes, ask patient to open his eyes and remove the strips of paper, taking care to note which strip was taken from the right and the left eyes. Measure the level of saturation on the strips in mm and record in notes '*y* mm after 5 minutes'. 6. Refer patient back to doctor ordering the test to explain the results and what it will mean in terms of further care. 7. If both tests I and II are being carried out, always do test I first, before instilling anaesthetic drops. (Check anaesthetic drops have not already been put in for another reason, e.g. applanation.)

Epilation

Ingrowing eyelashes are a recurring problem for some people. The constant irritation caused by these results in excessive lacrimation and they may cause actual damage to the ocular surface. One way to deal with these is removal, i.e. epilation.

Problem	Goal	Nursing intervention
Patient has watering eyes that are causing discomfort. This is due to ingrowing eye lashes. Potential risk of corneal abrasion.	To relieve discomfort and prevent further complications from occurring by epilating troublesome eyelashes.	1. Explain to the patient that the irritation and watering of his eyes is due to ingrowing lashes and that the only way to deal with these is to remove them. 2. Ask patient to sit back in chair with his head well supported. Ensure there is good illumination of the lids before commencing. 3. Explain that you are going to remove the lashes and that it will hurt slightly. Give him an estimate of how many lashes need to be removed. 4. Ask patient to sit still and look upwards. Wash hands, then hold lid firmly with one hand while removing the lash using an epilation forceps held in the other hand. Magnification may be needed to locate troublesome lashes and to check that all of these have been removed. 5. After removing all the lashes that appear to be ingrowing, ask patient to blink a few times and to say whether or not he can feel any more lashes. 6. Warn patient that these ingrowing lashes may grow back, in which case he should seek further treatment as soon as possible.

Strapping of Entropion

Entropion creates similar problems for the patient as ingrowing lashes, namely watering, discomfort and the risk of surface damage. Here, however, the whole lid (generally the lower one) is turning inwards and needs surgical correction. However, in the short term, symptoms can be relieved by simply strapping the lower lid to the cheek so that it regains its proper position.

Problem	Goal	Nursing intervention
Patient's eye is constantly irritated because of entropion.	To reposition lid so that proper drainage of tears and positioning of lashes is achieved.	1. Explain to patient that the problems he has had with his eye are due to the fact that his eyelid is turning inwards. Tell him that this can temporarily but simply be cured with tape, by strapping the lid to the cheek in the correct position.

Problem	Goal	Nursing intervention
		2. Ask patient to sit in a chair with his head well supported. Examine lids. Using approximately a 5 cm piece of tape, with one end stuck to the outer edge of the lower lid just below the lashes, pull lid gently away from the eye until it is in the correct position. Once this is achieved, strap the lid to the cheek. A more even pull of the lid margin may be obtained with a Y-shaped piece of strapping. 3. Ensure patient is aware that this treatment is only of a temporary nature and that the tape will need to be replaced regularly. Teach the patient or a relative how to reapply the tape to achieve the same result.

Patient Education

Patient education is becoming an increasingly important part of the ophthalmic nurse's role, and this applies as much in the outpatient department as in other areas. The majority of people attending as outpatients need some form of education. Examples of where, how and to whom this might apply are given below.

Problem	Goal	Nursing intervention
Patient placed on waiting list for admission. Worried about this as he has not been in hospital before.	To prepare patient for admission to the eye hospital. To relieve some of his anxiety about this.	1. Give patient a rough idea of how long it will be before he is admitted, or the actual date he is to be diary-booked. 2. Ask him if there is anything particularly concerning him about admission, or anything he would like to know about. 3. Give him a brief outline of likely ward routine and of the sort of thing that will happen to him when he is in hospital, e.g. pre- and postoperative care if a surgical admission. 4. Give advice on what he should bring into hospital with him, whether or not he will be wearing his own clothes while a patient, visiting hours, approximate length of stay, etc. Give him an information booklet on admission, if available, and discuss this with him. 5. Encourage patient to ask questions if he has any. Repeat more important pieces of information to him and try to give him written information to take home and read at his leisure.

Problem	Goal	Nursing intervention
Patient on first post-discharge outpatient visit following surgery. Worried whether or not he has been carrying out his treatment correctly.	To ensure patient is looking after himself properly at home. To reassure him and give the support and encouragement needed to carry on.	1. Talk to patient and ask him how he has been managing since he went home from hospital. Ask him if he has had any difficulty instilling his drops or remembering when to use them. If possible, check how well he manages this. 2. Ask whether he has had any difficulty with housework, support at home, etc. 3. Re-emphasize postoperative precautions of no rubbing or touching of eye, etc. 4. Answer any specific queries he may have. Give appropriate advice or suggestions in areas where it is needed. 5. If he appears to be managing well, give him plenty of encouragement and support to continue.

Problem	Goal	Nursing intervention
Patient on long-term treatment for chronic glaucoma. Potential problem of poor compliance with treatment because of its long-term nature.	To promote patient compliance with long-term treatment regime.	1. Measure IOP to check whether this is being satisfactorily controlled on current drop treatment. 2. Ask patient if he has any difficulty with instilling his drops or if there is anything worrying him about this, e.g. does he have difficulty remembering when to instil the drops; is there any difficulty with actually putting in the drops or doing so at the right times, etc. 3. If possible, check his drop technique. 4. Give advice in areas where you feel it is needed. Try to adapt drop schedule to fit in with patient's lifestyle as far as possible. 5. Encourage patient to continue with treatment by telling him, for example, that his glaucoma is well controlled, that he is doing well and that the treatment is stabilizing his condition (compliance has been shown to improve when someone, e.g. nurse, is supportive and encouraging). 6. Give him any new information or advice about glaucoma that has become available. Give written information if possible. 7. If relatives are present, involve them in teaching and emphasize to them the importance of complying with treatment.

Health Education

The outpatient department is an ideal environment in which to carry out general health education. Information about topical health issues, preventing accidents at work and in the home, first aid, etc. can be passed on in a variety of ways to the large numbers of people visiting the department every day.

Problem	Goal	Nursing intervention
Need to promote general health education within the outpatient department.	To make information about health education available to as many people as possible.	1. Display large colourful posters on topical subjects, such as heart disease, healthy eating, smoking, etc. in areas of the department where they can be seen by a large number of people. 2. Leave magazines and leaflets on health education topics in places where they can be picked up and read by people in waiting areas. 3. Consider having videos on current health issues for people to watch while they are waiting. 4. Ask patients for their comments on the subjects covered and also for their suggestions for other suitable topics. 5. Use any available opportunity to discuss relevant health issues with individual patients. 6. Update magazines, leaflets, videos, etc. on a regular basis. 7. Encourage patients to ask questions regarding general health issues.

Summary

Nursing care in the ophthalmic outpatient department is all about preparing the patient to care for himself. Changes in the organization and planning of nursing care that have been widely implemented in other areas have been slow to filter through to the outpatient department, and much of the nursing care given in this area has been carried out and initiated at the request of medical staff. Nurses have been assigned to work areas, so that the concept of patient-oriented care has been overlooked.

It is hoped that the suggestions made in this chapter will help to promote nursing care in the outpatient department that is planned, given and evaluated by nurses themselves. Implementation of some of these ideas provides a means of utilizing the skills of the ophthalmic-trained nurse in the outpatient department to the full.

Ophthalmic Day Surgery

Outpatient or day surgery is becoming increasingly popular in a number of areas of medicine, including ophthalmology. Patients usually dislike having to stay in hospital. Because of the increased effectiveness of surgical procedures and the advances in materials and instruments, surgeons are beginning to realize that there is a reduced need for postoperative therapy and supervision. It is also popular with patients. Importantly it cuts costs by allowing bed closures.

According to the Royal College of Ophthalmologists. appropriate operations can include cataract extraction, corneal transplant, procedures on the eye lid or tarsal plate, operations on the lacrimal apparatus, correction of strabismus, refractive surgery, laser surgery and glaucoma surgery.

Economics of Day Surgery

Day surgery is regarded by health service planners as an opportunity for reducing expenditure and, according to Department of Health and Social Security Circulars HM(73)32 and HSG(15)181, it is an expedient for reducing waiting lists. This is because day surgery allows for a potential increase in the volume of surgery and removes from the waiting list those whose admission is frequently delayed by the demands on beds of more 'urgent' cases.

In the Royal College of Surgeons of England's report *Guidelines for the Management of Waiting Lists* it is recommended that all patients who are listed for elective surgery should be given adequate notice of their admission date. Ideally a date for admission should be arranged at the time of outpatient consultation that is convenient to both hospital and patients, as this reduces the disruption to both working and domestic life.

In the treatment of many conditions day surgery is superior to inpatient surgery and it is satisfactory to both surgeon and nursing staff, which in turn leads to an improvement in the retention of staff, particularly those with outside commitments. This is probably due to more regular working hours and flexibility of part-time work, all in a satisfactory work environment. There are, after all, very few other areas of nursing where one nurse can follow a patient through from preoperative assessment to postoperative examination, education and discharge.

Facilities Required for Day Surgery

In general the provision of services takes three main forms:

1. **Day surgery unit**: This is the most ideal form, consisting of a self-contained unit with its own perioperative area, theatre and recovery area, together with its own administration facilities.
2. **Day ward**: This is the next best option, in which patients go from a specially designated area to the general theatre, where operating lists are made up entirely of day cases. Where the workload is less, or the capacity of the day ward smaller, planned day operations may be incorporated into routine operating lists.
3. **General ward with allocated day beds**: This arrangement is generally unsatisfactory, as beds can be blocked by emergency admissions. It also removes one of the main advantages of a day ward – that beds are closed at nights and weekends, thus reducing the cost of nursing care.

Design Features

The day ward is best designed on an open-plan basis, allowing for easier supervision of patients by fewer staff. Male and female changing rooms should be provided, with secure cupboards for outdoor clothes and belongings. Most ophthalmic patients can recover in chairs, although there should be some provision of beds to cater for the individual needs of the patients.

As the patients will have had either local anaesthesia or minimum general anaesthesia, and will be essentially fit, there is minimum need for facilities. Each patient area should have a nurse call system and a power point. There should be some availability of piped gases and access to a mobile resuscitation trolley.

Patient Selection for Day Surgery

Selection for day surgery requires careful assessment of the patient's health and social circumstances, particularly in selection for intraocular surgery.

The best approach requires the patient to attend a pre-admission clinic, where he can be interviewed by both nursing and medical staff before a final decision is made regarding day surgery and the type of anaesthesia required.

Presurgical Assessment Clinic

Patients should be invited to attend from the routine waiting list, for planned surgery, or from a clinic when the decision to operate is made. These assessment clinics should be planned so that patients are seen about 2–4 weeks prior to the time when they could be offered surgery; this requires careful co-ordination between medical, nursing and administration staff.

This is an important time, as there is a large amount of information that the nurse needs to glean from the patient and that the patient must absorb. It is therefore helpful if the patient can bring a friend or relative with him to this appointment. Information given to the patient must be clear, concise and supported by written materials, in a language familiar to him. A successful assessment depends on good communication using words that the patient understands and avoiding medical jargon. The patient should bring details of any current medication and a sample of urine.

During the assessment by the nurse the patient's pulse, blood pressure and respiration rate should be recorded and the urine sample should be tested. A brief social history should be taken, as well as details of medical history.

The patient will be seen by the nurse and then taken through to see the medical staff. If the decision is then taken to go ahead with day surgery the patient should sign a consent form and, together with the doctor, decide on a mutually acceptable date to come into hospital. The type of anaesthesia required will also be decided, and this will dictate any other tests or investigations the patient may need to undergo prior to admission.

These tests may include ECG, blood tests, chest/spine X-ray and biometry (for cataract patients). As many as possible of these should be carried out on the unit at the preadmission clinic by the nurse assessing the patient. As well as providing continuity of care, this also allows the nurse further time to inform the patient about what is going to happen to him.

Criteria for Day Surgery

Inclusion Criteria

1. Patient wants day surgery.
2. Patient understands and can be relied upon to follow instructions.

3. Transport to and from the hospital is available, especially if the follow-up appointment is the following day.
4. Telephone at home.
5. Support at home, constant for the first 24–36 hours and then available for shopping, etc. if necessary.
6. If patient needs a local anaesthetic, must be able to lie flat for the required period.

EXCLUSION CRITERIA

1. If the patient is to be padded following surgery, fellow eye has vision less than 6/60.
2. Insulin-dependent diabetes.
3. Any other medical condition, e.g. hypertension, that is out of control.

INSTRUCTIONS FOR PATIENTS

When all the details for admission have been made, the patient should be given clear written instructions about his attendance for surgery, possibly accompanied by a booklet explaining again the details of his condition and the surgery required.

Figure 8.1 is an example of these instructions, which clearly need to be adapted according to the surgery involved.

Patient's name:

The date of your operation is:

On that day please attend the Day Ward at ....

If you are taking any medicines, tablets or inhalers, please bring them with you and take them as normal before you come to hospital.

Please bring slippers and a dressing gown with you.

Please leave all valuables at home.

Ladies please do not wear make-up or nail varnish.

If you have a cold, feel unwell or for some reason cannot keep your appointment please phone .... as soon as possible.

Someone must be at home with you overnight following your operation.
The person who is going to escort you home after your operation should phone .... at about .... to arrange a time to come and collect you.

Figure 8.1 Instructions for patients requiring day cataract surgery under local anaesthesia.

Given that many of the patients involved in day ophthalmic surgery will have some visual impairment the clarity of the print used in giving these instructions should be carefully considered.

It may also be deemed necessary to inform the patient's general practitioner of the arrangements made for surgery.

Instillation of Drops – Patient Education

Many patients will require drops following surgery, instilled either by the patient themselves or by a friend or relative. Patient education regarding drop instillation is discussed at length in Chapter 7. Self-administration of drops following day surgery can only be successfully assessed at the preadmission clinic if the patient is already on eye medication.

If the relative or friend accompanying the patient is the one who will be instilling drops on discharge they can be shown, and observed performing, the technique during the preadmission appointment, with added emphasis placed on the need for hand hygiene, particularly following surgery. This can be done by using, for instance, hypromellose in order to help the patient or relative gain confidence, and can be repeated following surgery when the patient attends for his first dressing appointment.

Such education is time-consuming and each patient will have different problems. The nurse needs to adapt her care accordingly. An assessment form may include assessment of the relative as well as, or instead of, the patient themselves.

Admission for Day Surgery

The patient should be greeted on his arrival for surgery, his personal details checked and the postoperative requirements and expectations repeated to both him and his escort.

He should be shown where to put his outdoor clothes and, if necessary, assisted into a theatre gown and his dressing gown and slippers. Any medication should also be locked away securely.

If possible, the nurse who assessed the patient at the assessment clinic should care for him during his admission. She needs to recheck what he understands about what is going to happen to him and note any drugs he may have taken prior to admission. If the patient is to have a general anaesthetic she will also need to check when he last had anything to eat or drink and ensure that the results of any tests or investigations are filed in his notes and available to the medical staff. She needs also to be aware of his degree of visual impairment and arrange his immediate surroundings accordingly, ensuring his safety as she makes him comfortable in his chair. The patient should then be allowed to relax as much as possible while any preparation of the operating site, such as dilating the pupil, takes place. Premedication should be avoided except in children. She should then escort the patient to theatre.

Postoperative and Discharge Procedure

If the patient has had a general anaesthetic he will need to go to the recovery ward and undergo observation until he is ready to return to the day unit. Following local anaesthesia the patient can usually be returned to a comfortable, reclining chair where he can be offered a drink and refreshments. Adequate analgesia should be provided on the ward, and for discharge too, and any regular medication taken by the patient should be given to him, if required, during his recovery.

The timing of the first dressing and the first postoperative appointment will depend both on the surgeon's preference and the surgery undergone by the patient. Some first dressings can be performed 2–3 hours following surgery on the unit; many, however, will be done when the patient attends the unit for his first postoperative appointment.

In any case, the patient will need to be given further written instructions which the nurse should go through with him and the person who comes to collect him when the patient is ready to go home. He should also be given his required postoperative medication if he is not attending the following day. An example of these instructions, for cataract patients, is given in Figure 8.2

Outpatient Follow-up

Many patients will probably return to the ward the following day for the first dressing and this is the opportunity for the nurse involved to show either the patient or his carer again how to instil drops safely. This may also be the opportunity to give the patient his eye medication and any dressings or cartelle shield that the surgeon uses.

An appointment for an outpatient follow-up is given to the patient at this visit too, and the postoperative instructions given to him the day before on discharge are repeated, with particular emphasis placed on the importance of contacting the hospital at any time if the patient has any worries when he is at home. He may also be given a letter to take to his general practitioner.

Please rest quietly at home this evening and ensure that someone is staying with you overnight.

Do not disturb the plastic shield until you return to the hospital tomorrow and remember to wear it at night for 6 weeks.

Take care not to rub your eye.

You may notice that your face and mouth feel a little numb this evening. This is quite normal and should have worn off by tomorrow.

Slight discomfort may be experienced for a few days after the operation. This can be helped by taking paracetamol if you need to do so.

Sometimes your eye may be a little sticky, particularly first thing in the morning. If so, clean it as you were shown, using clean cotton wool and cooled boiled water.

Remember to wash your hands first.

Remember your eye drops are **very** important, and you must keep using them, as you have been shown, until the doctor in the clinic tells you to stop.

Healing takes 6–8 weeks, and sometimes it will take that long for your vision to really improve. It is possible that it will be blurred during that time too, and may not be as good as you expected for some time, so try not to be too disappointed if this is the case.

If you are worried about **anything** at all when you are at home, please do not hesitate to phone .... and someone on the ward will be happy to help you.

Figure 8.2 Information for patients following cataract surgery.

The same nurse who was involved with the patient at the assessment clinic and on his day of admission should attend to the patient at this appointment. By this time they will have a positive relationship and he will probably feel very able to discuss any worries or concerns he or his carer may have. This will be very rewarding for the nurse involved.

Children

The report on the welfare of children in hospital (Platt Committee, 1959) noted that special attention should be paid to devising methods of management of the sick child that avoid admission to hospital, and that once in hospital everything possible should be done to meet the special needs of the child and his family. Providing a service for day surgery on children is an excellent way of meeting those needs but it also requires some special planning.

Children require special facilities not shared with adults. A day unit for children will require a suitable reception area and playroom, as well as an area for parents to wait during the operation.

Children should therefore be admitted to a special children's unit or to a day unit reserved for use by children on one specific day. It may be possible to segregate children and adults in some units.

Children require special facilities and equipment in recovery rooms, and children's nurses must be available.

Presurgical assessment should be encouraged, although the time lapse between this appointment and surgery should be less than with adults as children are more susceptible to colds and other infections that cause surgery to be cancelled. It also allows the child, his parents and siblings to visit the area he will attend on admission, to meet the staff and to be introduced to the exciting toys that will be waiting for him when he comes into hospital!

References

Platt Committee (1959) *Report of the Platt Committee: The Welfare of Children in Hospital*, HMSO, London.

Royal College of Surgeons of England (1991) *Guidelines for the Management of Waiting Lists*, RCS, London.

Further Reading

Royal College of Surgeons of England (1992) *Report of the Working Party on Guidelines for Day Case Surgery*, RCS, London.

Traynor, M. (1990) Day case eye surgery. *Nursing Times*, **86**(39), 54–56.

9

Care of the Patient in the Operating Theatre

Janie M. Grabham

Chapter Summary

Principles of Care

The basic principles of care for ophthalmic patients are the same as for any patient undergoing surgery. The nurse in the theatre has to be acutely aware of the need for multidisciplinary team work between herself, the surgeons, anaesthetists, technicians and other support staff. This chapter will therefore concentrate on specific aspects of ophthalmic surgery. The skills and knowledge a nurse has to acquire to meet the needs of the ophthalmic theatre patient can be listed as follows:

1. provision of the optimum physical and psychological environment;
2. specific aims of surgery and potential complications, and the nurse's role in achieving a successful outcome;
3. provision of correct, sterile instruments and equipment in working order;
4. identification and solving of problems that may hinder a successful outcome.

In the past, the eye theatre was usually separate from the main operating theatre suites, often located close to the eye ward itself and staffed by the ward nurses in smaller units. Historically, this was because the patients often walked to theatre, climbed on to the table and then after surgery were transferred to the ward on a trolley. There was also a need for isolation from any source of potential infection. Quiet was needed for the surgeon performing delicate surgery and for the patient under local anaesthetic, a low noise level helping the patient to keep still during the procedure and lessening anxiety as to what might be going on around him. However, with the improvements in environmental ventilation and the advent of antibiotics, shared theatres are more common, but noise control has remained necessary. Shared theatres usually mean shared staff, but the nurse still requires specialized knowledge and skills to meet the needs of patients undergoing ophthalmic surgery. The Audit Commission and the Bevan Report both identify better utilization of day surgery and specialist theatres when the theatre is located next to patient areas.

Information Collection, Assessment and Preoperative Visiting

With information on the day's operating list and an in-depth knowledge of the requirements for specific surgical procedures, a generalized care plan can be agreed and discussed at the report session prior to the start of the list. However, more detailed information is required to give individual nursing care to the patient entering theatre. One way this information can be gained is by a member of the theatre staff visiting the patient on the ward before surgery. In circumstances where the theatre staff cannot make the visit it is possible for a theatre-orientated patient assessment to be made by other nursing staff and communicated to the theatre staff in an agreed written format.

There are many advantages in the theatre nurse making the visit.

1. The patient will become acquainted with the theatre nurse's attire.
2. The patient can gain assurance that his particular needs will be catered for.
3. The theatre nurse can plan care in conjunction with the patient, e.g. use of hearing aids, preferred positioning aid.

The first aim of the preoperative visit is to reduce the patient's anxiety about the forthcoming operation. Janis (1958) found that patients wished to know the things that directly involved them, and the sensations they are likely to experience. He went on to state that the patient might have adverse, emotional reactions upon encountering the unexpected, and he recommended giving detailed information. Lazarus (1960) described six psychologically stressful stimuli:

1. uncertainty about physical survival;
2. uncertainty about maintaining one's identity;

3. inability to control the immediate environment;
4. pain and privation;
5. loss of loved one;
6. disruption of community life.

Lazarus and Averill (1972) also described anxiety as 'an emotion based on the appraisal of threat' and stated that anxiety results when a person is unable fully to comprehend the world around him. The high percentage of older patients and patients having a local anaesthetic in ophthalmology make this particularly important. Ophthalmology also suffers from many old wives' tales, the most common being that the eye is taken out of the socket to be operated on. Many patients coming in for surgery also have vivid memories of visiting their relatives in the past when the absence of microsurgical techniques meant that the patient had to lie still for days until the wound healed, sometimes with sandbags at the side of his head to prevent movement. Disorientation and hallucination were also experienced due to the prolonged double padding and inappropriate sedation.

The preoperative visit is not a replacement for the ward nurse assessment and preparation of the patient for theatre; it is an addition. The nurse only has a short time in which to conduct the visit. Yet in this short interview, the nurse must be able to detect hidden anxiety in the patient. This can be identified by non-verbal signs such as restlessness, avoidance of eye contact and reluctance to talk freely. If particular worries are voiced then the nurse undertaking the visit must have sufficient skill and knowledge to reassure the patient and allay his fears. As well as the reassurance, the nurse must record this and note any action that the theatre staff may need to incorporate in their nursing care on the following day. The second aim of a preoperative visit is to assess potential problems so that care can be planned accordingly.

Assessment

Chronic bronchitis

Problem	Nursing intervention
Inability to lie flat for local anaesthetic.	1. Have additional wedges and pillows in theatre. 2. Adjustment of the microscope will be needed. 3. All staff must be aware of the problem. 4. Need for two runners during this case. 5. Place support over patient's chest to keep drapes away from his mouth. 6. Oxygen or air at low flow rate beneath the drapes to prevent feelings of closeness and smothering. Monitor or pulse oximeter as appropriate.
Possibility of coughing during operation while eye is open.	1. Detailed explanation that it is important not to move or cough, especially during the middle of the procedure. 2. Explain that if the patient feels a cough coming on he must tell the nurse and surgeon so that the surgeon can make the eye as safe as he can against a pressure rise during a cough.

Patient has an internal pacemaker

Interference by electrical current with action of the pacemaker.	1. Monitor patient during case using cardiac monitor. 2. Ensure no standard diathermy is used.

Hearing difficulties

Difficulty in communicating without hearing aid.	Ensure hearing aid is brought to theatre with patient. If GA patient, keep hearing aid safe (named and marked) and take to the recovery room.

Obese patient

Difficulty anticipated transferring patient to trolley and positioning.	Adequate numbers of porters to be sent to collect patient from the ward. Additional help in theatre to lift or use of patient transfer slide.

Patient does not speak English

1. Unable to communicate or understand. 2. Heightening of anxiety.	Ensure that relative or nurse who can translate prepares patient for the theatre and if possible escorts patient to theatre. Arrange translator if necessary.

Patient premature baby or elderly and thin adult

Difficulty in maintaining own body temperature.	1. Temperature control in theatre will need to be increased. 2. Additional blankets to hand and silver space blanket to reflect in body heat.

Patient premature baby or elderly and thin adult – *continued*

Problem	Nursing intervention
	3. Temperature monitor in use. 4. Heated water blanket available. Combination of one or more of these aids used as required.

Patient has recently developed very poor eyesight, therefore not adapted

Visual communications lost, unable to see smiling face.	Concentration on non-visual communications and reassurance, i.e. holding of hand, spoken reassurance and explanations of surroundings and events, keeping number of staff involved with patient to a minimum and ensuring their introductions to the patient.

Preoperative eye medication to dilate pupil

Decrease in vision from normal and increased sensitivity to light.	1. Explain what the eye drops are doing. 2. Explain that this is going to give easier access to the part of the eye that is requiring surgery. 3. Advise patient that keeping both eyes closed enhances the effect of the medication and prevents them feeling the sensitivity to the light.

Patient has a heart condition and is to undergo surgery with local anaesthetic which will probably contain adrenaline

Potential cardiac arrhythmias.	1. Ensure medication has been continued prior to surgery. 2. Use a cardiac monitor during surgery.

The increase in day surgery has made it essential to incorporate the preoperative assessment into the clinic.

The Anaesthetic Room

The reception into the anaesthetic room, whether it be for a general or local anaesthetic, should be a peaceful and confident time for the patient. The checks done reconfirming that it is the correct patient for the correct procedure in the correct theatre must not alarm the patient.

The use of a preoperative check sheet which is signed by ward and theatre nurses reduces the number of questions that have to be asked of the patient, thus allowing the optimum effect of a sedating premedication. In meeting the needs of the patient in the anaesthetic room and during the anaesthetic period, the nurse's assessment can again be made around the Roper, Logan and Tierney model (Roper, Logan and Tierney, 1990)

Maintaining a safe environment for the patient and breathing during the induction of general anaesthesia is outlined in the following points.

1. Patient must not have food for several hours so that there is reduced risk of vomit entering the respiratory tract while the cough reflex is suppressed.
2. Suction must be available to remove saliva, mucus, etc. from the patient's mouth and upper respiratory tract.
3. Dentures must be removed to prevent them obstructing the patient's airway once muscle tone has been lost.
4. Once drugs have induced sleep and muscle relaxation, maintaining the airway and breathing for the patient requires a plastic airway followed by the introduction of an endotracheal tube or laryngeal mask. The style of the tube and method of securing it in place with tape or ties is selected to provide security of the circuit once the head is draped, when the anaesthetist can no longer see or have easy access to the patient's face and mouth.
5. The patient needs to have loose clothing on as ECG monitoring leads will have to be attached to the chest. Also, the anaesthetist will need to use a stethoscope or observe chest movement to see that both sides are expanding when the breathing of the patient is taken over mechanically.
6. Oxygen, nitrous oxide, carbon dioxide and anaesthetic vapouring agents such as halothane or ethrane must be available on the anaesthetic machines.
7. It must be possible to change the patient quickly into a head-down position if he starts to vomit, by a tipping mechanism on the trolley.

A working party of the Royal College of Anaesthetists and the Royal College of Ophthalmologists has recommended that locally agreed protocols for local anaesthetic good practice are available.

Communicating

1. In the preparation and induction of the anaesthetic, it is easy to become involved in actions and forget the vital need of the patient to communicate. Communicate by touching – holding the patient's hand.
2. Whether to talk or not has to be judged on an individual basis. Some patients like the nurses to talk to them, to keep their mind off things. Always make sure you know the patient's name. Avoid handovers once the patient has been received into the anaesthetic room. Be aware of the information gleaned from the preoperative visit. The confidence a patient gains from realizing that the nurse

knows about him is enormous. The Patient's Charter gives the patient the right to expect continuity of care and a Named Nurse in the perioperative period.

3. Observe the patient's ability to communicate. A dry mouth from premedication or the embarrassment of not having his dentures may mean that the patient feels uncomfortable about talking.
4. Visual communication includes smiling and observing eye movements for guidance as to the patient's anxiety or calm. Assess a patient's lack of visual ability too: dilating drops in both eyes, say before a retinal detachment repair, will cause blurred vision and sensitivity to bright lights. This patient may require more explanation than a patient who can see the environment he has come into.
5. If a patient is to have a local anaesthetic, then establishing a form of communication before going into theatre is important. The nurse who is to hold the patient's hand can explain that moving the head and also talking should be avoided once the operation has started. (Even the movement of the mouth during a delicate stage of an intraocular procedure can defocus the surgical field for a moment. Try looking down the operating microscope and see how greatly any movement is magnified.) Often a prearranged sign, such as squeezing the nurse's hand if the patient wants to say something or if he is feeling some discomfort, allows the nurse to speak to the surgeon and, as soon as it it safe for the patient to speak, the surgeon or nurse can ask what the matter is.

Breathing

1. **Positional problems**: The patient cannot lie flat.
2. **Structural problems**: The patient has neck rigidity or loose teeth and crowns; additional aids may be needed at incubation such as an ET introducer.
3. **Airway maintenance**: Secure the endotracheal tube safely, as this area may be difficult to assess during the case.
4. **Assisted breathing**: Some anaesthetics involve paralysing the patient, so breathing has to be taken over mechanically.

Eating and Drinking

In fit patients this does not present real problems, given the short duration of most ophthalmic operations.

1. For general anaesthesia, checking that nothing has been taken by mouth during the allotted time prior to the anaesthetic is important.

2. Neonatal feeding varies from the standard nil by mouth period.
3. Certain categories of patients, such as diabetics, will have an intravenous infusion started so that easy control over blood glucose levels can be maintained during the anaesthetic.

ELIMINATING

Even though the patient will have been given the opportunity to empty the bladder before leaving the ward, some patients may feel they still need to do so. Problems may arise with:

1. patients given i.v. mannitol or diamox prior to surgery to lower intraocular pressure;
2. patients with a history of bladder problems;
3. any patient who has experienced a delay in the induction of anaesthetic for any reason;
4. children, who often have this need as a manifestation of anxiety.

Incontinence in theatre may be due to muscle relaxants and unemptied bladder. It is also due sometimes to a rise in the intra-abdominal pressure if the patient coughs at the end of the anaesthetic.

CONTROLLING BODY TEMPERATURE

Removing the patient's control over his own environment and body functions results in loss of overall control of his body temperature. Under normal conditions in theatre a fit adult should not present problems, but it is the responsibility of the anaesthetic team to monitor this.

Factors presenting potential problems are:

1. age – very young, very old;
2. physical condition – very thin or body temperature not normal at start of operation;
3. environment – unusually low/high air temperature in theatre;
4. long planned surgical procedure, or case with unexpected complications;
5. use of drugs in the anaesthetic or surgery that may alter the body's natural ability to control its own temperature, for example, the hypotensive drugs used during some orbital surgery.

The following actions should be employed to alleviate these problems:

1. continuous temperature monitoring, core or surface;
2. control of theatre temperature;
3. silver wrap/space blanket – reflects body heat;
4. additional blankets;
5. temperature-controlled water blanket;
6. use of intravenous infusion bath heater – heats infusion fluids to body temperature.

MOBILIZING

The patient is unable to move under a general anaesthetic and is asked to refrain from moving under local anaesthetic. Therefore the nurse must see that the patient suffers no ill effects from this restriction.

1. Legs must be positioned safely in such a way that they are not crossed and the calves of the legs are not taking undue weight. Heel pads and positioning pillows may be used.
2. Safe positioning of the arms, so that no undue pressure is taken by them. Padded arm retainers assist in this and also prevent damage.
3. Immobilization of the patient's head is required. This is achieved in ophthalmology by the use of:
   (a) Ruebens pillow;
   (b) head ring for children;
   (c) vacuum-pack positioning pillow which, when air is removed via a valve, retains the shape of the body part that it surrounds;
   (d) head-holding frame with wrist rests.

Care must be taken that the correct positioning aids are used for each patient and that there is no undue pressure at any point. The angle the head is positioned on each plane is important in some vitreoretinal procedures to help give the optimum view of the retina needing attention.

SLEEPING

Sleep induction is part of general anaesthesia, yet the anxiety about the operation may well have caused the patient problems with his sleep pattern. The patient needs to be informed that sleeping is part of the natural reaction of coming out of anaesthesia. It should always be remembered that, in sleep, hearing is about the last sense to be affected, so just because the patient appears to be asleep is no reason to start talking inappropriately. Lastly, if a patient is having a repair to an open eye wound, e.g. laceration of cornea or resuturing of corneal section, the nurse must point this out to the anaesthetist. In these cases, anaesthesia is induced without the use of scoline. This is because scoline causes a twitching of all the muscles as it acts and, although this lasts for just a short time, the squeezing of the eyelid muscles could cause herniation of the contents of the eye out through the wound.

Local Anaesthetic

It is not uncommon for an elderly patient who has had a premedication to go to sleep on the operating table during the operation. This is not as much of an advantage as it may first appear. The patient who wakes up suddenly often does not know exactly what is going on, and also tends to move or even sit up!

The patient who is having an ophthalmic procedure under local anaesthetic will, during the time in the anaesthetic room, have local anaesthetic eye drops instilled.

Goal	Intervention
To achieve anaesthesia of the eye surface, to allow an operation to take place without physical or psychological discomfort to the patient.	Prescribed anaesthetic eye drops are placed into the eye in such a way as to give surface anaesthesia. The patient is asked to look up and a drop is placed in the lower conjunctival fornix. After 30 seconds the patient is asked to look down and the nurse gently holds the upper lid and instils the next drop over the upper conjunctiva just above the limbus. This is to ensure anaesthesia at the usual site of the operation.

Most ophthalmic operations, however, require a retrobulbar or peribulbar injection to achieve adequate anaesthesia and akinesia (lack of movement). In addition, facial injections to prevent squeezing of the eyelids may be used. These injections can be given by the anaesthetist. The patient can experience a short period of discomfort during their administration. The nurse needs to have established a good rapport with the patient from his reception into theatre, in order to help him relax and co-operate at this time.

A complication of injection is that the needle may rupture a blood vessel in the orbit. The escaping blood (retrobulbar haemorrhage) collects in the enclosed space and

Goal	Intervention
Patient's gaze is fixed in the optimum direction to allow the safe passage of the needle as it is inserted through or close to the muscle cone where the major nerve supply runs.	The patient is asked to fix on an object, e.g. the nurse's hand. The nurse must encourage and observe that the patient's eyes do not move during this injection procedure. After the injection, to ensure the dispersal of the fluid and prevent an increase in the intraocular pressure, the nurse may be asked to keep pressure on the upper lid, or to apply a device to give optimum pressure.

causes a swelling. This can be seen as the lids bruise and swell. The nurse must observe the eye closely and inform the surgeon if she suspects that a retrobulbar haemorrhage has occurred. The operation may have to be cancelled if this complication arises, to avoid sight-threatening complications. The patient needs considerable comfort and support as it is explained to him that the operation has to be postponed. He will then usually have a pad and bandage applied to that eye to prevent further bleeding and reduce the amount of swelling. The patient will then be transferred to the care of the ward nurse, unfortunately in the knowledge that he will have to go home with a 'black-eye' and return for surgery at a later date.

During Surgery

It is vital in the organization of the theatre department that each person knows their role and what is expected of them. A short summary of the role of the scrub nurse and runner is therefore included here, which I hope will help a nurse who is starting an ophthalmic theatre allocation. There are many books dedicated entirely to theatre nursing, and permanent theatre staff will need to study these.

The Role of the Circulating Nurse

The circulating nurse, or 'runner' as she is often called, works in conjunction with the scrub nurse and the anaesthetic nurse/technician to form the essential non-medical component of the team. Together, the runner and scrub nurse should check the planned action for the operative procedure. A quick recheck of the plans made at the report prior to the list should be done.

1. The equipment needed is in the theatre and working.
2. There is nothing remaining in theatre from the previous case.
3. Instrument sets and extra instruments have been laid up in advance according to the information received about the case.

The runner is the 'unsterile hands' of the scrubbed team. Her place is in the theatre at all times during the case, and she needs to be one step ahead – opening the gowns and packs and being ready to tie the gowns of the scrub team. As the packets are opened and presented to the scrub nurse, the runner should always ensure that nothing unsterile ever passes over the sterile field where it might fall and contaminate it. Together with the scrub nurse, the preoperative count of swabs, needles and extras must be carried out and charted. As the patient enters the theatre, the runner may need to assist with the transfer of the patient to the table and positioning. A further check of patient details as the patient entered the theatre will be carried out. Then, after the patient is covered with sterile towels by the scrub nurse, the runner will position any lights and equipment needed, usually in close proximity to the patient, and check that leads are connected and tested. During the case the runner may be asked to alter settings on equipment such as the bipolar diathermy machine. If an instruction is not heard clearly, always ask for it to be repeated. Once the dial has been set to the new reading, say clearly, so that both the scrub nurse and surgeon can hear, 'diathermy set at (say) 5'. During the case additional items may be asked for. If something is required that is not in the theatre, and no intercom is available, check that another person in theatre, such as the anaesthetic nurse, is available before leaving and returning as quickly as possible. In cases that are long or complicated, a second runner will be needed.

Additional swabs and needles opened must be added to the count and charted. At the end of the case medication, dressings and strapping may need to be applied. A porter will be sent for and equipment moved back to allow clear access to the patient. A report in the patient's documentation or theatre information system may be dictated by the scrub nurse, who will sign it when she unscrubs. The final counts will be checked off. The runner needs to be ready to help with the transfer of the patient to the trolley, bed or wheelchair and then to clear the theatre.

As ophthalmic swabs and needles are very small, a careful check must be made to see that none are left behind in theatre as the scrub trolley is cleared. The runner is usually required to sign the register as a witness to the count. At the end of the list, the runner will help strip the theatre and restock items required for the next list.

It must be remembered that the duties and grade of staff who undertake the duties of the runner will vary. Never underestimate the importance of the runner's role. Once you scrub up you will realize how totally dependent the scrub nurse is on the runner. The skill of a good runner is an important acquisition in learning how to deliver the best patient care possible. It is vital that the runner is fully competent in the operation of the technical equipment that is increasingly in use in ophthalmic surgery, such as phacoemulsification or vitrectomy equipment.

The Role of the Scrub Nurse

The scrub nurse's main responsibility is to co-ordinate and implement the nursing care of the patient during the operation. She is assisted in this by the runner.

The scrub nurse needs to be fully aware of the predicted needs of the patient. This information will be gained from:

1. the operating list: name, age, proposed operation and name of the surgeon;
2. surgeon information: additional equipment used by this particular surgeon for this operation;
3. preoperative visit information, outlining any special needs this patient has;
4. direct discussion with the surgeon relating to any problems he anticipates that this patient may present;
5. the scrub nurse's knowledge of the step-by-step course of the operation. When a nurse in training is taking the role of the scrub nurse this information will be discussed with the trained nurse who is taking responsibility for the case. In the early stages of a theatre allocation, the senior member of the staff will scrub up and take the case, subsequently scrubbing up but allowing the nurse in training to play the main role, and only allowing her to scrub up alone when she is confident and able to do so.

It should also be noted that, although scrubbing and assisting is an accepted dual role for the nurse in microsurgery, a nurse in training should never be expected to do this. Specialized ophthalmic training recognizes that ophthalmic-trained nurses are competent to take on these responsibilities. Permanent theatre staff not holding an ophthalmic qualification may need to have this skill taught and competency documented in their 'Professional Profile'.

Armed with the information listed above, establish that all equipment needed for the case has been brought in and checked. Always scrub up in plenty of time to allow careful setting out of the trolley before the patient enters the theatre.

As the scrub nurse prepares the trolley, a careful check is made that each instrument is in good working order. Magnification should be available if necessary.

The circulating nurse will show the scrub nurse each pack and check with her that it is sterile before opening it. Nothing should be placed on the nurse's trolley without the scrub nurse either taking it or consenting to it being put there. In microsurgery costly damage can be caused if even small objects are dropped on to fine instruments. A check of swabs and needles is witnessed and recorded.

Once the patient is in the theatre a check of identification, notes, consent and allergies is made and the anaesthetist's permission is sought to start the case. The skin is cleansed using an antiseptic solution, starting along the lid margins and working out, taking care not to allow any of the solution to enter the eye. Drapes are then placed on the patient.

In a case in which an eye is to be removed, the surgeon is required to re-examine the eye (using indirect or direct ophthalmoscopy to identify the lesion) and confirm with witnesses the eye that is to be removed. Once the patient is on the operating table, his main need is for the surgery to proceed without delay and to a satisfactory conclusion. The scrub nurse assists in meeting the patient's need in the following way. The case must proceed smoothly, the scrub nurse anticipating the probable next step the surgeon is going to take and ensuring that the required instrument is ready to hand. Anticipation by the scrub nurse is a skill gained which is of particular importance when a case is being performed under local anaesthetic. Anticipation by the nurse avoids the need for the surgeon to ask for the next instrument. As the surgeon and nurse are at the patient's head (Figure 9.1), he may hear the request and find this adds to his anxiety. Anticipation by the scrub nurse, in requesting additional equipment to be on standby if complications start to develop, frees the surgeon to concentrate on the problems that are presenting and ensures minimal delay.

The way the scrub nurse passes instruments to the surgeon also has a bearing on the flow of the surgery. Most ophthalmic surgery is performed using the microscope. When you look down a microscope you have to adjust your vision and brain to function in this microenvironment. If your vision has then to readjust to the normal environment, this not only adds time to the procedure but also removes the surgeon's gaze from the operative field. The scrub nurse must aim to pass the instrument to the

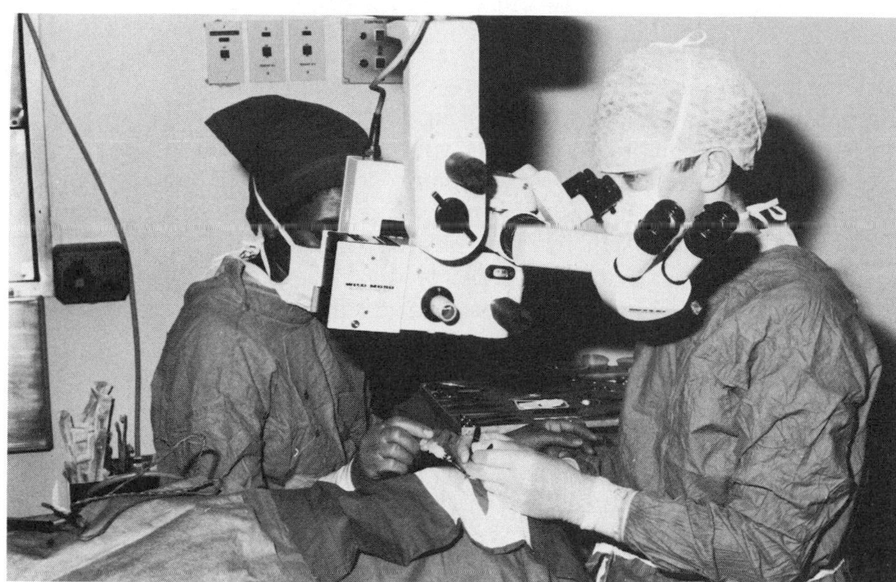

Figure 9.1 The usual approach to a microsurgical procedure. The surgeon is seated at the patient's head and the scrub nurse/surgical assistant on the same side as the operation. Note that the microscope is ceiling-mounted to maximize available space; additional eyepieces can be seen which are used for teaching/assistance.

surgeon's hand so that it can be used right away without needing to be readjusted. The scrub nurse notes the position where the surgeon's hand should grip the instrument (usually in the centre) and holds it just above or just below this point. She takes the last instrument from the surgeon with her free hand and places the next instrument gently in the surgeon's hand, not letting go until the surgeon has a secure grip on it. The scrub nurse can judge that she has been successful if the surgeon can use the instrument without looking away from the microscope or changing grip on the instrument.

During a vitrectomy the surgeon may wish to change one of the instruments entering the eye via the small incisions in the pars plana. With one instrument still in the vitreous cavity the surgeon should not have to look away from the microscope to receive the next instrument to be introduced. Likewise, during a dacrocystorhinostomy, the surgeon needs to be planning which bit of the lacrimal crest to remove next, so, as the bone punch is removed from the wound, it is the nurse who quickly wipes away the bone fragments and blood, leaving it clean.

If there is bleeding, any residual blood or tissue should be removed with a damp swab of an appropriate size as each instrument is returned to the swab nurse. For example, a small clot on a microtoothed or ring forceps can cause it not to grip the delicate edge of a partial-thickness incision into the cornea. An alternative to a damp swab is to dip the tip of the forceps in a small gallipot of saline, moving it gently from side to side. This is the best way of removing the small section of iris that often sticks to the forceps after an iridectomy. Surgeons tend to wipe instrument tips on their gown fronts or the drape, a practice which causes two problems. Firstly, the teeth of the delicate 2 into 2 forceps can be moved out of alignment and secondly, the teeth are likely to prick through the material, rendering the tip of the forceps unsterile.

Some uninformed nurses say the scrub nurse just passes instruments and query the nursing role involved. This can be compared with saying that in giving a drug you are just handing out pills, etc. at the doctor's bidding. The scrub nurse has a responsibility to meet the needs of the patient at whatever point she is involved with his care. Another aim of the scrub nurse is to minimize the risk of any contaminant entering the eye. This is the reason parts of instruments entering the eye should not be allowed to be touched by gloves or the trolley drape, where a speck of fibre or powder may be picked up. This is also one reason why needles should always be handled with the needle holder and forceps when being mounted ready for use. Another reason for this is that if a gloved hand touches the needle it may receive a needle prick, representing a risk to patient, surgeon and nurse. During the surgery the scrub nurse needs to know the whereabouts of the swabs and needles, doing checks as required. The trolley surface also has to be managed in a way that keeps instruments and other items in specific areas, segregated into unused items, used items ready for reuse and items that have been used and, although still sterile, should not be allowed to come into contact with an instrument re-entering the surgical field. The scrub nurse, once trained, may be required to cut sutures at the surgeon's request or hold a forceps to retract the conjunctival flap. The main skill that has to be learned is always to have your hand supported on some part of the patient's head for stability; experience of controlling hand action in a microscopic field is also necessary.

As the operation draws to a close, the scrub nurse must check that all swabs, needles and instruments are accounted for. She will supervise the dressing of the eye and ensure that the nursing report and theatre register are completed. The care of the patient is then transferred to the recovery area. The scrub nurse is then responsible for ensu the trolley is dismantled, that sharps are disposed of correctly and that instruments are placed ready for cleaning and resterilization. Saline is very corrosive, so rinsing of instruments in water is recommended if there is to be any delay in their decontamination. Finally, the scrub nurse should check that everything relating to the case just completed is removed from the theatre and that it is ready for the next case.

The nurse caring for the patient during the period of surgery must record, or dictate to be recorded, any specific nursing problems that presented and the action that was taken. This is so that continued nursing care is communicated to the Named Nurse who will be caring for this patient in recovery or back on the ward.

Documentation

In many hospitals the patient's ward nursing records accompany the patient to theatre. Other units use specific ward/theatre communication documents. These contain a resumé of the preoperative visit and preoperative ward and theatre check list. (Adaptations of those used in general surgery can be used, e.g. 'shave' or 'skin preparation' can be altered to 'dilating drops instilled'.) Then there is a section for anaesthetic nursing comment, theatre nursing comment and recovery nursing comment, with observation chart, and a section for evaluating care given. Lastly, there is a section for immediate postoperative instructions, problems and care plans. Some units use postoperative visits by theatre staff to evaluate operative care given, but this is not a widespread practice.

Recovery

Following surgery the patient will be transferred to the recovery area. Sample care plans for general theatre care and recovery can be found in *Learning to Care in the Theatre* by Kate Nightingale (1987).

Specific needs of the ophthalmic patient in the recovery area are summarized below.

Goal	Intervention
Calm passage to consciousness without causing direct or indirect pressure on the operated eye, which could cause complications.	1. Ensure that if a patient is being recovered in the lateral position the operated eye side of the patient is uppermost. Exceptions to this action are when positioning on a particular side or prone following retinal repair/vitrectomy. When surgery has been carried out on an infected eye or lacrimal sac, the patient may be required to lie with the operated eye on the lower side to prevent any infected fluid tracking down over the nose to the other eye and causing haemorrhage postenucleation. 2. Ensure that there is as little coughing or vomiting as possible, particularly in cases where the globe of the eye has been opened. This is achieved by careful, gentle suction and early administration of antiemetic injection if the patient is nauseated. Coughing and vomiting cause indirect pressure on the eye. 3. Ensure that the patient does not rub or poke the operated eye. Gently hold patient's arm or tuck it under the blanket and continually encourage relaxation and remind the patient that the operation is over, so the eye must not be touched. 4. Avoid using any particular stimulus to encourage the patient to come round from anaesthetic as this causes the patient to screw up his eyes and thereby cause pressure.

It should be noted that most patients recovering from ophthalmic surgery have discomfort but not outright pain. An exception to this is the use of an encircling scleral band for repair of retinal detachment. These patients more often suffer from pain and nausea than the average ophthalmic case. Severe pain in the eye in the immediate postoperative period should be reported to the surgeon and anaesthetist.

Optimal positioning of the patient as soon as possible following injection into the eye of air, gas or silicon oil is usually required. When an air bubble is placed in the anterior chamber of the eye following cataract surgery, the surgeon usually wishes the patient to be nursed supine to prevent the bubble slipping through the pupil and iridectomy behind the iris.

Following vitrectomy an air-plus-sulphahexa-fluoride (SF6) gas mixture or a silicon oil bubble may be left in the vitreous cavity (internal tamponade). In order for the bubble to function the patient may need to be as far into the prone or exaggerated lateral position as possible. The preferred side will be given by the surgeon in the operation notes. Most patients are already prepared for postoperative positioning, but if complications arise at surgery which need to be treated by internal tamponade then as soon as the patient is able to understand verbal communications the recovery nurse must start to explain and encourage the patient to remain in the position required.

References

Janis, I. L. (1958) cited in Boore, J. R. P. (1978) *Prescription for Recovery*, Royal College of Nursing, London, pp. 19–21.

Lazarus, R. S. (1960) cited in Boore, J. R. P. (1978) *Prescription for Recovery*, Royal College of Nursing, London, pp. 19–21.

Lazarus, R. S. and Averill, J. R. (1972) cited in Boore, J. R. P. (1978) *Prescription for Recovery*, Royal College of Nursing, London, pp. 19–21.

Nightingale, K. (1987) *Learning to Care in the Theatre*, Hodder and Stoughton, London.

Roper, N., Logan, W. W. and Tierney, A. J. (1990) *The Elements of Nursing*, 3rd edn, Churchill Livingstone, Edinburgh.

Further reading

Berry, E. and Koan, M. (1979) *Introduction to Operating Room Technique*, McGraw-Hill, New York.

Codes of Practice (1981,1983) *Health and Safety in the Operating Theatre*, National Association of Theatre Nurses, London.

Greaves, F. T. (1979) *Seeing Theatre Nursing*, Heinemann, London.

Theatre Safeguards (1987) NATN, MDU, RCN.

Part Two

Applied Ocular Physiology and Pathology

10

Examination of the Eye

Ian Rennie

Chapter Summary

Before learning how to examine the integrity of the visual system, we must be familiar with its basic anatomy and physiology.

Anatomy

In simple terms, the eyeball can be considered as a round globe approximately 24 mm in diameter, with a wall composed of three concentric layers (Fig. 10.1). The outer layer is a tough, fibrous tunic approximately 1 mm thick. This consists of the white, opaque sclera and the transparent cornea. The middle coat is a vascular layer consisting of the choroid, iris and ciliary body collectively termed the uveal tract. The innermost layer is the retina, which contains several million light-sensitive cells, the photoreceptors. These cells are responsible for converting the light into electrical impulses. Inside the globe, suspended from the ciliary body by a myriad small fibres known collectively as the zonule, is the transparent crystalline lens. By virtue of its own elasticity, the lens can change shape, becoming more or less concave depending on the tension exerted by the zonular fibres. The lens and zonule divide the eye into two compartments. The posterior cavity is filled with an avascular, jelly-like substance known as vitreous humour. The anterior compartment is bathed in a fluid called aqueous humour, which provides nutrients to the lens and cornea and is produced by the epithelium of the ciliary body. The aqueous flows between the lens and the posterior surface of the iris (posterior chamber), through the pupil into the anterior chamber. It then leaves the eye through a drainage system located in the angle between the base of the iris and the cornea. The drainage system consists of a sieve-like network of fibrous tissue known as the trabecular meshwork,

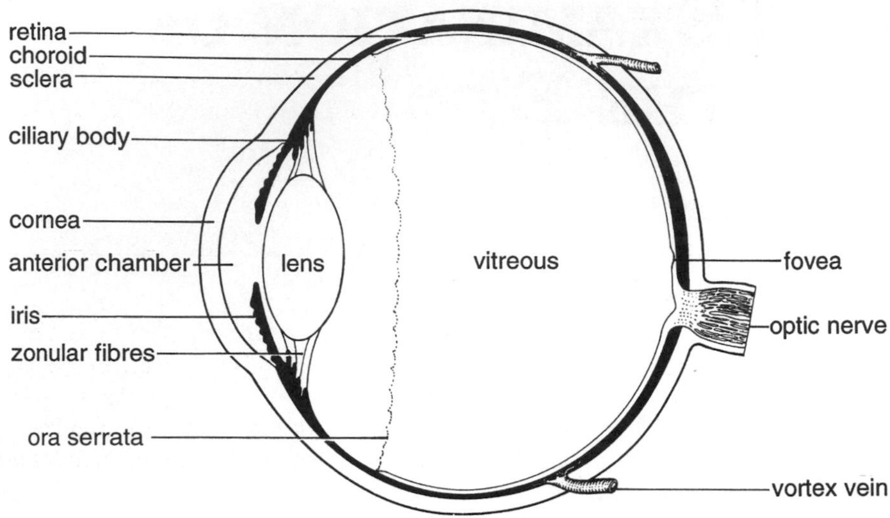

Figure 10.1 The basic structure of the eye.

connected to the canal of Schlemm; this runs as an incomplete ring around the circumference of the globe between the cornea and the sclera. In turn, this structure is connected to a number of small modified veins which perforate the globe and drain into the systemic circulation.

The eyeball lies in the anterior aspect of a pyramid-shape cavity, the orbit. This structure is enclosed by four bony walls (roof, floor, medial and lateral walls) which converge posteriorly to form the orbital apex. The orbital contents include the globe, lacrimal apparatus, muscles, fatty tissue, blood vessels and nerves. The surface of the globe is bathed in tears, which originate from the lacrimal gland and pass in a medial direction towards the punctae and then via the canaliculi and lacrimal sac into the nose. There are six striated muscles responsible for moving the eye: the medial, lateral, superior and inferior recti, and the superior and inferior oblique muscles. The optic nerve runs from the posterior aspect of the globe to the orbital apex where it enters the cranial cavity via the optic foramen. Running in the opposite direction the ophthalmic artery, a branch of the internal carotid artery, enters the orbit through the foramen. The remaining blood vessels and nerves gain access to the orbit via two clefts in the posterior/lateral wall known as the superior and inferior orbital fissures. Anteriorly the orbit is enclosed by the eyelids. The upper lid, which is the most mobile of the two, is elevated by a combination of smooth and striated muscles, known as Müller's muscle and levator palpebrae superioris, respectively.

Physiology

In order for a clear image of an object to be perceived, light rays from it must be precisely focused on to the retina. This focusing of the light involves bending of the light rays, i.e. refraction. This will be discussed in greater detail in Chapter 12. For the present, all we need to know is that refraction occurs at two principal points within the eye: at the anterior surface of the cornea and at the crystalline lens. Contrary to popular belief, it is the cornea and not the lens which is responsible for most of the refracting power of the eye. Indeed, the cornea is responsible for approximately two thirds of the total. Unless some pathological change occurs to the corneal surface, the amount by which it can refract light is constant. However, the lens, by virtue of its ability to change shape, can vary the amount of refraction it produces; this is necessary if we are to visualize objects close to and in the distance with equal clarity. The normal eye in its 'relaxed' state will bring rays of light from distant objects into sharp focus. If we wish to view an object which is close to us, for example when reading a book, we must increase the total refractive power of the eye. To achieve this the lens alters shape, becoming more spherical. This process, known as accommodation, is initiated by contraction of the ciliary muscle in the ciliary body. This causes the ciliary body to change shape slightly, releasing the tension on the zonular fibres, allowing the lens to become more spherical by virtue of its elasticity. The ciliary muscle is under the control of the parasympathetic part of the autonomic nervous system. Accommodation forms one part of an autonomic reflex known as the synkinetic near reflex. The other parts of this reflex are constriction of the pupils (miosis) and inturning of the eyes (convergence), i.e. all the events that occur when a near object is observed.

Once the rays of light have been focused on to the retina their energy is converted into electrical energy by the photoreceptors. This is the first part of the neurological process of seeing. The photoreceptors, i.e. the rods and cones, connect (synapse) with other neural cells within the retina, principally bipolar cells, which in turn relay the neural impulse to the nerve fibre layer. The nerve fibres leave the globe via the optic nerve and travel towards the brain until they reach the lateral geniculate body. Now the visual system is able to put together images formed in each eye. In order that binocular vision is achieved it is necessary for the nerve fibres from the nasal half of each retina to cross over to the other side of the brain. This decussation occurs at the optic chiasm. Thus, each lateral geniculate body receives nerve fibres from the temporal retina of the eye on the same side and fibres from the nasal retina from the opposite eye. A further relay occurs at the lateral geniculate body from where the fibres travel to the occipital lobes of the brain. Here the nervous signals are processed into images of the object. The visual cortex, within the occipital lobe, is well connected to higher centres in the brain so that we can, for example, recognize the images that we are seeing.

Examination

Visual Acuity

An accurate assessment of visual acuity is the most important part of any ophthalmic examination. Under normal circumstances it is desirable to test the patient's distance and near visual acuities. It is extremely important that, when testing visual acuity, the test type or reading material is correctly illuminated. It is also important to remember that some adult patients are illiterate or have reading difficulties, and this must be taken into consideration when testing the patient's acuity. If the patient is illiterate, or does not speak English, their acuities may be assessed using a special chart such as the Snellen E chart. Various tests are also available for young children who have not reached a reading age, e.g. the Kay Picture Test or Sheridan Gardiner test. If a patient normally wears spectacles to correct a refractive error then he should be tested both with and without glasses. This applies to both distance and near reading correction. In either case it should always be clearly indicated in the notes whether glasses were worn or not. It is also important to record if a patient uses contact lenses and if they were being worn at the time of the test. It is essential to test both eyes separately, using an opaque plastic occluder or card to cover the other eye. It is important that the patient does not use his fingers as an occluder because he may be able to see through the gaps between the fingers.

Distance Visual Acuity

The Snellen test chart is the method most commonly employed for testing distance visual acuity. In order for a reproducible result to be obtained, there should be a standard distance between the patient and the chart. If the surroundings permit, the chart is viewed directly at a distance of 6 metres; if, however, the examination area is too small to permit this, the patient may view a reversed chart through a mirror placed 3 metres away. The Snellen chart consists of a series of lines of black letters on a uniform white back-

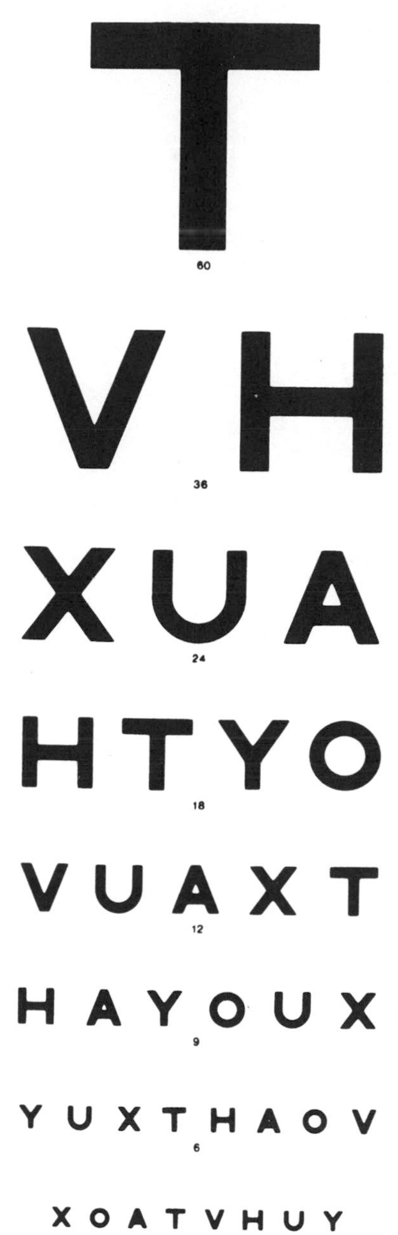

Figure 10.2 The Snellen chart. This is the standard equipment for measuring the distance visual acuity.

ground (Fig. 10.2). At the top of the chart there is a single large letter and on subsequent lines the letters become progressively smaller, with an extra letter being added on each line. Adjacent to or below each line there is a number which represents the distance in metres at which a patient with normal vision would be expected to read letters of that size. Thus when the patient is tested at 6 metres, he should be able to read down to the line with '6' corresponding to it. Thus 6/6 means that the patient has read at 6 metres the letters that were designed to be read at 6 metres and has a 'normal' visual acuity. If for example a patient has 6/36 vision, this means that the patient has read at six metres the line at which a person with a normal vision would read at 36 metres.

When using the test chart the patient is instructed to start with the top letter and then read each subsequent line below until they can no longer clearly identify the letters. This is then recorded as described above. Quite frequently, a patient can identify some but not all of the letters on an individual line clearly, which may be recorded as 6/9 part. Alternatively, it is possible to record the number of letters incorrectly described on a given line by using a minus sign, e.g. $6/9^{-2}$. If the patient only correctly identifies one or two of the letters on a line it is better to add these to the line above, e.g. $6/12^{+2}$.

Many patients with poor vision will be unable to read clearly even the top letter of the Snellen chart at 6 metres. In these cases it is permissible to move the patient closer to the chart at 1 metre intervals until the top letter can be read. Thus, if a patient is capable of reading the top letter at 3 metres from the chart, his visual acuity would be recorded as 3/60. If the patient is unable to read the chart when he is only 1 metre from it, then some other method of assessing visual acuity must be employed. Usually the next method is to ask the patient to count the number of fingers presented by the observer on an outstretched hand at 1 metre against a contrasting background. If the responses are accurate this is recorded as 'count fingers' (CF). If the patient is unable to count fingers then the hand should be moved to and fro in front of him. If the patient is able to perceive the movements of the hand, they should be recorded as having 'hand movement' (HM) vision. Should the patient be unable to visualize a hand moving in front of his eye then a bright pen torch should be shone in the eye intermittently and the patient should be instructed to state whether he thinks the light is on or off. If the patient can discern the light shining into the eye, this is recorded as 'perception of light' (PL). Finally, should the patient be unable to see the bright light shining into the eye, then the eye is blind, and should be recorded as 'no perception of light' (NPL). It is extremely important to differentiate accurately between perception of light and no perception of light because an eye which still retains perception of light has retained at least some function and, with appropriate treatment, it may be possible to obtain some improvement.

The Pinhole Test

The most accurate way of differentiating between visual loss secondary to a refractive error and pathological processes is to test patients for spectacles and provide them with the appropriate prescription before proceeding to test their visual acuity. This is time-consuming and, in many clinical situations, may be impossible. One simple method of differentiating between refractive and pathological visual loss is to use the pinhole test. As the name implies, this consists of using an occluder with a small pinhole (usually about 1 mm in diameter) in the centre of it. The patient is instructed to hold the pinhole close to the eye and move it to and fro slightly until the test chart can be seen through it. With the other eye covered, the patient should then read down the test chart in the standard manner. If the reduced visual acuity is related to a refractive error then the patient will usually be able to read considerably further down the chart with the aid of the pinhole. The pinhole works by only allowing the rays of light close to the principal axis through to the retina. These rays require very little refraction and are relatively unaffected by errors in the patient's optical system. It is customary to use the pinhole test routinely in all situations where a visual acuity of 6/9 or less is recorded.

Patients who have frequent visual acuity tests may be suspected of memorizing the letters and in these situations, a chart with a different letter mix may be used or the patient asked to read their final line backwards. Alternatively, further encouragement can improve a visual acuity recording.

Near Visual Acuity

In most instances, it is also desirable to evaluate the patient's near, or reading vision. Again the patient should use their reading glasses, if this is their normal habit.

Although a variety of test types have been used for testing reading vision, the one most commonly employed was designed by the Faculty of Ophthalmologists of Great Britain in 1952 (Fig. 10.3). This consists of a card or book containing short passages of text printed using ascending sizes of typeface. The smallest print is 5 point and is desig-

N.5.

The streets of London are better paved and better lighted than those of any metropolis in Europe: there are lamps on both sides of every street, in the mean proportion of one lamp to three doors. The effect produced by these double rows of lights in many streets is remarkably pleasing: of this Oxford Street and especially Bond Street, afford striking examples. We have few street robberies, and rarely indeed a midnight assassination. This last circumstance is owing to the benevolent spirit of the people; for whatever crimes the lowest orders of society are tempted to commit, those of a sanguinary nature are less frequent here than in any other country. Yet it is singular, where the police are so ably regulated, that the watchmen, our guardians of the night, are generally old decrepit men, who have scarcely strength to use the alarm which is their signal of distress in cases of emergency. It does credit, however, to the morals of the people, and to the national spirit, and evinces that the brave are always benevolent, when we reflect that, during a period when almost all kingdoms exhibited the horrors of massacre and the outrages of anarchy, when blood had contaminated the standard of liberty, and defaced the long established laws of nations, while it overwhelmed the freedom it pretended to establish, this island maintained the throne of reason, erected on the firm basis of genius, valour and philanthropy.

cave acorn veneer succour

N.6.

This amusing personage generally draws a crowd around him in whatever street he fixes his movable pantomime, as children who cannot afford the penny or halfpenny insight into the show-box are yet greatly entertained with his descriptive harangues, and the perpetual climbing of the squirrels in the round wire cage above the box, by whose incessant motion the row of bells on the top are constantly rung. The show consists of a series of coloured pictures, which the spectator views through a magnifying glass, while the exhibitor rehearses the story, and shifts the scenes by the aid of strings. These Showmen carry their box on their backs, and frequently travel into the country.

ears raven course essence

N.8.

Water Cresses are sold in small bunches, one penny each, or three bunches for twopence. The crier of Water Cresses frequently travels seven or eight miles before the hour of breakfast to gather them fresh; but there is generally a pretty good supply of them in Covent Garden market, brought, along with other vegetables, from the gardens adjacent to the Metropolis, where they are planted and cultivated like other garden stuff. They are, however, from this circumstance, very inferior from those that grow in the natural state in a running brook, wanting that pungency of taste which makes them very wholesome; and a weed very dissimilar in quality is often imposed upon an unsuspecting purchaser.

rose sauce cannon reverse

N.10.

Hearth Brooms, Brushes, Sieves, Bowls, Clothes-horses, and Lines, and almost every household article of turnery, are cried in the streets. Some of these walking turners travel with a cart, by which they can extend their trade and their profit; but the greater number carry their shop on their shoulders, and find customers sufficient to afford them a decent subsistence, the profit of turnery being considerable, and the consumption certain.

neon verse runner caravan

Figure 10.3 Test type. This is the standard text for measuring the near visual acuity.

nated N5 and the largest print is 48 point, and similarly, designated N48. When being tested, the patient should be seated and instructed to hold the test type at a comfortable reading distance. They should then be asked to indicate which is the smallest print they can read comfortably.

Colour Vision

Colour vision depends on the retinal cones. As many as 7% of the male population are born with defective colour vision, some of whom will be unaware of this defect. In addition, however, defective colour vision may be acquired and is sufficiently characteristic of some conditions to be helpful in diagnosis. These include optic neuritis and certain macular disorders.

Ishihara colour plates are the most commonly used method of testing colour vision, being simple and quick. They consist of numbers made up of red and green dots against a background of different coloured dots. More detailed and informative is the Farnsworth-Munsell test, where 84 coloured chips have to be arranged according to changing hue.

External Examination of the Eye and Related Structures

When examining the eye and related structures it is important to remember a few general principles. Good illumination is essential and some form of magnification often beneficial. A bright pen torch and small × 10 magnifying loupe will often provide all the illumination and magnification necessary. It is strongly recommended, as in all forms of clinical examination, that the eye and related structures are examined in an orderly sequence. In this respect it is probably best to examine the periocular structures, eye movements, the lids and finally the globe itself.

Periocular Tissues

A cursory examination of the skin, bony landmarks and position of the globe within the orbit should be made. It is not uncommon for generalized or local skin problems, such as acne rosacea, to affect the eyes. Furthermore, a localized area of inflamed excoriated skin involving the eyelids and immediate periocular tissue may indicate that the patient is allergic to a topical ocular medication. A comparison of the relative positions of the eyes within the orbits should be made. One or both eyes may appear excessively prominent. If the eye or eyes have been pushed forward by a disease process within the orbit, it is termed **proptosis** (**exophthalmos**). The amount of protrusion may be measured using an exophthalmometer (Fig. 10.4). When using this instrument both the patient and the observer should be seated with their eyes at approximately the same level. The exophthal-

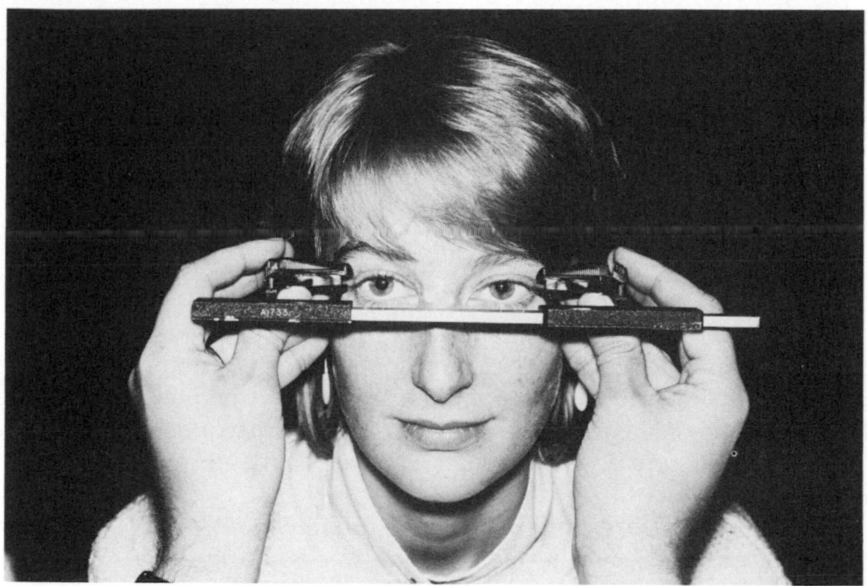

Figure 10.4 Exophthalmometry. Mirrors at the side of each eye allow the observer to measure how far the eyes protrude.

mometer is not only used for making the diagnosis of proptosis but also, on occasion, for monitoring its progress. A rough guide as to the presence and degree of any protrusion may be obtained by standing behind the patient, retracting the upper lid slightly and viewing the relative positions of the globes.

Eye Movements

This subject is covered in detail in Chapter 22.

The Eyelids

Normal eyelid function is essential if the integrity of the anterior surface of the eye is to be preserved. The relative positions of the eyelids should be noted. Under normal circumstances the upper lid just covers the corneoscleral junction at 12 o'clock. If an area of sclera is visible between the upper lid and the cornea then this usually means that either the lid is pathologically retracted, or the globe is proptosed. Alternatively, the upper lid may cover an appreciable portion of the cornea. This excessive drooping of the eyelid or eyelids is termed **ptosis** and is due to abnormalities of the levator muscles or their innervation.

Both upper and lower lids should remain in contact with the globe at all times; abnormalities of apposition, particularly of the lower lid, are common. Excessive lid laxity may lead to turning out of the lower lid (**ectropion**). The converse may also occur with an inturning of the eyelid (**entropion**). Occasionally this condition may be intermittent; if suspected, the patient should be asked to tightly close his eyes and then open them. As the patient opens his eyes the inturned eyelid may be observed.

In addition to malpositions of the eyelids, a careful inspection of the eyelashes should also be made. Under normal circumstances the eyelashes point away from the globe. However, as a consequence of a variety of pathological conditions, the eyelashes may become misdirected and turn towards the globe. This condition is termed **trichiasis**. Frequently the lashes are finer than normal; in consequence their detection may be facilitated by the use of a magnifying loupe.

In patients who are complaining of a foreign body sensation, the upper lid should be everted as this will allow the examiner to inspect the palpebral conjunctiva and fornix of the upper lid. To do this the patient should be instructed to look down; the eyelashes of the upper lid are then grasped between the examiner's thumb and first finger. Using a cotton bud in the other hand, pressure is applied to the lid above the tarsal plate and then the lid is gently everted over the bud (Figs 10.5 and 10.6). The lid is repositioned by asking the patient to look up and blink. Care must be taken when performing this procedure on patients wearing contact lenses.

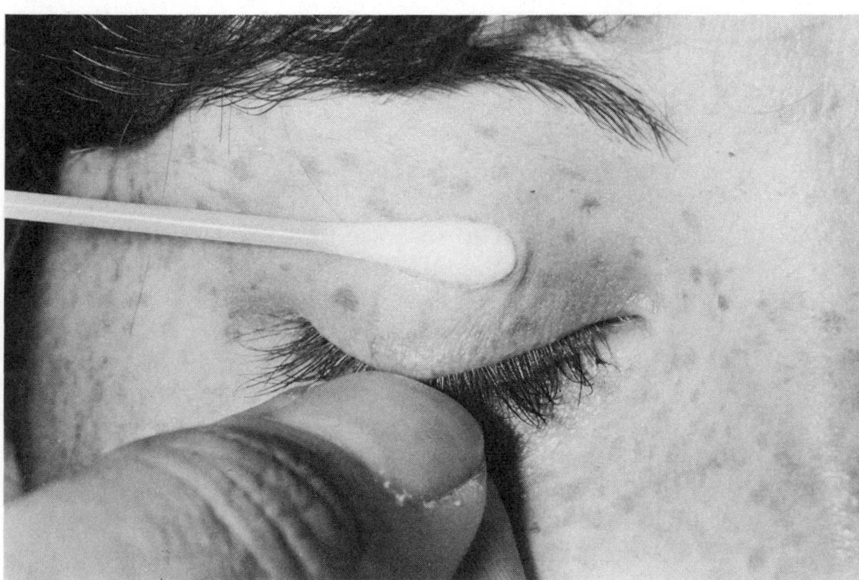

Figure 10.5 The first stage of lid eversion.

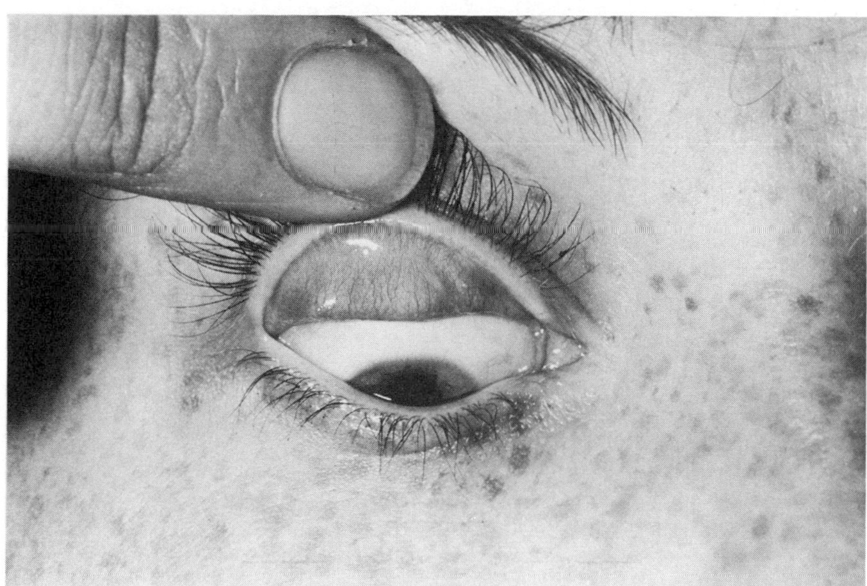

Figure 10.6 The everted lid, exposing the tarsal conjuctiva.

External Examination of the Globe

The palpebral conjunctiva, visible sclera and cornea must be examined carefully in a good light with the aid of some magnification. Th examination of the cornea is facilitated by the use of a stain such as sodium fluorescein. This stain, which is available on sterile paper strips or in solution, will, if the integrity of the corneal epithelium has been breached, stain the underlying stroma a bright green. Thus small abrasions or ulcers, which would otherwise be invisible, may be detected. When using sodium fluorescein it is best to view the cornea with the aid of a blue light. The simplest way to do this is to use a cobalt blue filter on a standard pen torch.

If a patient finds it difficult to open his eyes during the examination due to photophobia or irritation, a drop of topical anaesthetic should be instilled, which, by relieving the symptoms, will permit the patient to open his eyes.

The presence of blood (hyphaema), or white cells (hypopyon) (Plates 1 and 2) in the anterior chamber may be visible to the naked eye, as is the depth or distance between iris and cornea. However, full evaluation of both the cornea and anterior chamber requires slit-lamp examination.

Examination of the Pupils

Before testing the pupil reflexes, it is important to compare the size and shape of each pupil. While small differences in size between pupils may be normal (**physiological anisocoria**), marked differences in pupil size and shape are always abnormal and should be carefully documented (Plate 3).

Under normal circumstances, when a bright light is shone in one eye the pupil rapidly constricts. This is called the direct light response. In addition, at precisely the same time, the pupil in the fellow eye will also constrict. This is termed the consensual light response. When testing the pupils the patient should be seated in subdued lighting looking into the distance. Using a bright pen torch, held approximately 15 cm from the eye inferiorly and slightly temporally to the line of fixation, the direct reaction of the pupil is noted. The process is then repeated and the response of the other pupil (consensual response) is noted. The pen torch should then be positioned in a similar fashion on the other side and the procedure repeated.

While the simple light reflex may detect gross abnormalities in the pupil nerve pathways, subtle damage to the different pathways may go undetected. The swinging flashlight test is a more sensitive method of detecting subtle optic nerve disease. In this test a pen torch is used to illuminate the pupil in a similar fashion to that used for the normal light reflex; however, once the pupil has constricted the torch is 'swung over' to illuminate the fellow eye. During the transit of the pen torch from one side to the other, its light will not shine on either pupil and they will both start to dilate. Normally, as soon as the light impinges on the fellow pupil it will start to constrict; however, if significant optic nerve disease is present, the pupil continues to dilate. Thus when the observer moves the pen torch from one side to the other, if retinal or optic nerve damage is present on this second side, the pupil will initially dilate.

The near reflex should then be tested. The simplest way to do this is to place a pencil in the midline approximately 15 cm away from the patient's face with its tip level with the pupils. The patient is then instructed to look at a distant object and then to look at the tip of the pencil. Under normal circumstances this will cause the pupils to constrict and, in addition, the eyes to turn inwards.

The Red Reflex

A pen torch shone into the dilated pupil will elicit a red reflex, similar in appearance to that seen in flash photography. An absence of this reflex may indicate gross pathology such as dense lens opacity or vitreous haemorrhage. Full use of the red reflex is discussed later in this chapter under Ophthalmoscopy.

Slit-lamp Microscopy

The slit-lamp is the most versatile instrument used in ophthalmology. By careful attention to illumination and the use of a limited number of accessories the ophthalmologist or ophthalmic nurse can examine the eye in great detail. Furthermore, by using the microscope in combination with an applanation tonometer, the intraocular pressure can be measured. As the name implies, the slit-lamp microscope consists of two basic elements: a light source with a variable slit beam and a binocular lower-power microscope (Fig. 10.7). By altering the width of the beam, or its angle incident to the eye, it is possible to highlight certain structures and examine them in detail. For example, in cases of anterior uveitis, by using direct illumination with an extremely fine beam of light it is possible to see white blood cells circulating within the aqueous. Alternatively, by critically altering the incident angle of the beam it is possible to make the inner surface of the cornea act like a mirror and produce a reflection of the endothelial cells on its surface. This technique, termed specular reflection, permits the ophthalmologist to examine the corneal endothelium for signs of disease. With the advent of intraocular lenses following cataract extraction the examination of the corneal endothelium has become increasingly important and specially designed specular microscopes are now available that permit not only viewing of the endothelium, but also its photography.

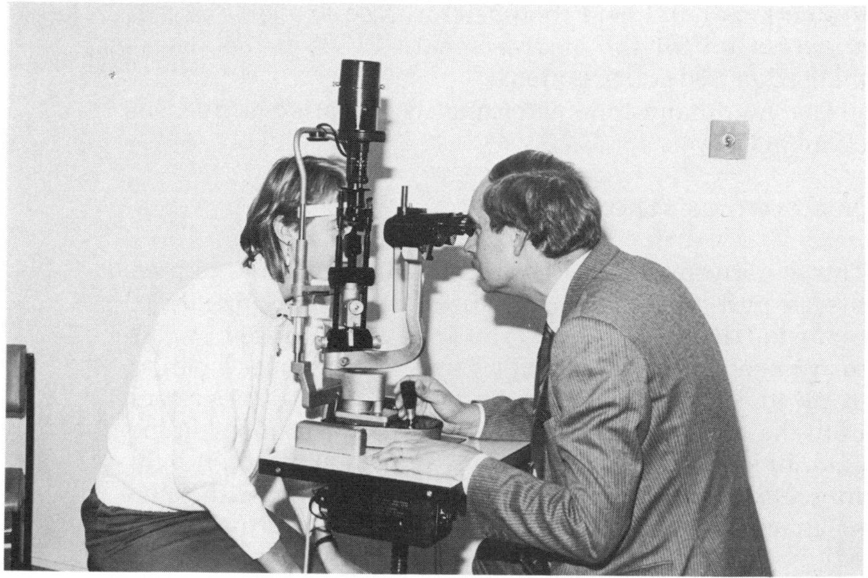

Figure 10.7 Slit-lamp examination.

Measurement of Intraocular Pressure

The accurate measurement of the intraocular pressure (IOP) is an important and everyday part of ophthalmic examination. While digital palpation of the eye provides the experienced examiner with a crude estimate of intraocular pressure, this method has little to recommend it.

Indentation Tonometry

Indentation tonometry is based on the principle that a known force will indent a fluid-filled sphere to a greater or lesser extent depending on the internal pressure. For many years, the Schiotz tonometer was employed to measure IOP on this principle. Unfortunately, several readings had to be obtained using different weights before the pressure could be calculated from standardized tables; this made the use of this instrument time-consuming. Applanation tonometry is now the method of choice for measuring IOP.

Applanation Tonometry

Applanation tonometry employs the principle that the force required to flatten a fixed area of the normally convex cornea is proportional to the IOP. In 1954 Goldmann designed a tonometer that employs this principle, which has since become the standard instrument for routinely measuring IOP. This tonometer is used in combination with the slit-lamp microscope. A modification of this instrument, the Perkins hand-held tonometer, is also available and is widely used for the measurement of IOP in the anaesthetized or bedridden patient.

The Goldmann tonometer and its use are described in detail in Chapter 18.

Non-contact Tonometry

This is performed using an instrument, sometimes termed the 'air puff' tonometer, which uses a fine, high-pressure jet of air to flatten the cornea. The jet of air produced by this instrument has a force that increases linearly over a period of up to 8 ms. The increase in force of this jet progresses until the cornea becomes perfectly flat. At this moment the anterior surface of the cornea acts as a plane mirror. A light source and photoelectric sensor are positioned within the machine in such a way that rays of light from the source will be reflected from the cornea into the sensor when the corneal surface behaves like a plane mirror. When the sensor receives the light impulse the jet of air is immediately switched off, and the force required to flatten the cornea is recorded and converted into an intraocular pressure reading. Although this machine has the great advantage of not having to touch the cornea, it is expensive. Furthermore, many patients dislike the sensation of a jet of air striking the cornea. This makes them apprehensive and tense, which in turn may give rise to inappropriately high pressure readings.

The Gonioscope

Another accessory for the slit-lamp is a contact lens incorporating a single inclined mirror (or sometimes two identically inclined mirrors) for examining the iridocorneal angle. This lens, called a gonioscope, allows the ophthalmologist to observe in detail the drainage angle of the eye; this is of value in the diagnosis and management of glaucoma.

Examination of the Media and Ocular Fundus

For the purposes of examination the aqueous humour, lens and vitreous humour are often collectively called the ocular media. The other tissues that can be examined by ophthalmoscopy are the retina, optic disc and, to a lesser extent, the choroid. The ophthalmologist can make use of two basic types of ophthalmoscope to visualize these structures.

Direct Ophthalmoscopy

The direct ophthalmoscope is the instrument most commonly used to examine the ocular media and fundus. The ophthalmoscope consists of a bright light source and a mirror with a central hole in its reflecting surface. The mirror is inclined at approximately 45° to the light source, which means that the rays of light from this source are reflected through 90° into the patient's eye. Some of the rays of light returning from the patient's eye pass through the central hole in the mirror and can be viewed by the observer. In view of the fact that either the observer or the patient (or both) may have a refractive error, a set of concave and convex lenses of increasing power is placed in a circular wheel behind the mirror. This wheel can be moved by the observer's finger in order to obtain a focused image of the patient's ocular fundus. For the right eye the examiner uses his right hand with his first finger controlling the lens selection. With the lens setting at zero, light from the ophthalmoscope is directed into the patient's pupil from a distance of about 15–23 cm from the eye. Opacities in the ocular media, particularly those in the crystalline lens, will appear as black shadows within the red reflex. With experience, scrutiny of this reflex can provide the observer with a great deal of information regarding the presence and relative density of cataractous change and vitreous opacities. Once the red reflex has been examined, the observer moves the ophthalmoscope towards the patient's eye until it is about 1 cm away from it. Adjustments are then made to the power of the lens within the ophthalmoscope aperture until the retinal detail is brought into sharp focus. Almost inevitably, a retinal vessel or vessels will be immediately visible to the observer. The observer can then follow one of the vessels back to the optic disc. When moving from one point to another within the retina, coaxial illumination must be maintained at all times. To do this the observer must move his head synchronously with the ophthalmoscope. Once the optic disc has been visualized, its contour, colour, cup and circulation can be assessed. When the optic disc has been adequately examined, the peripheral retina and the macula may be examined. It must be noted that, while a limited examination of the ocular fundus may be obtained through an undilated pupil, for proper evaluation pupil dilation is a prerequisite.

The direct ophthalmoscope provides the observer with an erect magnified image of the ocular fundus; it does not, however, provide the observer with a good view of the peripheral retina. Moreover, if there are significant opacities in the media the resultant view of the retina may be poor or non-existent.

Indirect Ophthalmoscopy

The indirect ophthalmoscope provides the observer with a low magnification view of a large area of the ocular fundus. This permits the observer to view the peripheral parts of the retina and, by virtue of its stereoscopic effect, allow him to assess elevated lesions.

The instrument is, at least to begin with, difficult to use, in that the observer must position himself and a condensing lens (+20 or +28 dioptres) accurately in order to obtain a view of the ocular fundus (Fig. 10.8). To make life even more difficult, because of the optics of the system, the image is inverted. If, however, the patient is examined from above the head the image is turned the right way up! Nevertheless, this instrument is very useful in the visualization of the retina through relatively dense opacities in the media.

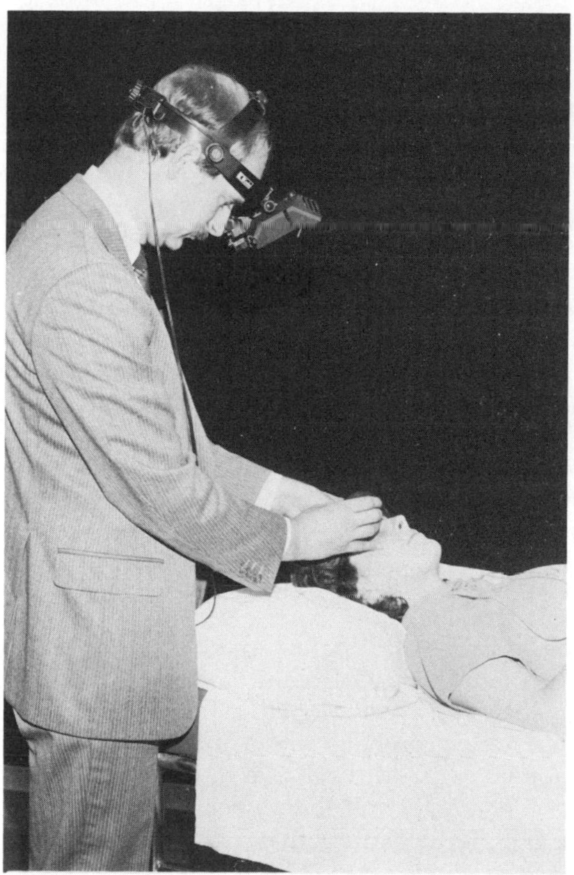

Figure 10.8 Indirect ophthalmoscopy, best achieved with the patient lying down.

Slit-lamp Examination of the Fundus

The Hruby lens is a concave lens of high refractive power (usually –55 dioptres). By carefully placing this lens between the patient's eye and the objective of the slit-lamp microscope it is possible to view the patient's fundus. When using the Hruby lens it is essential to have a dilated pupil. Although with the standard slit-lamp microscope the size of the image is only equivalent to that seen with the direct ophthalmoscope, the Hruby lens permits a stereoscopic view of the retina and optic disc. This can be extremely useful for detecting subtle changes to the macula or optic disc. Convex lenses of high refractive power (+90 and +78 dioptres) are now available which are also placed between the patient's eye and the slit-lamp objective; this is actually a form of indirect ophthalmoscopy.

An alternative method for viewing the ocular fundus with the slit-lamp microscope is to use a contact lens. A number of lenses have been devised to facilitate this technique. The simplest contact lens resembles the Hruby lens in that it has one concave surface, which fits over the cornea, the other surface being flat. Again, when using this lens, pupil dilation is essential and the examination is restricted to the central (posterior) part of the retina. In order to view the more peripheral parts of the retina with the slit-lamp, a lens has been devised which incorporates three mirrors inclined at varying angles. By viewing the fundus through one of the inclined mirrors it is possible to visualize the extreme periphery of the retina. This technique is particularly useful for examining the peripheral retina for small areas of retinal degeneration which may cause, or may already have caused, a retinal detachment.

Examination of the Visual Field

If you close one eye and look at an object directly in front, you will become aware of being able to see many other things at which you are not looking. This is because they all cast light on your peripheral retina; in other words they fall within your visual field. Each eye has its own visual field which has a characteristic shape, being larger on the temporal side (Fig. 10.9). With both eyes open the more medial parts of the two fields overlap. An object in this area lies in the binocular field of vision, that is, it forms an image in both eyes. Hold a pencil about a foot in front of your nose. Move the pencil 1 cm to the right, but continue to look ahead. If you close your left eye the pencil is seen because of the image formed on the nasal retina of your right eye. If, however, the right eye is closed the pencil is seen because an image is formed on the temporal retina of your left eye. Both images come together in the visual cortex, using the nervous pathways already described.

Damage to any part of the visual pathway from retina to visual cortex can result in a defect in the visual field even though the visual acuity may be normal. If the damage is in front of the optic chiasm the defect will be found only in the visual field of that eye. If the damage is behind or actually at the chiasm the defect will appear in both visual fields. As we have seen above both visual fields are represented behind the chiasm because here the fibres from the nasal retina cross over to the opposite side.

An accurate record of the visual field is an essential part of the diagnosis and monitoring of several conditions. For example, tumours of the pituitary gland may press on the

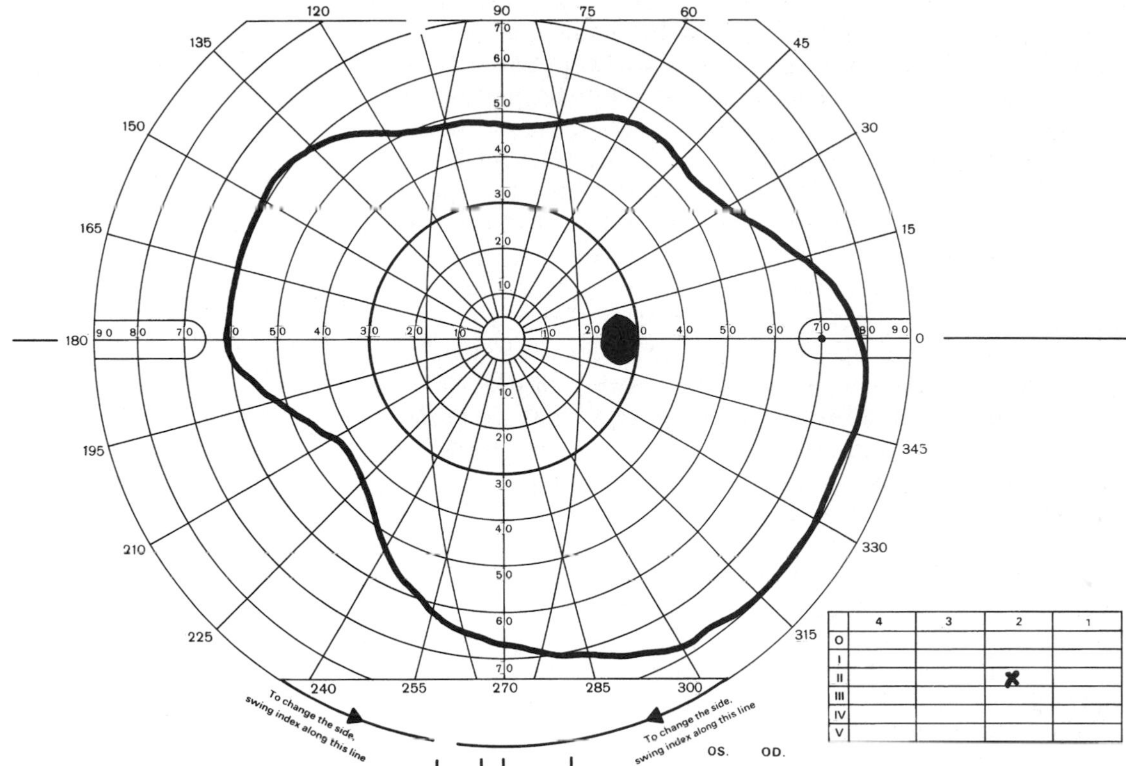

Figure 10.9 The right visual field from a Goldmann perimeter, showing a normal blind spot.

chiasm and cause defects in both peripheral visual fields. The patient may actually present with a complaint of bumping into things which they did not see, for instance when parking the car. Other conditions, such as glaucoma, may result in 'scotomas'; these are patches of visual field which are missing.

The method of field assessment ranges from the rapid qualitative screening test of 'confrontation', which requires no equipment, to the new and highly sophisticated systems, such as the Humphrey system, which are semi-automated.

The two basic forms of field analysis are kinetic perimetry, when a moving target is used, and static perimetry, when a stationary target is presented intermittently. When the visual field is plotted the patient is asked to fixate the eye being tested on a central target. Moving or flashing targets of different size or brightness are then presented in the visual field. The various points at which a target can first be seen are joined up in a line called an isoptre. In this way constriction of the field or scotomas are recorded. Everyone has a normal scotoma in each visual field – the blind spot.

An object in space that casts an image on the optic disc, where there are no photoreceptors, is not seen.

The two best examples of visual field equipment are the Goldmann perimeter, which is used for kinetic perimetry, and the Friedman Analyser, which is for static perimetry. The Bjerrum screen is a large flat black cloth hung on a wall which is used in particular for measuring central fields. Another test of central visual field using a flat (or tangent) screen is the Amsler chart (Fig. 10.10).

Where a rapid, qualitative screen test for the visual fields is required, the confrontation test may be used. This test is useful in demonstrating field loss due to intracranial lesions or gross retinal disease and is described here. It is of little value in demonstrating small isolated scotomas, as may be found in early chronic simple glaucoma. The examiner and the patient should be seated 'confronting' each other approximately a yard apart; the patient is then instructed to look at the examiner's nose. The examiner then holds up both hands with the palms facing the patient and approximately 30 cm apart. The patient is then asked, while still looking at the examiner's nose, to state how many hands are being held up. If the patient informs the examiner that he can see both hands, he should be then questioned as to whether both hands appear the same. Should the patient fail to see one of the examiner's hands, or if they state that they cannot see one hand as clearly as the other, this may indicate loss of half of the visual field (hemianopia). The test is then repeated with the patient covering each eye in turn. More detailed information can be elicited using less crude targets, such as the fingers and white or red targets, usually 'hatpins'.

AMSLER RECORDING CHART
A replica of Chart No. 1, printed black on white for convenience of recording

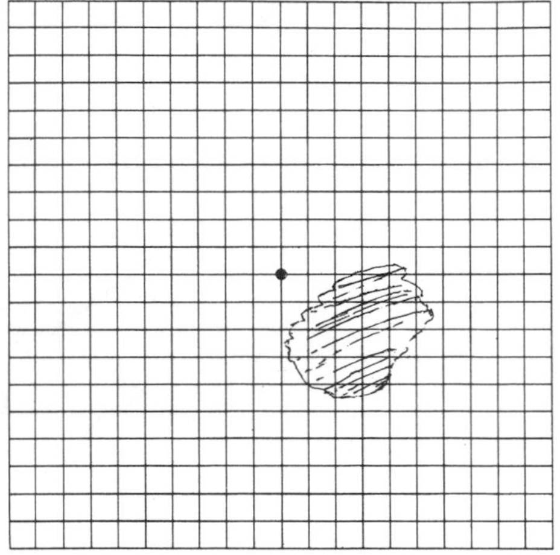

Figure 10.10 The Amsler chart, showing an area shaded in by the patient (while fixing on the central point) indicating an area of distortion corresponding to a lesion close to the fovea.

Goldmann Perimeter

The Goldmann perimeter or one of its modifications still remains one of the most popular perimeters (see Chapter 18). The perimeter consists of an illuminated hemispherical bowl on to which a small spot of light can be projected. This light source can be varied in size, intensity and sometimes colour. The position of the stimulus inside the bowl is controlled by a pantograph handle. Moving the handle across a chart of the patient's visual field will accurately reflect the position of the illuminated target within the perimeter bowl. In the centre of the bowl there is a small fixation target for the patient. Behind this fixation point is a small viewing porthole which allows the observer to check that the patient is fixing at all times on this target. Although the perimeter uses mechanical methods, in essence its mode of action is similar to that of the tangent screen.

The Tangent Screen

The simplest type of perimeter is a matt black cloth screen with a white central fixation target. The screen is marked by stitching, indicating the radial meridians and the degrees from fixation. The patient is seated 2 metres away from the screen and one eye is covered. The patient is then instructed to look at the central target while the examiner moves a smaller target on the end of a matt black stick in from the periphery. The patient tells the examiner every time he can see the target appear out of the 'corner of his eye'; its position is then marked on the screen with a faint chalk mark or small pin. The observer moves the target inwards along each radial meridian until the complete circumference of the field has been charted. The blind spot or pathological scotomas may be detected by the observer moving the target along each meridian towards the central fixation spot and instructing the patient to indicate if the target disappears from view at any point. Should the target disappear, indicating the possible presence of a scotoma, the observer should try to map out the non-seeing area. This is usually done by placing the target in the non-seeing area and then moving it outwards from this area until the patient notes its reappearance. The size and colour of the target may be varied to increase the sensitivity of the test. The advantages of the tangent screen are that it is inexpensive and easy to use; its disadvantages are that it is time-consuming and may produce variable results if meticulous care is not taken when positioning the patient and lighting the screen. It is inappropriate for testing the peripheral visual field.

The Friedman Visual Field Analyser

This is an example of a static perimeter and consists of a stroboscopic light source that flashes for about 0.5 ms and evenly illuminates a translucent screen. The intensity of the flash is controlled using a variety of filters. A pair of black opaque screens, perforated by 98 small holes, are situated in front of a diffuser screen. The outermost plate is viewed by the patient. A lever controlling the rear plate can be placed in 31 different positions. In each position two, three or four holes can be opened so that, when the strobe flashes, the patient will perceive an equivalent number of spots of light. Thus, by moving the rear plate two, three or four spots of light can be presented to the patient in 31 different configurations. In operation, the examiner moves sequentially through the 31 different positions, requesting that the observer inform him in each position the number of lights visible. If in any position the observer fails to perceive the number of lights correctly, the operator discerns the spot which the patient did not see and records it.

This method of testing visual fields provides the operator with a rapid method of screening for visual field loss.

There is now a generation of sophisticated and largely automated methods of field analysis. They are increasingly used in daily practice and one such system is briefly described here.

The Octopus Perimeter System

This is a fully automated system of static perimetry that uses a computer to monitor both the stimulus presented by the perimeter and the patient's response to it. Patient fixation is monitored by using a video system which allows the operator to see any eye movement. On completion of the examination, the computer will print out a scatter plot of the relative intensities of the targets used by the computer. Although over 2800 points are represented on the scatter plot, only a certain number of points (usually 72) are actually tested and all the other points are assumed values calculated by the computer from the known points nearby. The Octopus is particularly useful in the detection of early field defects. One of several programmes is selected according to what kind of field defect is suspected.

Special Investigations

Fluorescein Angiography (see also Chapter 20)

Fluorescein angiography of the fundus provides the clinician with a method of examining the retinal and choroidal microcirculation. It can also be of considerable value in evaluating the health and integrity of the retinal pigment epithelium and optic disc. The technique consists of injecting a small amount of fluorescein dye into the circulation and then taking multiple photographs of its transit through the ocular circulation. Normally, 500 mg of fluorescein is injected as a 10% solution into a vein in the antecubital fossa. The injection is rapid to ensure that there is a single bolus of fluorescein travelling through the circulation. Great care should be taken when injecting this dye to ensure that none extravasates into the surrounding tissues; if this occurs, it will produce considerable irritation. Within a matter of seconds the dye will reach the ocular circulation, and

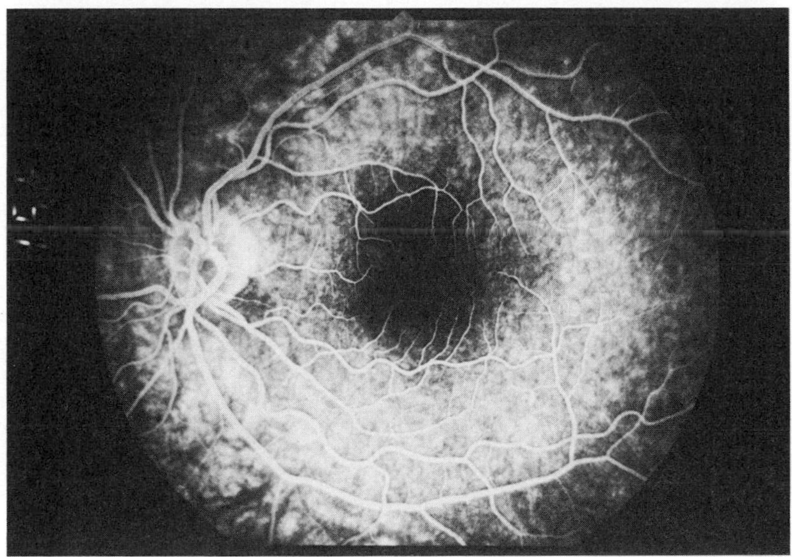

Figure 10.11 The appearance of a normal fluorescein angiogram approximately 30 seconds after the injection of dye. The smaller, more tortuous vessels are arteries, the larger ones veins. There are no areas of leakage, which would show up as bright white patches.

for this reason the patient is already seated at the fundus camera. Because the fluorescence achieved is relatively faint, the fundus camera contains special filters that remove wave lengths of light other than those emitted by the fluorescein.

When a fluorescein angiogram is viewed two separate circulations can be seen. Under normal circumstances the retinal vessels are sharply defined against the background because their configuration does not permit leakage of the dye. Conversely, choroidal vessels allow the fluorescein to leak profusely and consequently, rather than seeing clearly defined vessels, a generalized fluorescence is seen. The view of this choroidal fluorescence is modified by the retinal pigment epithelium, which acts as a barrier to the fluorescence. The normal retinal pigment epithelium is more intensely pigmented at the macula and consequently this area appears as an area of hypofluorescence (Figure 10.11).

In general this technique is extremely safe; patients may sometimes experience transient nausea and even vomiting, particularly if they have previously had a fluorescein angiogram. Caution should be exercised if the patient has severe cardiovascular disease or a history of allergy. Although severe reactions are rare, a resuscitation trolley or box containing emergency medications, methods of maintaining an airway and oxygen should always be readily available.

ULTRASONOGRAPHY

Ultrasound consists of sound waves that are inaudible to the human ear. These sound waves are produced by passing an electrical current through a small quartz crystal. This causes the crystal to vibrate and emit a high frequency sound wave (8–10 $\times$ 10^{16} Hz). The crystal and its electrical connections are known as a transducer and are located in the tip of a probe. Because the sound waves have a high frequency they can penetrate tissue. In many ways sound waves will behave in a similar way to light waves in that they will continue in a straight line until they hit a surface. If the surface is at right angles to the wave front the waves will be reflected back towards their source. The returning sound waves are detected by the probe and in turn can be converted into an image on the screen. As an analogy, one could imagine bouncing a ball against a wall, with the player's hand representing the probe tip and the wall the reflecting surface. Obviously, the further away from the wall the player stands the longer it takes for the ball to return to their hand. Structures with smooth surfaces that are perpendicular to the sound wave will reflect a greater percentage of the sound back than will irregular surfaces placed obliquely. By a combination of these two features it is possible to visualize structures within the globe.

Ophthalmic ultrasound can be used in one of two modes. In A scan mode the image is a series of vertical spikes displayed on a horizontal axis. The height of the spike represents the amount of reflectivity from a surface and the horizontal axis represents the time elapsed, which in turn is a function of tissue depth. A modification of the A scan is used to measure accurately the length of the eye (biometry) and is essential for calculating the power of intraocular lens implants.

By moving the transducer rapidly to and fro within the head of the probe it is possible to take multiple recordings from the eye and surrounding structures; when displayed visually, they appear to give a two-dimensional slice through the eye and orbital structures. This is called B scan mode, and is particularly useful for evaluating the retina and vitreous, particularly when opacities in the anterior media make direct visualization impossible.

In practice, a variety of ultrasound probes are available. Some may be used through the closed eyelid (Figure 10.12) whereas others need to make contact with the cornea or conjunctiva. Occasionally, particularly if detailed visualization of the anterior segment is required, the probe must be placed in a waterbath that has been created to cover the eye.

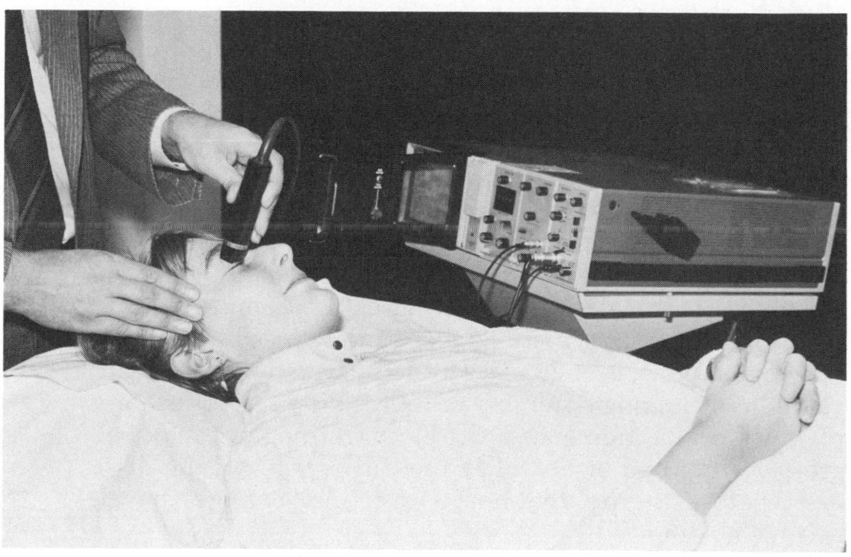

Figure 10.12 Ultrasonography. Jelly is normally placed on the eyelid prior to the application of the probe.

Computerized Tomography (CT)

This is a sophisticated form of X-ray. The CT scanner has dramatically improved our ability to visualize intracranial structures. In ophthalmology the CT scanner is particularly useful for evaluating intraorbital lesions (see Figure 21.2).

Magnetic Resonance Imaging

Magnetic resonance imaging (MRI) is a revolutionary technique used to examine a wide range of anatomical structures. Although the final images in some ways resemble those produced by CT scanning, this method uses a powerful magnetic field rather than conventional X-rays. MRI scanning has proved particularly useful for examining the orbit and intracranial visual pathways. In particular, this technique has proved valuable in imaging vascular orbital lesions and pathology situated at the orbital apex. Further refinements will undoubtedly enhance the usefulness of the technique.

Electrodiagnostic Investigations (see also Chapter 20)

When discussing the basic physiology of the eye in the introduction to this chapter, it was noted that light energy is converted into electrical energy by the photoreceptors within the retina, and that these impulses were in turn transmitted through a complex network of nerves to the brain via the optic nerve. Although these electrical currents are extremely small, by using sensitive detectors and amplification they can be measured. The electroretinogram is a method of measuring these signals. A contact lens containing an electrode is placed on the cornea and a second electrode is applied to the forehead. By stimulating the retina with a bright flash or flickering light a complex wave pattern, representing the total electrical changes occurring within the retina, is obtained. This technique can be of great value in evaluating a number of retinal diseases; for example, in retinitis pigmentosa the electroretinogram may be grossly abnormal or absent in the early stages of the disease, before the ophthalmoscopic retinal changes have become obvious.

It has been observed that, even when the retina is not being stimulated, an electrical potential difference exists between the cornea and the ocular fundus. This can be measured and forms the basis of the electro-oculogram. The electrical potential is measured in bright conditions and then in darkness; the difference between these two potentials is then calculated. This difference, usually expressed as a ratio (the Arden ratio), is reduced in a number of hereditary retinal diseases.

11

PHARMACOLOGY

Patrick W. Joyce

CHAPTER SUMMARY

Pharmacology is the study of how drugs act in the body as a whole. This chapter is concerned with the action and interaction of drugs on the eye. In order to appreciate these effects some aspects of general pharmacology will be discussed. An overview of the drugs affecting the eye will be presented, as well as reference to the preparations, formulation and dosage regimens. In addition the major adverse reactions will be mentioned.

DRUG ACTIONS

Drug action can be considered broadly under two headings: pharmacodynamics and pharmacokinetics.

PHARMACODYNAMICS

Drugs are given to produce an effect at a particular site. However, not only are the expected responses seen but there may also be adverse effects, including allergic reactions. The subject which relates to these aspects of pharmacology is called **pharmacodynamics.**

To achieve their effects drugs act on receptors. These can be inside the cells or on the cell membranes. The receptors are believed to be proteins, such as enzymes, which can be stimulated or inhibited by the drug. The effect will be determined by the concentration of the drug, its strength of attachment to the receptors (affinity) and the presence of other drugs.

As stated above, drugs can have unwanted side effects elsewhere in the body, for example paraesthesiae with acetazolamide and dyspnoea after topical timolol. Delayed adverse effects can also occur with chronic dosage, for example blood dyscrasias, or upon reintroduction of a drug, for example penicillin allergy and contact dermatitis from atropine drops.

PHARMACOKINETICS

The response to a drug and any adverse effects will vary from person to person. This is related to the absorption, metabolism, distribution and excretion of the drug. To a lesser extent age, general health, genetic background and the presence of other drugs are influential. These are all considered under the heading of **pharmacokinetics**. In relation to the eye there are two basic groups of drugs, 1) systemically administered drugs and 2) locally applied medication.

SYSTEMICALLY ADMINISTERED DRUGS

ABSORPTION

The route of administration will have a major role in the absorption of a drug. Most drugs are given orally and are absorbed mainly in the stomach and small intestine. However, such factors as the solubility of the drug, the dissolution of the tablet or capsule, the gastrointestinal enzymes and the presence of food will determine the degree of absorption.

Some drugs are given by injection (i.e. intravenously, intramuscularly or subcutaneously). The total amount of drug reaches the bloodstream with the intravenous mode of injection and to a lesser extent with the latter two. Nevertheless, higher and more constant plasma levels can be maintained by these routes than by oral administration.

DISTRIBUTION

Many drugs bind to plasma proteins, e.g. albumen, and establish an equilibrium between bound and unbound forms. Only the free (unbound) drug is able to move out of the bloodstream. Most drugs can penetrate from the bloodstream into extracellular tissues, except for the brain, aqueous humour and retina where they must be fat-soluble.

METABOLISM

The majority of drugs administered systemically are broken down in the liver, either by a process called conjugation or by various chemical reactions such as oxidation and reduction. Some drugs, such as acetazolamide, on the other hand, are not metabolized at all. They are excreted in the urine unchanged.

Excretion

The kidneys excrete most water-soluble drugs and the biliary system the large molecular weight compounds. Some drugs appear in the tears (e.g. tetracycline and aspirin), saliva and breast milk which, though small in quantity, may affect the breast-fed baby.

Following absorption, the time for one-half of the plasma concentration of the drug to be eliminated is called the biological half-life or $T_{\frac{1}{2}}$. This has important implications in relation to dose frequency.

Local Agents

Topical Application

Topical drugs for extraocular conditions such as conjunctivitis are effective if their concentration is maintained. The concentration is diluted by tears, drainage through the nasolacrimal duct and loss through conjunctival and eyelid blood vessels.

Other topical drugs are required to penetrate into the eye, in glaucoma, for instance. They therefore have to cross the cornea. To do this they have to cross the precorneal film, the corneal epithelium, stroma and endothelium.

Initially (Figure 11.1) the drug has to be in the unionized form (lipid-soluble) to pass through the corneal epithelium. It must then move back into the ionized form (water-soluble)

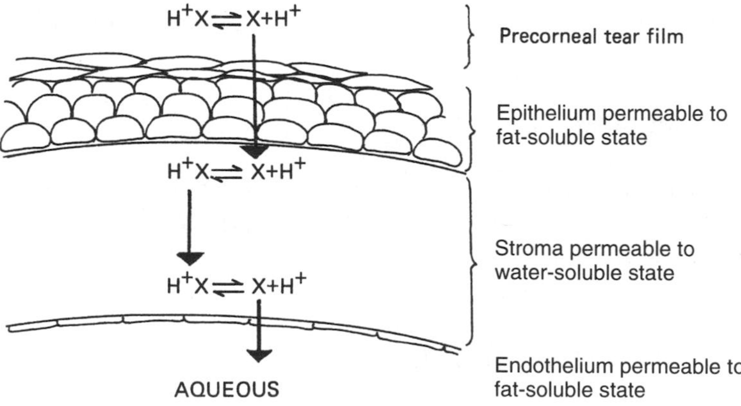

H^+= hydrogen ion
H^+X= ionized from of drug (water-soluble)
X = unionized from of drug (fat-soluble)

Figure 11.1 Passage of drugs across the cornea.

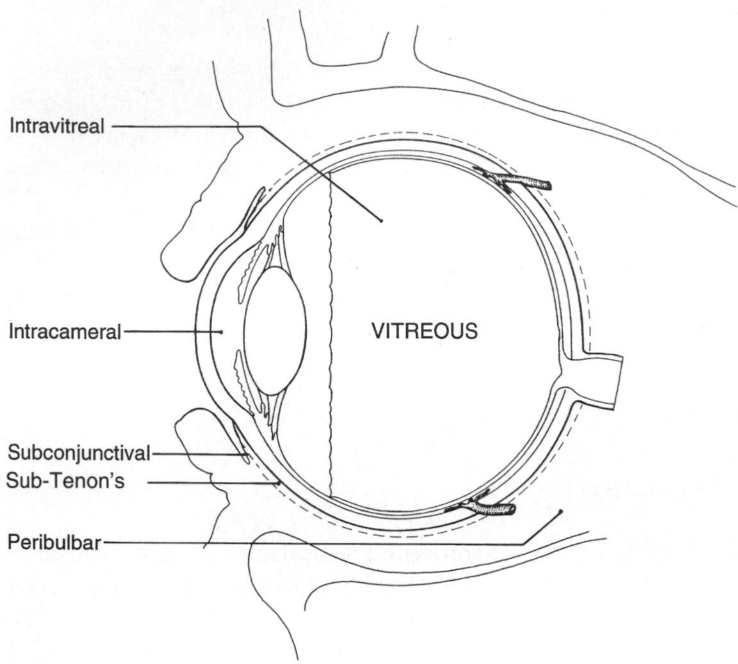

Figure 11.2 Possible sites for injection of drugs.

to pass through the stroma, and return again to the union-ized form to pass through the endothelium to the aqueous.

Subconjunctival, Sub-Tenon's and Peribulbar Injections (Figure 11.2)

In these situations drug penetration is by local diffusion through the tissues.

Metabolism

Local agents applied to the eye are metabolized by enzymes within the globe, although the exact sequence of events is not yet known.

Drugs Affecting the Eye

Before discussing the various groups of drugs it is appropriate to mention routes of administration, as there are several into the eye.

1. Direct routes
   (a) Topical
      (i) Drops
      (ii) Ointments
      (iii) Special delivery systems, e.g. soft contact lenses

(b) Injections (Figure 11.2)
 (i) Subconjunctival
 Sub-Tenon's
 Peribulbar
 (ii) Intracameral, i.e. into the anterior chamber
 (iii) Intravitreal
2. Indirect routes (systemic)
 (a) Oral
 (b) Intravenous
 (c) Intramuscular

TOPICAL DRUGS

These have several requirements.

PRESERVATIVES

Benzalkonium chloride, thiomersal, chlorbutol and phenylmercuric nitrate are germicidal at very weak concentrations. They thus preserve the sterility of eye drops. In a single-drop dispenser unit, such as Minims, a preservative is unnecessary as the unit is disposable.

ISOTONICITY

Isotonicity with tear fluid is desirable as it facilitates the acceptance of the eye drop by the patient. To achieve this sodium chloride is added.

OXIDATION

Some substances, for instance phenylephrine, are oxidized and so a reducing agent is added. Sodium metabisulphite is one such agent.

HYDROGEN ION CONCENTRATION (PH)

The hydrogen ion concentration is expressed as the pH and the 'neutral' value is 7.4. The eye can withstand a pH range of 4.5–10. However, extremes are to be avoided, so solutions known as buffers (e.g. sodium citrate) are used to remove excess hydrogen ions. It is not only for ocular comfort that a desirable pH is needed. Some drugs are physiologically active only at a particular pH, so that a balance has to be struck between comfort and activity, hence the need for buffers.

VISCOSITY

Because of drainage of tear fluid, overflow and blinking, a topical agent only remains in the lower fornix for a short time. In order to prolong the presence of a drug and enhance corneal uptake substances with a higher viscosity than tear fluid are added to drops. Examples of such agents include polyvinyl alcohol and methylcellulose.

Light

Light may cause oxidation or hydrolysis. Dark containers are therefore needed for some products, such as adrenaline drops.

Sterility

Drops

These are autoclaved (heated at 121°C for 15 min at 103.5 kPa 15 psi), passed through a bacterial filter, or subjected to bactericides with heat (100°C for 30 min). The drops must be filtered to remove particles and aseptically transferred to containers.

Ointments

These consist of a base (liquid paraffin, wool fat and yellow soft paraffin) and the medicament. The base is prepared first, sterilized for one hour at 150°C in dry heat and filtered, and the drug is then added. Ointments are rarely contaminated as micro-organisms do not grow easily in the greasy base.

Drugs for Injection

These come in ampoules, either in the drug form for reconstitution with water (e.g. acetazolamide, hyaluronidase, alpha-chymotrypsin and antibiotics such as methicillin and ticarcillin) or in liquid form (e.g. gentamicin and atropine). All of these have to be prepared aseptically, filtered and sterilized.

It should be pointed out that all drops, ointments and drugs for injections prepared must match the recommended regulations as set down in the British Pharmaceutical Codex (BPC) with regard to quality and sterility (Table 11.1).

Table 11.1 Recommended expiry dates for drugs (BPC) – eye drops

For domiciliary use – one month.
For hospital (ward or outpatient) use – one week.
For hospital (theatre) use – use once and discard remainder.

NB. Eye drops for use during surgical procedures should contain no preservatives.

Classification of Ophthalmic Drugs

Drugs affecting the eye may be considered under a variety of headings and in the following text they have been classified as:

1. antimicrobial agents – antibiotics, antiviral and antifungal agents;
2. anti-inflammatory agents – steroids, antiprostaglandins and antihistamines;
3. drugs affecting the autonomic nervous system;
4. systemic agents in glaucoma;
5. ocular lubricants;
6. local anaesthetic agents;
7. diagnostic agents.

This list is not intended to be exhaustive and will only cover the general principles of the major areas of ocular pharmacology. Specific drugs will not be covered in detail, but named examples will be given as appropriate. Up-to-date information on specific drugs can be obtained from the British National Formulary, ABPI Data Sheet Compendia or specific drug data sheets as issued by the pharmaceutical companies in compliance with the Medicines Act 1968.

Antimicrobial Agents

Antibiotics (Including Sulphonamides)

Some of these drugs are produced by micro-organisms and others made synthetically. They are said to be **bactericidal** when they destroy bacteria during active multiplication, and **bacteriostatic** when they diminish the rate of multiplication.

The mechanism by which each antibiotic acts may be one or more of the following:

1. interference with the synthesis of the cell wall of the bacterium, e.g. penicillin and cephalosporins;
2. prevention of protein synthesis inside the micro-organism, e.g. erythromycin, chloramphenicol and tetracycline;
3. disturbance of cell wall permeability so that the bacterium lyses, e.g. polymyxin B;
4. by inhibiting DNA gyrase, the enzyme responsible for supercoiling of the DNA helix, e.g. ofloxacin.

Antibiotics are said to have a narrow or broad spectrum of activity. Antibiotics with a narrow spectrum of activity are effective against either Gram-positive or Gram-negative bacteria. Broad-spectrum antibiotics are effective against both. Resistance to antibiotics can develop quite quickly. Certain bacteria produce enzymes which break down antibiotics; for example certain staphylococci produce penicillinases which make them resistant to many penicillins. Some bacteria undergo chromosomal mutation, which confers resistance and which can be passed on to the next generation of bacteria.

Very few drugs act without some adverse effects and the antibiotics are no exception. For example, gentamicin is toxic to the ear and the kidney and the penicillins may cause allergic reactions in susceptible cases. Local toxic responses may also result from the preservative, especially after prolonged usage. The corneal epithelium is a formidable barrier to topical agents and both the blood/retinal and blood/aqueous barriers are hardly breached by systemically administered drugs. However, when the eye is inflamed the situation changes and more systemically administered drug is capable of entering the eye. A damaged corneal epithelium also allows for greater penetration of topical agents. Individual drugs have different abilities to cross the cornea. If they are lipophilic (soluble in fat), like chloramphenicol, they enter the epithelium easily. To enhance the concentration of the antibiotic passing into the eye subconjunctival and sub-Tenon's injections may be given.

When prescribing systemic antibiotics the age of the patient, presence of liver or kidney disorders and the possibility of pregnancy should be taken into account. Certain general principles are also worth bearing in mind – two bactericidal drugs are additive, two bacteriostatic drugs are additive, but a bacteriostatic and a bactericidal drug together are antagonistic.

The choice of antibiotic for topical use should ideally be based on swab reports. In practice a broad-spectrum antibiotic such as chloramphenicol is usually prescribed for any presumed bacterial condition in the first instance. If a corneal ulcer/abscess is present, the taking of a corneal scrape for culture and Gram staining is mandatory before any treatment.

Antiviral Agents

Viruses proliferate inside cells. Therefore antiviral agents must penetrate the cells to prevent the multiplication of virus particles. There are several viruses which can affect the eye but it is only against herpes viruses that there is any effective drug therapy. The drugs work by inhibiting viral deoxyribonucleic acid (DNA) synthesis. They include idoxuridine (IDU), adenine arabinoside (Vira A, Ara-A) and trifluorothymidine (F_3T), which bring about substitution of a base in the chain for DNA synthesis. However, they act on normal cells too, and therefore are toxic.

Acyclovir, the most recent addition, acts by blocking viral replication within the infected cells only. The drug acts specifically in cells containing virus, because it needs an enzyme produced by the virus to convert the drug into its active form. It is the treatment of choice in ointment form for herpes simplex keratitis. Foscarnet and ganciclovir are the two drugs used for treating cytomegalovirus (CMV) retinitis.

Antifungal Agents

These are rarely required for eye disease. However, when a fungal infection occurs in the eye early effective treatment is important. There are a number of drugs available. These include amphotericin B, nystatin, 5-flucytosine, the imidazoles and pimaricin.

Antiamoebic Agents

Propamidine, neomycin and chlorhexidine are all used for acanthamoeba keratitis.

Anti-Inflammatory Drugs

Corticosteroids

Steroids are substances that are normally produced in the cortex of the adrenal gland. There are three kinds of steroid: glucocorticoids, mineralocorticoids and sex hormones. It is the glucocorticoids that concern us most here. The particular substance which is important is called **cortisol** or **hydrocortisone** and is released in response to a pituitary hormone, ACTH. There is a negative feedback between the level of hydrocortisone and the level of ACTH in the circulation, which is monitored in the hypothalamus.

Hydrocortisone has many physiological effects but the one that is of most importance here is the anti-inflammatory effect. This effect is exploited in the treatment of many inflammatory disorders. However, large doses have to be used. Normally the body produces 25 mg of hydrocortisone per day. Doses well in excess of this are used therapeutically. In addition, many new agents have been developed with a far greater potency than hydrocortisone. Unfortunately they do have side effects.

Local and systemic steroids are used in the treatment of eye disease. The local agents comprise topical drops, ointment, skin lotions and injections around the eye. The systemic steroids are made up of oral and parenteral preparations. The drugs used in local therapy are primarily used to treat disease anterior to the lens. However, there is some overlap with the treatment of posterior segment disorders in respect of periocular injections. This part of the eye and the tissues behind it are treated primarily by oral therapy along with sub-Tenon's or retrobulbar injections if clinically necessary, for example in choroiditis.

Local Steroids

Drops: In ascending order of potency, prednisolone, betamethasone, dexamethasone and prednisolone acetate are available. The last two are isomers and are reckoned to have equal potency. Fluorometholone (0.1%) appears least likely to cause a rise in intraocular pressure when used in the long term. Prednisolone acetate penetrates the eye exceptionally well and is recommended for corneal graft rejection. A steroid preparation can be combined with an antibiotic, for example prednisolone and neomycin (Predsol N).

Ointments: The commercially available ointments are hydrocortisone, betamethasone and dexamethasone. Some are combined with an antibiotic (e.g. hydrocortisone and chloramphenicol). Ointment stays longer on the ocular surface, increasing the effect of the drug, though some temporary disturbance of vision can be experienced.

Skin lotions and creams: Hydrocortisone lotion in a 1% strength or higher is a useful preparation for allergic reactions in the eyelids in the short term. Steroid creams are also available.

Subconjunctival/sub-Tenon's/retrobulbar injections: There are two preparations used commonly, betamethasone (Betnesol) (4 mg) and methylprednisolone (Depo-Medrone) (40 mg/ml). The former is colourless, the latter white. Betamethasone is useful for short-term effect (24 h) and methylprednisolone for longer treatment. Its effect lasts approximately 10 days or more.

Systemic Steroids

Oral: Prednisolone is the mainstay of oral anti-inflammatory treatment in ocular inflammation. The starting dose in some conditions is high: up to 80 mg daily in giant cell arteritis. Enteric-coated tablets are available to minimize intestinal ulceration. Reduction in treatment has to be gradual, perhaps 10 mg per day with larger doses and

2–5 mg with smaller doses every 3–5 days, according to clinical response.

Parenteral: Not many ocular conditions are treated with systemic steroids by injection. Two exceptions are the initial treatment of arteritis with intravenous hydrocortisone and the occasional use of ACTH intramuscularly to treat manifestations of multiple sclerosis such as repeated episodes of optic neuritis.

ADVERSE EFFECTS

Both local and systemic treatments are complicated by side effects. The local and systemic treatments can give rise to open-angle glaucoma in susceptible individuals. Thus the intraocular pressure must be monitored if patients are on long-term steroid treatment. Among topical treatments fluorometholone and clobetasone are known to raise the intraocular pressure less than other steroid preparations.

Topical steroid therapy can predispose an eye to bacterial, viral and fungal infection if used for a long time.

Withdrawal of topical steroids should be gradual if a relapse or rebound effects are not to be seen, for instance after anterior uveitis. In particular, withdrawal of steroid used in herpetic stromal disease of the cornea must be very gradual. Indeed a gradual titrated reduction of the concentration of steroid is possible down to very weak strengths such as 0.0001% prednisolone. Some patients may have to remain on such a weak preparation indefinitely. Steroids are strictly contraindicated for herpes simplex dendritic ulcers, and herpes zoster neurotrophic ulceration.

Finally, prolonged systemic treatment will be accompanied by exaggerated physiological effects of steroids (the effects on glucose and lipid metabolism lead to raised blood sugar, a cushingoid appearance and hypertension due to fluid and electrolyte imbalance). There may also be mood changes, causing euphoria or depression. The high level of steroid in the circulation leads to disruption of the negative feedback mechanism between the adrenal cortex and the anterior pituitary. This leads to atrophy of the adrenal cortex if treatment is prolonged. This could necessitate lifelong replacement therapy. Other adverse effects include osteoporosis, peptic ulcers, reactivation of tuberculosis and diminished growth in children. Thus a careful history must be taken before steroids are given.

NON-STEROIDAL ANTI-INFLAMMATORY DRUGS

These are principally drugs that block the effects of prostaglandins, which are found in almost all tissues, including the eye. Prostaglandins are released in inflammatory reactions and are deemed to be mediators in this process.

Several drugs have been shown to block the synthesis of prostaglandins. The earliest one of note was salicylate (aspirin). Some recent additions have been indomethacin and flurbiprofen. They are the initial treatment of choice in scleritis. Like steroid tablets they can cause peptic ulceration.

Topical indomethacin drops are available in addition to the standard oral preparation. Studies have shown that both forms of treatment can reduce the incidence of cystoid macular oedema and inflammation after cataract surgery.

Antihistamines

Allergy is a common cause of conjunctivitis, the bulk of which is treated in general practice. The cause of symptoms and signs is principally the release of histamine. Treatment may be affected by: 1) using drops that block histamine receptors, such as Otrivine-Antistin, which contains antazoline and xylometazoline, and Vasocon-A, which contains antazoline and naphazoline – the first drug in each combination is the antihistamine and the second is a vasoconstrictor; or 2) using drops that prevent the release of histamine, such as sodium cromoglycate. This is a mast cell stabilizer, which means it will prevent the release of histamine and other substances involved in allergic reactions. Thus in atopic individuals and those who suffer from hay fever and asthma it has proved to be a very helpful prophylactic agent. The topical preparation comes as a 2% solution and as a 4% ointment. Lodoxamide is another mast cell stabilizer.

Drugs Affecting the Autonomic Nervous System

Anatomy

The autonomic nervous system is divided into sympathetic and parasympathetic pathways (Fig. 11.3).

The sympathetic pathway originates in the hypothalamus, passes down the spinal cord and emerges in the thorax. The fibres then pass upwards towards the superior cervical ganglion lying at the carotid bifurcation where they synapse. The transmitter here is acetylcholine. The postganglionic fibres run towards the eye wrapped round the internal carotid artery and finally reach the eye via the ophthalmic artery. They supply the dilator pupillae, the trabecular meshwork and the blood vessels in the eye.

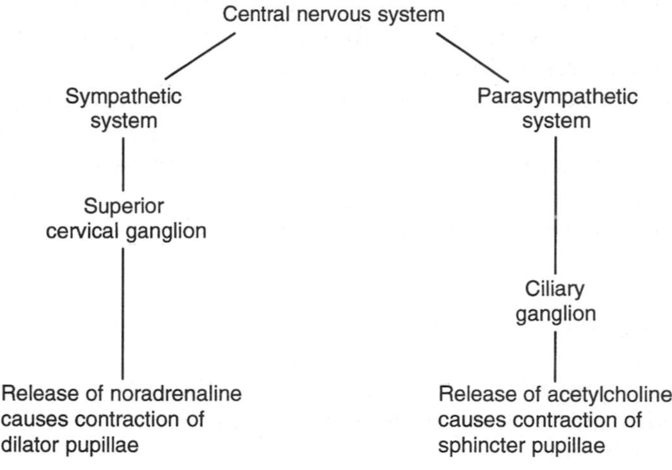

A drug which mimics the action of the chemical transmitter of the sympathetic nervous system is called a sympathomimetic e.g. adrenaline.

A drug which blocks the action of the sympatholytic e.g. guanethidine.

A drug which mimics the action of the chemical transmitter of the parasympathetic nervous system is called a parasympathomimetic, e.g. pilocarpine.

A drug which biocks the action of the parasympathetic nervous system is called parasympatholytic e.g. atropine.

Figure 11.3 Drug action on the sympathetic and parasympathetic nervous system.

The chemical transmitter is noradrenaline which acts on both alpha- and beta-receptors.

The parasympathetic pathway originates in the midbrain; fibres run in the IIIrd nerve towards the eye and synapse in the ciliary ganglion, which lies within the muscle cone between the lateral rectus muscle and the optic nerve. The chemical transmitter is acetylcholine. The postganglionic fibres then innervate the constrictor pupillae and ciliary muscle as well as sending branches to the lacrimal gland and trabecular meshwork. The chemical transmitter is also acetylcholine.

Drugs Affecting the Sympathetic System

If a drug mimics the transmitter in its actions it is called a sympathomimetic agent.

If a drug blocks the effect of the system it is a sympatholytic agent. Thus a sympathomimetic will produce some or all of the following:

1. dilation of the pupil;
2. decreased secretion of aqueous;
3. lower outflow resistance;
4. constriction of the conjunctival vessels.

Examples of this are adrenaline and phenylephrine.

The only sympatholytic agent of note is guanethidine, which is present in Ganda eye drops.

In fact because there are two sorts of adrenergic receptor (alpha- and beta-) the effects of these drugs may be complex, especially with regard to intraocular pressure control. Timolol blocks beta-receptors and reduces aqueous output. Adrenaline acts by increasing aqueous outflow.

Drugs Affecting the Parasympathetic System

A parasympathomimetic agent mimics the effects of acetylcholine and a parasympatholytic agent blocks the effect of acetylcholine.

The parasympathomimetics may work: 1) directly – examples are pilocarpine, which causes miosis, accommodation and increased outflow of aqueous, and acetylcholine chloride (Miochol), which is used for rapid pupil constriction during intraocular surgery; or 2) indirectly, by acting on enzymes that normally metabolize acetylcholine and therefore potentiate its action. An example is neostigmine, which is used in myasthenia gravis.

Parasympatholytic agents work by blocking acetylcholine from its receptors. They cause pupil dilation and varying degrees of cycloplegia. Atropine is the most powerful long-acting agent and is now used infrequently. Tropicamide is a short-acting drug which dilates the pupil but has limited effect on accommodation and is therefore an ideal drug for examining the fundus. Cyclopentolate (0.5/1%) dilates the pupil and causes cycloplegia for up to 24 hours.

Systemic Agents in Glaucoma

These include oral and intravenous drugs.

Carbonic Anhydrase Inhibitors

This group of drugs blocks the enzyme carbonic anhydrase (CA) in the following reaction:

$$H_2O + CO_2 \overset{CA}{\rightleftharpoons} H_2CO_3 \rightleftharpoons HCO_3 + H^+$$

Note that these are reversible reactions and that carbonic anhydrase plays no part in the second reaction. The enzyme is found in abundance in the body but especially in the epithelium of the ciliary body, the red blood cells, the central nervous system and the kidney, where the actions of the members of this group of drugs are seen to have most effect.

In the UK the two agents available are acetazolamide and dichlorphenamide.

Osmotic Agents

These substances reduce intraocular pressure very effectively in the short term. They increase the osmotic pressure of plasma in relation to aqueous and vitreous, the effect of which is to draw fluid out of the eye. The possible agents available are urea, mannitol and glycerol. In practice only the last two are used, and then only occasionally in acute glaucoma.

Ocular Lubricants

The precorneal tear film is made up of lipid, aqueous and mucous components. The lipid layer is on the outside, the aqueous layer is in the middle and the mucous layer is on the epithelium (Chapter 14). Disturbance in any one of these layers affects the function of the others. This leads to a dry eye state. The drugs available to treat this problem are designed to alleviate symptoms and reform the tear film.

The ideal solution should be one that increases the tear fluid volume and also effectively performs what the mucous layer does by increasing the length of time the aqueous layer remains on the cornea and conjunctiva, in other words increasing the tear breakup time (BUT). Further, the drops should not interfere with the lipid layer because it is involved in diminishing evaporation of the aqueous layer.

There are many drugs available – some commercially and others that have to be prepared in the pharmacy to order – which are all designed with the above principles in mind.

Hydroxypropylmethylcellulose (hypromellose) is the most commonly used. This type of tear supplement can be made more viscous with the addition of dextran or polyvinyl alcohol. Paraffin-based ointments such as simple eye ointment or Lacri-Lube may be used at night.

Local Anaesthetic Agents

These are administered topically or by injection. The topical agents are all useful for examination and treatment – for example applanation tonometry, contact lens examination and simple procedures such as removal of foreign bodies from the cornea.

The injected drugs are useful for a number of procedures. These include eyelid procedures such as repair of entropion or ectropion and incision and curettage of meibomian cysts. Subconjunctival injections of local anaesthetic can be given to ease delivery of antibiotics or steroids by this route. Peribulbar injections for sensory and motor blockade around the eye can be given for operations such as cataract extraction and for laser photocoagulation if required.

The addition of hyaluronidase to local anaesthetic solutions has meant that additional injections are now rarely necessary to achieve a facial block and thus prevent squeezing.

Diagnostic Agents (Dyes)

There are several preparations available but only two are in regular clinical use. These are sodium fluorescein and rose Bengal. Other agents are available for special applications; these include alcian blue, trypan blue and methylene blue. Only very small quantities of these agents need be placed on the eye.

Sodium Fluorescein

This is the most commonly used diagnostic agent in ophthalmology. It is presented in a number of forms:

1. dry paper impregnated with 1 mg of fluorescein;
2. a 2% solution for topical use;
3. in combination with lignocaine for tonometry;
4. an intravenous form which can be obtained in different strengths.

The principle on which its use is based stems from the fact that it absorbs light of a certain wavelength and emits light of a longer wavelength; in other words it fluoresces.

The principal clinical uses are as follows:

1. demonstrating surface defects – on the cornea and conjunctiva;
2. applanation tonometry;
3. demonstrating potency of nasolacrimal ducts;
4. demonstrating leaking wounds (Seidel's test);
5. checking the fit of a hard contact lens;
6. fluorescein angiography, both of the retina and iris (this technique has been associated with side effects due to fluorescein).

It is also used as a research tool to measure rates of aqueous flow with the fluorophotometer. This machine is also used to measure the early leakage of fluorescein in the retina in certain disease processes, for example diabetic retinopathy.

Rose Bengal

This is a vital dye, in other words it stains damaged cells and tissues. It also stains mucus. Although it has a deep red colour, it is a derivative of fluorescein. It is available in a single dispenser unit (Minims Rose Bengal). The principal clinical uses are as follows:

1. diagnosis of keratoconjunctivitis sicca;
2. acute dendritic ulcers, as well as the infected cells surrounding geographic ulcers;
3. exposure keratitis.

It causes considerable irritation, more so in those with severe dryness.

Adverse Effects of Systemic Drugs

Several important drugs used in general medicine may be deposited in or damage the eye. They are considered according to the part of the eye that is affected.

The Cornea

The antimalarials, of which chloroquine is the best known, are also used to treat rheumatoid arthritis, systemic lupus erythematosus and other connective tissue diseases in higher doses than are effective in malaria. They can cause a whorl-like disturbance of the epithelium, which disappears if the drug is stopped. Amiodarone, which is an antiarrhythmic drug, and tamoxifen, used in breast cancer, cause similar changes. Other drugs, such as gold salts and indomethacin, also cause corneal deposits.

The Lens

Corticosteroids can cause cataracts if given in high dose (10 mg/d or more) for long periods. These are posterior subcapsular in character. Gold salts will cause deposits on the anterior surface of the lens. The phenothiazines will cause anterior cortical opacities.

The Conjunctiva

Oral practolol has been withdrawn because of the devastating cicatrizing effect it had on the conjunctiva of some patients.

The Pupil

Several groups of drugs can affect the pupil if taken systemically. These include the phenothiazines, antihistamines, anticholinergics and amphetamines, which dilate the pupil. Morphine and its derivatives (e.g. pethidine) and anticholinesterases will cause constriction.

The Retina

Many drugs affect the retina. Most affect the retinal pigment epithelium. They include the following.

Chloroquine and its Derivative, Hydroxychloroquine

It is in relation to their use in the collagen-vascular disorders, such as rheumatoid arthritis and systemic lupus erythematosus, that problems arise. The recommended maximum dosage range is 200–400 mg per day for hydroxychloroquine and 250 mg for chloroquine. For chloroquine the total cumulative dose must exceed 300 g before signs of retinal toxicity appear. Thus regular checkups are necessary for anyone on long-term therapy. The sign of damage in the early stages is diminished visual acuity. Pigmentary changes occur at the macula and are irreversible.

Thioridazine

This is a drug used in psychotic states. It can cause reversible retinal toxicity during its initial use (first 30–60 days). Generally a dose of 1200 mg per day for 30 days is needed to produce damage. It reduces visual acuity initially and may be followed by night blindness. Early fundus appearances include scattered peripheral pigment clumping. Interestingly, the more commonly used phenothiazine chlorpromazine is generally free of retinal toxicity.

Quinine

This damages the retinal ganglion cells and also the retinal arterioles in susceptible cases or in excess dosage. Overdose can result in sudden reduction of vision in both eyes, and recovery of visual field may not be full. The defect is thought to be due to ischaemia.

Other Drugs

Digitalis

Toxicity causes transient visual disturbances, particularly abnormalities of colour vision (e.g. objects appear yellow or green). Visual acuity may be diminished as well.

Tamoxifen

This is a drug used to treat breast cancer and may cause retinal toxicity with a reduction in visual acuity due to macular lesions. These take the form of yellow, glistening deposits.

Oral Contraceptives

These are associated with vascular occlusive episodes which include branch vein occlusion and, rarely, arterial occlusion.

Optic Nerve

Ethambutol is used to treat tuberculosis. It affects the optic nerve if the dose is greater than 15 mg/kg per day over a period of months. It causes a retrobulbar neuritis with an associated red-green colour defect. There is also a decrease in visual acuity, so testing every 6 months is necessary. The higher the dose the more regular the checks should be. Cessation of treatment causes the effect to disappear in most patients.

Methanol

This is highly toxic to the optic nerve. Optic atrophy and blindness will ensue even with minimal abuse.

Administration of Drugs

The large majority of drugs used in ocular diagnosis and therapeutics are given topically. The nurse must remember that drops are drugs and should be administered with the same deference that is given to oral, intramuscular or intravenous drugs. While the act of administering drugs is usually governed by local policy and procedure, the nurse must be aware of her professional accountability when doing so. As a guideline, before a nurse administers a drug she should be aware of the following information about the drug:

1. the non-proprietary or other proprietary names;
2. presentation, e.g. drops, ointment, tablets;
3. normally accepted dosages;
4. mode of action and resultant effects;
5. possible side effects;
6. indications for use;
7. the information required by the patient.

The increase in patient turnover in hospitals has resulted in a shorter inpatient period, with the preparation for self-care on discharge commencing earlier. This means that the nurse is usually administering ophthalmic drugs for shorter periods but is instructing and supervising the patient or parent/relative in administration.

The nurse must remember that being able to instil the medication does not necessarily mean the patient is reliable. Davidson and Akingbehin (1980) point out that the more complex the treatment regime, the more likely it is that non-compliance will occur. Norrell (1979) suggests that compliance can be improved by motivating the patient with improved knowledge and helping him adapt the regime to his normal routine as well as teaching the patient how to administer the drug. Where self-administration is necessary for discharge the nurse should evaluate the patient's skill and, in conjunction with the doctor, plan the discharge when adequate competency is achieved.

Drugs given topically in the eye will drain through the lacrimal system and be absorbed through the nasopharyngeal mucosa into the systemic circulation. While the amount may be small and have little or no effect in the healthy adult, this may not necessarily apply to children or adults with renal or hepatic impairment. To minimize systemic absorption while ensuring adequate local medication, the lower punctum can be occluded with the index finger after the instillation of drops.

In order that the patient obtains the desired effects of ocular medication it must be used in a particular way, which usually demands regular compliance to administration, and the nurse has a major role in achieving this.

References

Davidson, S. I. and Akingbehin, T. (1980) Compliance in ophthalmology. *Transactions of the Ophthalmology Society*, **100**, 26.

Norrell, S. E. (1979) Improving medication compliance – randomised clinical trial. *British Medical Journal*, **64**, 137–141.

12

OPTICS

Peter Cole and John Storey

CHAPTER SUMMARY

Basic optics

The eye as an optical system

Measurement of refractive error (refraction)

Correction of refractive error

The correction of aphakia, including intraocular lenses

BASIC OPTICS

Light can be considered as a stream of energy passing along a ray. Light is an electromagnetic radiation that produces the sensation of sight. Other radiations that travel at the same speed (186 000 miles per second) include gamma rays, X-rays, ultraviolet and infra-red rays, microwaves and radio waves. This explains why X-rays and infra-red rays can be filmed and how a radio telescope (e.g. Jodrell Bank) can be used to visualize stars beyond the reach of optical instruments.

Light may be polarized or made truly directional so that a second polarizer set at right angles will extinguish all light. Such a property is used in sunglasses to reduce or eliminate glare. The term 'laser' is an acronym for **l**ight **a**mplification by **s**timulated **e**mission of **r**adiation. By changing the random phases of light emission found normally so that the light-emitting atoms are in step, extremely powerful and truly parallel light is produced. This has found applications in ophthalmology, with different forms of laser for different parts of the eye.

The speed of light changes at the division between two media so that a light ray is reflected to a degree which depends on the transparency of the new medium and its reflective properties, together with the angle of incidence (Figure 12.1). Mirrors reflect the most, whilst transparent surfaces such as spectacle lenses reflect only about 8% of light. Refraction (transmission) of light generally means that the light is bent according to the refractive index of the medium, the direction of the incident ray (Figure 12.1) and the quality and shape of the surface. In Figure 12.2 we find two positive or convex surface powers producing convergence to a focal point. Surface powers, lens powers and vergences are measured in dioptres (D), which are reciprocal measurements of metres. So the spectacle lens illustrated has a total power of 4 D and a focal length of 25 m. Equally, a lens might have concave surfaces, in which case light would diverge instead.

The Eye as an Optical System

The axial length of an eye averages 23.3 mm, which means that a power of just about 60 dioptres is needed to focus light on the retinal receptors. This is achieved with the cornea, of some 43 dioptres in power, and the crystalline lens, of about 20 dioptres in power in the relaxed state, if emmetropia (no refractive error) is to be achieved. The cornea has a positive outer surface of high curvature (mean radius 7.8 mm), which accounts for its high power. The negative back surface power is largely neutralized by the aqueous humour. In front of the lens a variable aperture or pupil (controlled by the iris) plays a vital role in the regulation of light, which passes through the lens to the retina. Where it is small the better depth of focus can assist the person greatly, particularly near to. The crystalline lens has focusing properties (accommodation) that are highly developed in children but reduce with age, so that reading glasses different from the distance refraction may be needed as early as 40 years of age in some people, while others may cope well until they are over 50. Those who read closer or who have pupils that do not contract enough during accommodation will inevitably need reading spectacles earlier.

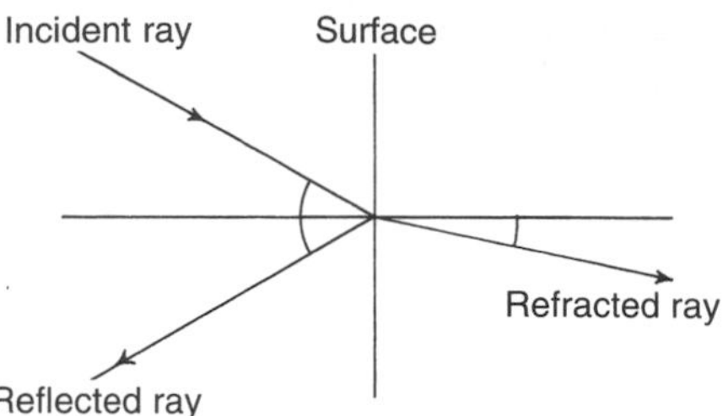

Figure 12.1 Basic ray diagram showing reflection and refraction.

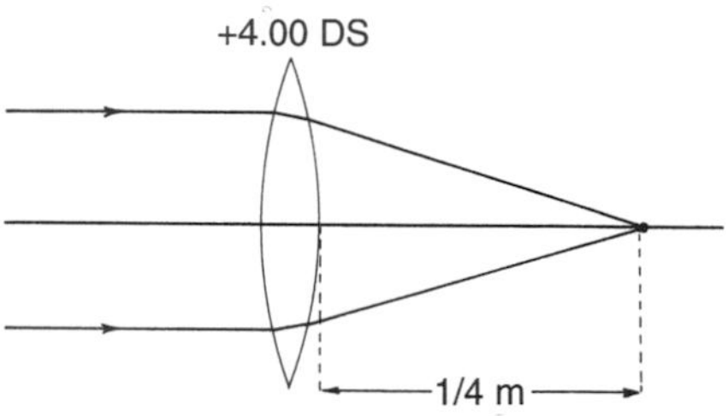

Figure 12.2 Convergence of rays by a +4 dioptre convex lens.

Drugs called mydriatics (e.g. tropicamide) increase pupil size. More powerful drugs called cycloplegics (e.g. cyclopentolate and atropine) increase pupil size and abolish accommodation. Miotic drugs (e.g. pilocarpine) reduce pupil size and can cause a spasm of accommodation.

The ability of the crystalline lens to alter its power is called accommodation. This enables an image to be focused on the retina when viewing objects at different distances. The accommodative power is from 15–23 dioptres; it is age-dependent and when the accommodative range has declined to about 4 dioptres the eye becomes **presbyopic**.

Emmetropia and Ametropia

In an unaccommodated eye, parallel light from a distant object will produce an image at the eye's second principal focus. If this focus and the retinal receptor layer (the back of the retina) are coincident, then the eye is **emmetropic** and no refractive error is present. If they are not coincident the eye is **ametropic** and a refractive error exists. A focus in front of the retina (in the vitreous) gives **myopia** (short-sightedness), which may be due to a longer eye than average, or too powerful a focusing system, or both. The maximum axial length ever recorded at Manchester Royal Eye Hospital to date was 37.3 mm and this eye had a refractive error of about –50.00 D! Conversely, if the focus is behind the retina, then the eye is **hypermetropic**, or long-sighted. However, if accommodation is sufficient the image can be 'pulled forward' into focus on the retina. Hypermetropia is due either to a short axial length or a weak focusing system or both. The shortest axial length ever recorded at this hospital was 11.00 mm in a baby with a growth deficiency syndrome.

On average, at birth the eye is 16 mm in axial length and this increases to 23 mm by three years of age. The cornea and lens are particularly steep in curvature at birth so that hopefully only a small amount of hypermetropia exists, but as the eye grows in length these curvatures flatten out to avoid a highly myopic situation. If a distribution curve of refractive errors is plotted and compared to a normal distribution then an excess of near emmetropes is found. So clearly, in nature, an attempt is made to avoid ametropia. Lower degrees of ametropia are due to inadequate compensation in general, whereas large degrees are mainly related to abnormal axial lengths.

Myopia

In myopia, the patient usually complains of poor or blurred distance vision. In contrast, the near vision is often quite good. Sometimes, in an attempt to overcome the blurred vision, the patient 'screws up' his eyes. This creates a 'pinhole effect', which increases the depth of field, producing a clearer image.

Myopia can be categorized into three groups: simple, pathological and others.

Simple Myopia

Simple myopia is the most common form. It usually develops in childhood and adolescence and it is important that it is corrected in order for the child to progress satisfactorily at school (for example, to work from a blackboard). The progression of the myopia is not usually fast, but it is sufficient to require an eye examination at 6-monthly intervals for the purpose of updating the spectacle correction. The myopia often stabilizes in the late teens and twenties.

Pathological Myopia

Pathological myopia is due to an abnormal component. Often, high degrees of myopia are produced if there is a hereditary factor. The axial length increases progressively and degenerative retinal and vitreous changes occur.

Other Myopia

Metabolic changes can cause index changes to the crystalline lens and this can produce a myopic shift in the refractive error. An example of this occurs in diabetes when the blood sugar level changes. A diabetic patient might complain of blurred distance vision, and that he can see to read in his distance vision spectacles.

Hypermetropia

Patients with low or medium degrees of hypermetropia and with sufficient accommodation usually have quite good distance and near vision. However, if the accommodation is insufficient, the patient may experience near vision difficulty and sometimes reduced distance acuity. High degrees of hypermetropia result in poor vision for both distance and near. Although a patient may have good vision he may experience asthenopic symptoms such as headaches associated with reading, general fatigue and difficulty changing focus from near to distance.

The majority of hypermetropia is 'simple'. However, pathological hypermetropia is due to such conditions as microphthalmos, reduced axial length due to raising of the retina (e.g. by macular oedema) and, of course, aphakia.

Astigmatism

Astigmatism occurs when the refractive power in one meridian is different from the power in another meridian. These meridians are usually at 90° to each other (regular astigmatism). Astigmatism can occur in conjunction with myopia, 'emmetropia' and hypermetropia.

Astigmatism is usually produced by the anterior corneal surface. Corneal astigmatism is mainly classified as simple, but other factors may induce it. These include lid pressure (due to, for instance, a lid tumour), corneal scarring from trauma or ulceration, surgery for cataract, corneal transplantation and even squint. Astigmatism can also be produced by the crystalline lens (or intraocular lens implant) being tilted. Not surprisingly, highly irregular astigmatism occurs in keratoconus.

Anisometropia

The condition in which the refractive error in one eye differs from that of its fellow by a sizeable amount is termed anisometropia. This can be brought about by a difference in the refracting components or in the axial lengths, or by a combination of both. Monocular aphakia is an example of refractive anisometropia. The correction of anisometropia is problematic and is discussed later in the chapter. Significant anisometropia in childhood can lead to amblyopia in the less normal eye.

Measurement of Refractive Error (Refraction)

The refractive error can be determined either subjectively or objectively. Subjective techniques rely entirely on a response to various tests. If a patient is able to comprehend the tests and co-operate in giving repeatable and accurate responses a satisfactory result can be obtained. However, such conditions are not always possible, for instance in babies, younger children and senile or unco-operative patients. Therefore it is essential to be able to obtain results by objective methods that do not rely on patients' responses. In most cases, a combination of objective and subjective methods is used.

Subjective Techniques

The basic tools of subjective assessment are visual acuity charts for distance and near vision. Visual acuity is the ability of the eye to distinguish form or fine detail. The most commonly used charts are based on Snellen letters to determine the minimum recognizable visual acuity (VA) for distance.

The Snellen test distance is standardized at 6 metres. The size of the letters is calibrated according to distances at which their unit widths subtend an angle of 1 minute of arc. Just as the charts are standardized, the luminance of the chart and the ambient illumination in the test room should be standardized (see Chapter 10).

The Snellen acuity itself does not indicate the type of magnitude of the ametropia. However, it can demonstrate what type of error is not involved. For instance, a visual acuity of 6/5 precludes myopia or moderate astigmatism.

In myopia alone, however, the magnitude of the error can be estimated from the visual acuity as shown in Table 12.1, assuming an average size of pupil.

Astigmatism causes a reduction in visual acuity but its orientation creates a variable influence. The visual acuity is reduced least if the astigmatic axis is vertical or horizontal, where 1.00 dioptre of cylinder power reduces the visual acuity to 6/9.

Table 12.1 Relationship of degree of myopia to acuity

Acuity	Degree of myopia
6/18	1.00 D
6/36	2.00 D
6/60	2.50 D

A pinhole disc may be used to negate approximately ±3.00 D (or its equivalent astigmatic error) by increasing the range of the depth of field. Hence, an improvement in monocular visual acuity with a pinhole indicates that the acuity may improve with spectacles. It is best, if possible, to allow the patient to centre the pinhole, as an improvement is only achieved if the pinhole is accurately aligned along the visual axis.

Most subjective methods rely on placing spectacle lenses (trial lenses) in front of the patient's eyes and obtaining the subsequent change in visual acuity. Initially, an overcorrection of convex lenses or an undercorrection of concave lenses is used to 'fog' or reduce the visual acuity. This is done for two reasons:

1. to relax accommodation if the patient is hypermetropic;
2. to render the combined spectacle lens/eye system artificially myopic, enabling an estimate to be made of the combined refractive error from the fogged visual acuity.

The aim is to determine the least powerful lens capable of giving the fullest visual acuity for that eye.

When astigmatism is present, the visual acuity is still reduced and it is necessary to employ an astigmatic or cylindrical power lens to neutralize the astigmatism. The spherical power components are then finally adjusted to give optimum acuity as before.

As mentioned previously, the near acuity is recorded with the aid of a near vision reading chart. The chart consists of several passages of text in different 'N' point size print. If a patient has reading spectacles, they should be worn and the chart is held at the distance that gives the best acuity. The result is recorded, for example, as N5 at 25 cm.

The reading spectacle correction is determined by the addition of extra positive power to the distance refractive correction. This extra 'reading add' is calculated according to the patient's amplitude of accommodation and the most useful and comfortable reading distance for that particular person.

Objective Methods

The most commonly used technique is retinoscopy, which depends on the refractionist's skill to obtain an accurate result. Automatic refractometers are now available and, when used on eyes which have clear media and undistorted corneas, they produce results that are accurate.

Retinoscopy

In reduced illumination the patient, wearing a trial frame, views an object (usually a spot of light) at 6 metres, and the refractionist directs light from a retinoscope into one eye of the patient. The light illuminates an area of retina, which acts as an 'object'. Rays from this object retroverse through the eye, and focus either in front of or behind the sight hole of the retinoscope through which the refractionist is looking. The refractionist sees an area of the patient's pupil illuminated (the retinoscopic reflex), and with small movements of the retinoscope mirror the reflex moves. The shape of the reflex and the direction of its movement indicate to the refractionist the type and power of the trial lens to insert in the trial frame.

Eventually, a situation occurs when the reflex totally fills the pupil and no apparent movement is observed. At that point, the sight hole position is conjugate with the patient's retina. The trial lens power is then reduced by the 'working distance'. This retinoscopic result, if required, can then be used as a starting point for a subjective refraction.

Retinoscopy tends to give the full refractive correction and as such it is especially useful when dealing with children. Usually, it is necessary to employ cycloplegia to relax a child's accommodation fully, and to employ retinoscopy to obtain the absolute refractive correction.

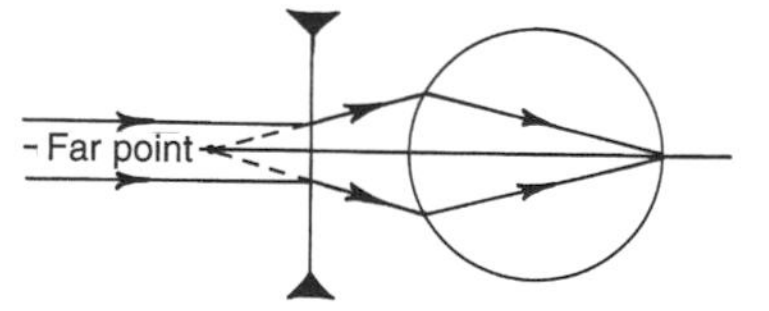

Figure 12.3 Position of far point in myopia.

Correction of Refractive Error

In ametropia, the point which is conjugate with the retina is termed the eye's far point. In myopia, the far point is in front of the cornea, and in hypermeropia it is behind the retina (Figures 12.3 and 12.4).

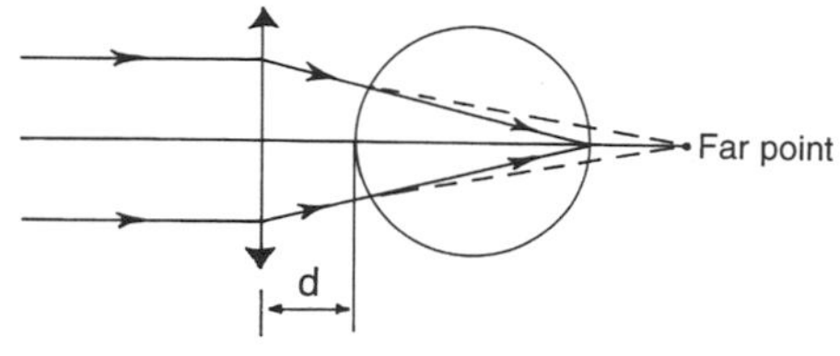

Figure 12.4 Position of far point in hypermetropia. 'd' is the back vertex distance.

If the power of the spectacle lens is over 4.00 D the distance of the spectacle lens from the corneal vertex (the back vertex distance) is important. This is especially important in 'aphakic' spectacle corrections, where lenses of 10.00 D or more are used. It is a common cause of complaint for a patient wearing glasses of this kind that are not correctly fitted.

Spectacle Lenses

Spectacle lenses are made in glass or plastic material. Glass lenses tend to be thinner and heavier than plastic lenses. Plastic lenses scratch much more easily, but they are much safer in the case of an accident. For this reason monocular patients must have plastic spectacle lenses. Lenses prescribed predominantly for one distance (reading or distance vision) are termed single vision lenses. Bifocal lenses have a distance power portion and a reading portion (the bifocal segment). Varifocal lenses have a distance correction in the superior portion of the lens and then a region of gradually changing intermediate distance power and a stabilized reading zone inferiorly. In high-powered corrections, lenses are often lenticular in form in order to reduce weight and thickness. These have to be fitted as close to the face as possible in order to give a reasonable field of view. Lenses should be centred both horizontally and vertically otherwise unwanted prismatic effects are produced. For instance, a tilted pair of spectacles may produce a vertical prism effect, which may cause diplopia. The interpupillary distance must also be taken into account.

Contact Lenses

Contact lenses have several important optical advantages over spectacle lenses. The field of view with a centred contact lens is approximately 100°, but with a spectacle lens it is reduced to about 80°. Oblique optical aberrations are minimized as the contact lens remains almost centred over the pupil, and prismatic effects due to decentration are minimal. Hence, in anisometropic correction, the induced differential prism does not occur unless there is excessive contact lens movement due to a loose fit. Because of the close proximity of the contact lens to the principal planes of the eye, magnification is minimal. In myopia, the retinal image size is increased compared to spectacles and hence an improvement in visual acuity with contact lenses may result. Conversely, contact lens correction of hypermetropia produces a smaller retinal image. This result is important in correcting refractive anisometropia. Perhaps the most important advantage of a contact lens is the ability to replace irregularities of the corneal surface with a smooth refracting surface. Finally, the physical weight and encumbrance of spectacles are removed by the use of contact lenses.

Contact lenses may be classified according to size and material.

1. 'Corneal lenses' are the smallest, the overall size being less than the corneal diameter. The usual range of size is from 8.20–9.60 mm. Three basic types of material are employed: polymethyl methacrylate (PMMA), gas permeables (GP) made of methyl siloxane, and silicone rubber. All three types are referred to as 'hard' lenses.
2. 'Soft' lenses are made from a variety of hydrogen polymers, which are hydrophilic. They vary in size from 12–15.50 mm. The central portion of the lens rests on the cornea and the peripheral zone rests on the bulbar conjunctiva.
3. Scleral or haptic lenses are the largest type of contact lenses and are usually horizontal oval in shape, the horizontal dimension being about 22–25 mm. The central 'dome' of the lens just vaults the corneal diameter and the haptic 'flange' rests on the scleral conjunctiva. They are made from PMMA, though recently a gas-permeable design has been introduced.

Each type of contact lens functions in a different way. A rigid corneal lens rests on a layer of tears, which forms a tear lens. It is the 'contact lens/tear lens' system which corrects the ametropia. As the refractive indices of the tears and cornea are very similar (cornea 1.376, tears 1.336), 90% of the anterior corneal astigmatism is effectively neutralized. Any spherical power contact lens is able in addition to correct astigmatism of up to 2 dioptres. Above this value, lens instability becomes a problem and toric back surface contact lenses are required. The use of a rigid corneal contact lens in early keratoconus demonstrates the benefit of replacing an irregular corneal surface with a smooth refracting surface. As a hard PMMA lens is impervious to oxygen the design of the lens must facilitate a good tear exchange in the retrocentral space. This enables an adequate supply of oxygen to reach the cornea, and for debris to be removed. This oxygen supply may be insufficient to prevent corneal oedema. Because of the long-term ill effects of PMMA lenses, GP hard lenses with good surface wetting characteristics are recommended. A good disinfectant cleaner is essential for all lenses.

Soft lenses are used for both refractive correction and therapeutic purposes. There is a wide range of materials, all of which are hydrophilic, and their water content ranges from 38–85%. The higher water content materials have greater oxygen transmission rates. As the lenses are flexible they adopt the corneal shape so that most of any astigmatism is regenerated on the front surface of the lens. Hence, toric soft lenses are required to correct astigmatic eyes. As the oxygen transmission through a lens is a function of the material and lens thickness, high-powered plus lenses of a greater centre thickness require materials of high water content. Likewise, extended-wear lenses need high oxygen transmission in order to prevent corneal damage. Extended-wear lenses are employed when a patient is incapable of handling daily-wear lenses, or when a patient's form of work makes it essential. A high water content lens is used to soak up excessive tears in a 'wet' eye. On a drier eye a lower water content and a low surface evaporation rate of material are appropriate, together with the use of saline or artificial tear eye drops. In general, soft lenses are contraindicated on dry eyes. For cosmetic purposes, soft lenses can be tinted or even have iris prints incorporated and, as their movement on the eye is minimal, good results can be obtained. All hydrogen lenses are prone to surface deposits of mucus, lipids, proteins and calcium and again proper cleaning is imperative.

Scleral lenses usually have at least one fenestration. The overall lens size permits ease of handling by patients who are incapable of handling or seeing corneal or semiscleral lenses. They are useful in several conditions. For disfigured or shrunken eyes, a painted eye will restore the cosmetic balance and even 'correct' an inoperable squint. Scleral lenses are able to protect the cornea from damage due to trauma or from drying. In advanced keratoconus, it may be impossible and dangerous to fit corneal lenses, and sclerals provide the best form of optical correction. Modified scleral lenses are occasionally used in cases of ptosis to raise the upper lid.

Insertion, Removal and Care of Lenses

In order for any type of contact lens to be worn successfully it must be maintained in optimum condition. This necessitates safe handling (insertion and removal) techniques, suitable cleaning procedures and storage methods that ensure sterility.

Prior to touching lenses, hands must be washed carefully with soap and water and dried on a clean paper towel. Antiseptic hand scrubs must be thoroughly removed and hands dried. Finger nails should be kept as short and smooth as possible. If practical, insertion and removal of lenses should be performed over a clean paper towel on a work surface. This helps reduce the risk of scratching or losing a lens. PMMA and GP lenses may be wiped with very soft tissues (medical wipes), but soft lenses should not. Lenses generally should not be held by their edges. On removal of a lens from its case, it should be carefully examined to ensure that there are no chips or tears and that its surfaces are clean. Wetting solution should then be applied to the surfaces of PMMA or GP lenses. Soft lenses do not require wetting solutions. The wetted lens is placed concave side up on the right forefinger, if the lens is to be inserted into the right eye; the left hand is used to hold the upper right lid well up clear of the cornea. The middle finger of the right hand pulls down the lower right lid and the lens is placed on the cornea, with the eye looking straight forward. Alternatively the lens may be placed on the bulbar conjunctiva and then recentred on the cornea with the use of the lids. The removal techniques for soft lenses and rigid corneal lenses are different. Soft lenses are removed by sliding the lenses on to the bulbar conjunctiva and then pinching off using the thumb and forefinger. The cornea is turned away, usually upwards or nasally, while the lens is pinched off. Rigid corneal lenses can be removed by opening the lids as wide as possible and beyond the lens edges. With the eye looking straight forward, the lids are pulled towards the top of the ear and a blink should release the lens. If not, the forefinger of each hand is positioned firmly on both lid margins and one lid margin is manipulated to free the lens.

On removal the lenses should be cleaned with a cleaning solution in the palm of the hand, and then thoroughly rinsed off with either sterile saline or soaking solution. PMMA and GP lenses have their own solutions, which contain stronger preservatives than those for soft contact lenses. Some users are allergic to even the preservative used for hydrophilic soft lens solutions and if the lens has a low water content it can be boiled after careful cleaning and rinsing in unpreserved, sterile saline. It is vital that aerosols or that which contain such solutions are never used for storage unless the lens has been boiled in the solution using a commercially available boiling unit. In recent years we have seen a dramatic increase in serious and damaging corneal infection (e.g. ulcers), which may partly be due to incorrect use of solutions. In addition to surfactant cleaners, some patients use enzyme cleaners but care must be exercised with these in view of the possibility of an allergic conjunctivitis from minute traces of the compound.

It is important that lenses cases must be kept clean and sterile and regularly changed. Soaking solutions should be changed daily. Solutions for hard or GP lenses must not be used with soft lenses.

If a patient is to have fluorescein instilled into the eyes prior to slit-lamp examination, it is essential to remove soft lenses beforehand to avoid lens staining. The fluorescein must be irrigated away using sterile saline and, after a further waiting period of at least half an hour, the lenses may be reinserted. Occasionally, difficulty may be experienced on attempting to remove an extended-wear or bandage soft lens and then a few drops of sterile saline should be instilled so that the lens becomes mobile. Similarly, a few drops of saline gently instilled on a soft lens helps it to settle if an air bubble is trapped beneath the lens following insertion.

The Correction of Aphakia, Including Intraocular Lenses

Aphakia

In aphakia, the lack of the crystalline lens produces hypermetropia in the region of 12 D, in an eye that was previously emmetropic.

If a patient is a binocular aphakic, or a monocular aphakic with poor or no useful vision in the other eye, then spectacles may provide a practical form of optical correction. Plastic spectacle lenses made in lenticular form with one surface aspherical give the safest and best type of spectacle solution. The lenses have to be fitted close to the eyes in order to increase the field of view. However, the spectacle magnification is of the order of 20%. This magnification of the external world gives rise to false spatial perception, which initially is quite disorientating for the patient. Objects appear much closer than they actually are, and objects suddenly jump into view in the peripheral visual field because of the high prismatic effect at the lenticular margin on the lens. Eventually, however, the patient becomes accustomed to his new visual environment. No such problems occur with contact lenses or intraocular lenses.

However, if the patient is a unilateral aphakic with potential binocular vision, spectacles cannot provide an acceptable solution, because of the large differential prismatic effect and retinal image sizes. The form of correction then must be a choice between a contact lens and an intraocular lens. From an economic and patient management viewpoint intraocular lenses are now the first choice. Contact lenses have to be replaced and solutions are required. If an extended-wear lens is required regular check-ups are essential to ensure that no damage to the cornea is occurring.

Intraocular lenses, properly located, give image magnifications of the order of 3%, and with contact lenses the image magnification is between 6% and 12%, depending on the type of contact lens. However, the power of a contact lens can be very accurately prescribed and simply obtained, and adjusted if required. Ultrasonic biometry is commonly used to help decide the power of an intraocular lens and in the majority of cases the resultant refraction is within a dioptre of the prediction.

Both contact lens correction and intraocular lens correction, therefore, often require spectacles to be worn by the patient in order to correct any residual ametropia.

Intraocular Lenses

There are three basic types of intraocular lens.

1. **Anterior chamber lenses** are positioned in front of the iris, within the 'feet' in the angle, and are principally used for secondary implantation.
2. **Iris-fixated lenses**, in which the optic is situated in the anterior or posterior chamber, are now infrequently used.
3. **Posterior chamber lenses** are supported by the capsular envelope or ciliary sulcus, after extracapsular lens extraction (Chapter 19). These are by far the most commonly used.

In order to be able to calculate the required lens power of implant, the central corneal radius ('K' reading) is measured on a keratometer and the axial length is determined by A scan ultrasonography (biometry). Using a formula which includes the A constant of the implant to be used, the power of the implant can be calculated to give the desired effect.

13 Eyelids and Adnexa

Brian Leatherbarrow and Jane Fox

Chapter Summary

Functional Anatomy

The eyelids are specialized folds of skin that protect the eye and, by blinking, distribute the tear film, preventing drying of the cornea and conjunctiva. The horizontal opening forms the palpebral aperture, which is slightly higher at its lateral end. The eyelids consist of two lamellae (layers), an anterior lamella formed by skin and muscle and a posterior lamella formed by tarsal plates and the conjunctiva (Figure 13.1). The conjunctiva is very firmly adherent to the tarsal plate in both the upper and lower eyelids.

The skin of the eyelids is thin and loosely attached, allowing large collections of subcutaneous oedema and blood to occur. Excess upper eyelid skin is useful for small full-thickness skin grafts in the periorbital region. The upper lid skin crease is formed by the insertion of the levator aponeurosis between the orbicularis oculi muscle bundles. Incisions in the upper lid are made in the skin crease wherever possible. In the lower eyelid it is important to excise skin lesions as vertically as possible to avoid an ectropion.

The orbicularis oculi muscle comprises an oval sheet of striated muscle, innervated by the facial nerve, which is artificially divided into an orbital portion surrounding the orbital rim and a palpebral portion that is in turn divided into a preseptal and pretarsal portion. The orbital portion is responsible for forced voluntary closures of the eyelids, whereas the palpebral portion is responsible for reflex blinking.

Pretarsal muscle takes its origin from the superficial part of the lateral canthal tendon and inserts by two heads, a superficial and a deep head. The superficial heads form the superficial limb of the medial canthal tendon, while the deep heads insert on to the posterior lacrimal crest, forming the posterior limb of the medial canthal tendon. The posterior limb of the medial canthal tendon plays an important role in the structural integrity of the medial canthus and it is important to repair it precisely following lacerations of the medial canthal tendon.

Preseptal muscle arises from the lateral palpebral raphe and similarly inserts by a superficial and deep head. The superficial heads form the superficial part of the medial canthal tendon and the deep heads insert into the lacrimal fascia on the lateral side of the lacrimal sac. When the muscle contracts the lacrimal fascia is drawn laterally, creating a relative vacuum in the lacrimal sac as the pretarsal muscle simultaneously draws the puncta medially into the lacus lacrimalis. Tears thereby enter the lacrimal sac. As the muscles relax, the lacrimal fascia returns to normal and tears pass down the nasolacrimal duct.

The tarsal plates consist of dense fibrous tissue and give form and stability to the free margin of each eyelid. The upper lid tarsal plate is usually 9–11 mm in height, whereas the lower lid tarsal plate is only 3–4 mm in height. The stability of the upper lid margin can be maintained with only 4 mm of tarsus, allowing the rest of the upper lid tarsus to be used in eyelid reconstruction.

Each tarsal plate contains approximately 20 vertical orientated meibomian glands whose ducts open on to the eyelid margin immediately posterior to the grey line. The grey line marks the junction between the moist conjunctiva and skin.

The eyelashes grow in two or three rows anterior to the grey line. They are more numerous in the upper eyelid and take approximately 10 weeks to grow. Opening into the follicle of each eyelash are ducts of sebaceous glands.

The orbital septum is a tough sheet of fibrous connective tissue which arises from the orbital rim and inserts into the upper and lower lid retractors a short distance from the tarsal plates. It separates the eyelids from the orbital contents. Lying immediately behind the orbital septum is the preaponeurotic fat. The fat lies in front of the eyelid retractors and aids in the identification of the upper and lower eyelid retractors at surgery.

The upper eyelid retractors are the striated levator palpebrae superioris muscle and the smooth Müller's muscle. The levator muscle is innervated by the superior division of the oculomotor nerve and is under voluntary control. The levator aponeurosis is a sheet of fibrous tissue which arises from the levator muscle as this approaches Whitnall's ligament. The aponeurosis has a vertical orientation and inserts on to the anterior surface of the tarsal plate and between the orbicularis muscle bundles to form the skin crease (Figure 13.1).

Müller's muscle arises from the undersurface of the levator in the region of Whitnall's ligament and inserts on to the

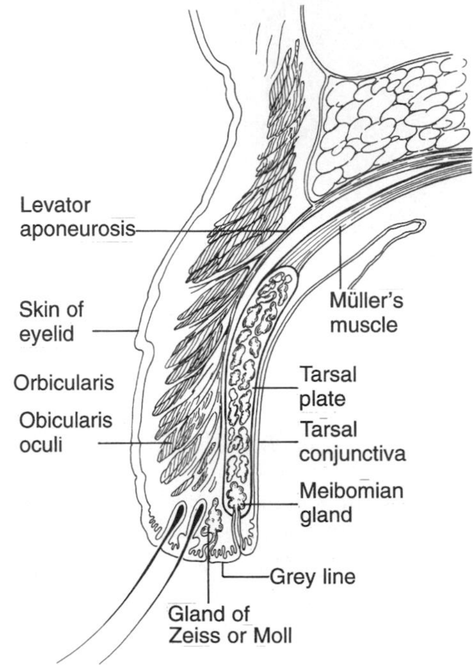

Figure 13.1 A cross-sectional diagram of the normal upper eyelid.

upper border of the tarsal plate (Figure 13.1). It is highly vascular and is innervated by sympathetic nerves, loss of which causes the ptosis of Horner's syndrome.

The lower eyelid retractors consist of a sheet of fibrous tissue, analogous to the levator aponeurosis, which extends from the inferior rectus muscle to the lower border of the tarsal plate, and a sheet of smooth muscle, analogous to Müller's muscle in the upper lid. The retractors are responsible for the downward movement of the lower lid on downgaze.

The eyelids receive a rich blood supply from the palpebral arteries arising from branches of the ophthalmic and external carotid arteries. In the upper eyelids there are two main palpebral arcades, the lower one lying on the tarsus and the upper lying at the upper border of the tarsus. In the lower eyelid the palpebral artery lies on the tarsus approximately 2–4 mm from the eyelid margin.

The sensory nerve supply to the upper eyelid is from branches of the ophthalmic division of the trigeminal nerve and the supply to the lower eyelid from branches of the maxillary division of the trigeminal nerve.

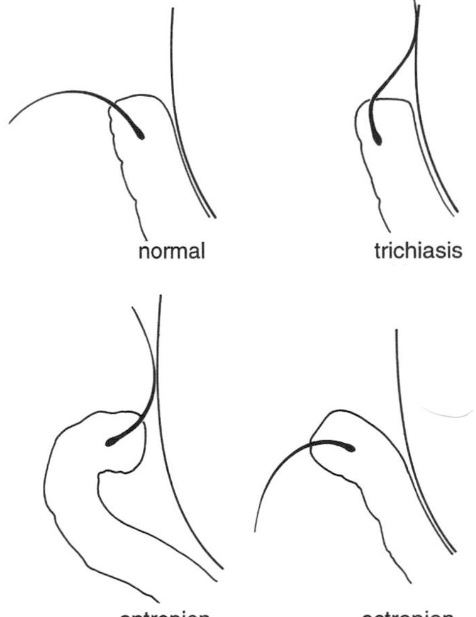

Figure 13.2 Positional disorders.

Eyelid Malpositions

Entropion

This is a malposition of the eyelid in which the eyelid margin is inturned, causing the eyelashes to abrade the cornea, leading to irritation, tearing and ultimately corneal ulceration (Figure 13.2).

Lower Lid Entropion

A lower lid entropion may be congenital or acquired. It may be classified as involutional, spastic or cicatricial (caused by scarring).

Involutional

An involutional entropion is the most common variety of entropion. The entropion results from a number of aetiological factors: overriding of the pretarsal orbicularis muscle by the preseptal orbicularis muscle, laxity of the lower eyelid retractors and horizontal laxity of the eyelid. A wide range of surgical procedures have been described to deal with the eyelid malposition.

The procedure of choice should attempt to address the underlying aetiological factors involved. This is best achieved by using an inferior retractor reinsertion procedure combined with a lateral tarsal strip procedure. This can usually be performed under local anaesthesia on a day surgery basis.

Problem	Goal	Nursing intervention
Surgical wound of the lower eyelid.	A healed surgical wound.	Advice – cleanse with normal saline if required, avoiding unnecessary contact. Instruct the patient on the use of dressings and the application of drops/ointment as prescribed. Instruct re-removal of sutures.
Potential problem of postoperative bleeding.	Early detection and treatment should potential complications occur.	1. Maintain firm dressing until oozing has stopped. 2. Instruct patient to apply firm dressing and hand pressure should bleeding occur. 3. Advise patient to return to the hospital immediately if bleeding does not stop or becomes excessive.

The lid may be taped to the cheek to afford some relief from symptoms while awaiting surgery. Strapping (taping) the eyelid margin to the cheek can be used as a temporary measure prior to surgical correction (Chapter 8).

Problem	Goal	Nursing intervention
Irritation and discomfort from inturning eyelid.	Eyelid temporarily returned to the normal position and patient free from irritation and complications.	Teach/demonstrate strapping of the eyelid. Involve district nurse/relatives if necessary. Explain that this is a temporary measure prior to surgery. Promote eyelid hygiene. Instruct patient on applications of drops/ointment as prescribed.

For patients who are bedbound or otherwise unfit for surgery, the lid malposition may be temporarily corrected by means of simple everting sutures, which can be inserted at the bedside.

Cicatricial

A cicatricial entropion results from a scarring process affecting the posterior lamella of the eyelid, such as mucous membrane pemphigoid, Stevens–Johnson syndrome or chemical burns. The surgical management depends on the underlying cause and the severity of the entropion. This may involve a simple tarsal fracture procedure, a retractor reinsertion procedure, where surgery involving the posterior lamella needs to be avoided, or mucous membrane grafting.

Ectropion

Ectropion is a malposition of the eyelid in which the margin is turned away from the globe (Figure 13.2). This results in abnormal eyelid closure and a poor distribution of the tear film, leading to exposure keratopathy and conjunctival thickening and keratinization. The malposition of the inferior punctum results in chronic epiphora (watering). Patients can be helped to cope with the problems while awaiting surgery.

Problem	Goal	Nursing intervention
Continuously watering sore eye with the potential risk of corneal and conjunctival pathology from exposure.	Acceptable discomfort while awaiting surgery and the prevention of complications.	Instruct the patient to: 1. massage the lower eyelid; 2. correctly wipe away tears; 3. instil drops/ointment as prescribed; 4. undertake eyelid hygiene as required; 5. wear dark glasses in windy and dusty environments.

Lower Lid Ectropion

This may be classified as involutional, cicatricial, mechanical or paralytic.

Involutional

An involutional ectropion is the most common variety seen. It results from increasing laxity of all the eyelid structures. It may affect only the medial aspect of the lower eyelid or its whole extent. The choice of surgical procedure for this eyelid malposition depends on the extent of the ectropion and the degree of associated laxity of the medial canthal tendon.

Cicatricial

A cicatricial ectropion results from a shortage of skin, which may be due to a variety of causes, for example congenital, as seen occasionally in Down's syndrome, dermatological disorders and allergies to topical medications. The management depends on the underlying cause. Medical management is required in the case of dermatological disorders although surgery may also be required in these cases. The surgical management usually involves either local skin transposition, as in a Z-plasty, or skin replacement in the form of a full-thickness skin graft.

Mechanical

A mechanical ectropion results from a tumour near the lid margin mechanically everting the lid. The management involves the surgical excision of the cause, and horizontal lid shortening if the lesion is associated with horizontal eyelid laxity.

Paralytic

A paralytic ectropion results from a lower motor neurone facial palsy. The surgical management depends on the severity of the ectropion, the prognosis for recovery of facial nerve function, the severity of the associated exposure keratopathy and the presence or absence of corneal sensation, the cosmetic appearance, and the age and general health of the patient. The ectropion is usually best managed by means of a lateral tarsal strip procedure combined with a medial canthoplasty.

Ptosis

Ptosis is a drooping of the upper eyelid which can affect all age groups and may be congenital or acquired, unilateral or bilateral. It may cause a functional visual deficit or merely represent a cosmetic defect. It is important to recognize that ptosis itself is merely a physical sign and before therapeutic decisions are made it is essential to make every effort to determine the underlying cause. The causes of ptosis are numerous. In considering them it is useful to use a classification of ptosis based upon aetiological factors. This aims to provide some insight into the pathological processes involved, and classifies ptosis as pseudoptosis, neurogenic, myogenic, aponeurotic or mechanical.

Pseudoptosis

Pseudoptosis refers to a condition that mimics a true ptosis. An example is abnormal reinnervation of the facial nerve after injury and the postenucleation socket syndrome.

True ptosis may result from neurological disorders or from specific defects in the innervation of the levator palpebrae superioris muscle, from disorders affecting the levator muscle itself, from defects in the levator aponeurosis or in the attachment of the aponeurosis to the tarsal plate (much the commonest), or from mechanical factors that restrict normal movement of the eyelid. These aetiological mechanisms may be found in all age groups with varying frequency.

Neurogenic Ptosis

Oculomotor Nerve Palsy

Oculomotor nerve palsy is characterized by a variable degree of ptosis associated with deficits of adduction, elevation and depression of the eye due to weakness of the levator muscle, the superior, inferior and medial rectus muscles and the inferior oblique muscle. The pupillary fibres of the oculomotor nerve may be affected or spared, depending on the underlying cause. The Bell's phenomenon is typically absent or poor.

Treatment of the ptosis is problematic due to the impaired Bell's phenomenon with a risk of exposure keratopathy.

Horner's Syndrome

Horner's syndrome is characterized by a ptosis of 1–2 mm with good levator function and a raised skin crease, miosis and an apparent enophthalmos, and is occasionally associated with facial anhydrosis. The features are due to interference with the sympathetic nerve supply to Müller's muscle in the upper eyelid, its smooth muscle counterpart in the lower eyelid and the dilator pupillae muscle. The resultant anisocoria is accentuated in dim illumination. The apparent enophthalmos is due to the decrease in size of the palpebral aperture.

The ptosis may be treated surgically, by either a Fasanella–Servat procedure or a levator aponeurosis advancement procedure.

Myasthenia Gravis

Myasthenia gravis is an autoimmune disorder caused by antibodies to the acetylcholine receptors of the motor endplate of voluntary muscle. The antibodies block access of the neurotransmitter acetylcholine to the receptors. The hallmarks of the disorder are variable muscular weakness and fatigue on exercise. Myasthenia may be generalized, and may threaten the muscles of respiration, or it may be localized to the eyes (ocular myasthenia). Approximately 30% of patients present with ocular signs and symptoms (ptosis and diplopia), while 80–90% of patients have ocular signs at the time of diagnosis. If the symptoms and signs remain confined to the eyes for 3 years, progress to generalized myasthenia is unlikely. Ptosis is the most common clinical manifestation of myasthenia. It may be unilateral or bilateral.

Synkinetic Ptosis

Marcus Gunn jaw-wink phenomenon. In this disorder there is a central anomalous innervational pattern between the oculomotor and trigeminal nerves. The phenomenon is characterized by eyelid synkinesis with jaw movement. Characteristically, a unilateral ptosis of variable degree is noted shortly after birth. The ptotic eyelid is noted to open and close as the infant feeds. The phenomenon accounts for approximately 5% of congenital ptosis cases and may be associated with amblyopia, anisometropia and strabismus. It may also be associated with a superior rectus palsy or a double elevator palsy. The treatment of this phenomenon is very complex and a discussion of it is beyond the scope of this text.

Aberrant reinnervation of the oculomotor nerve. In this disorder there is an innervational anomaly within the neural sheath between the eyelid and other targets of the oculomotor nerve. It is characterized by inappropriate eyelid and extraocular muscle synkinesis. The disorder typically follows trauma or compression of the oculomotor nerve.

Myogenic Ptosis

This can be classified as congenital localized dystrophy, myotonic dystrophy or chronic progressive external ophthalmoplegia.

Congenital Localized Dystrophy

This is caused by a development defect of the levator muscle. The levator function is typically fair to poor. Typically, there is lid lag on downgaze. It may be associated with a weakness of the superior rectus muscle. Many cases simply pose a cosmetic problem but in severe unilateral cases sensory deprivation amblyopia may ensue if treatment is not carried out at the appropriate time. In these cases a temporary frontalis sling procedure is performed. Otherwise, surgery is best deferred until the child is old enough to cooperate with an accurate assessment of the levator function. This is usually after the age of 4 years.

Myotonic Dystrophy

Myotonic dystrophy is a rare myopathic process, which may be associated with a mild degree of symmetrical ptosis with a fair to poor degree of levator function. It is characterized by progressive symmetrical external ophthalmoplegia, myopathy with atrophy affecting the musculature of the face, neck and limbs, and classic cataracts.

Chronic Progressive External Ophthalmoplegia

This condition, which is now regarded as a neurogenic disorder, is characterized by a progressive, symmetric paralysis of the extraocular muscles, which do not respond to oculocephalic movement nor to caloric stimulation. The levator muscle is also affected, resulting in a degree of ptosis related to the degree of severity of the disorder. The levator function is usually poor, as is the Bell's phenomenon. The orbicularis function is usually good.

Aponeurotic Ptosis

This results from defects in the levator aponeurosis or in the attachment of the aponeurosis to the tarsal plate. It may be caused by involutional changes or may be seen following various ophthalmic surgical procedures, following episodes of upper lid oedema or in contact lens wearers. Typically the patients have a good levator function and respond well to a levator aponeurosis advancement procedure in which the levator aponeurosis is identified and advanced on to the tarsal plate. The results of the procedure are enhanced if this is done under local anaesthesia with the patient's co-operation.

Mechanical Ptosis

This is caused by mechanical factors which restrict normal movement of the eyelid. This may be seen with eyelid tumours, excess upper eyelid skin (dermatochalasis) or conjunctival scarring.

Patient Assessment

An accurate and detailed history should be obtained. Particular note should be made of the length of history, predisposing factors (e.g. trauma, variability), associated symptoms (e.g. diplopia, dysphagia) and the family history.

The degree of ptosis should be measured, together with the levator function. This is performed by asking the patient to look down while a millimetre rule is placed before the eyelids, noting the position of the upper lid margin. A thumb is placed over the eyebrow to eliminate the frontalis action. The patient is asked to look up and down. The difference in measurements is the levator function. The normal levator function is between 15 and 18 mm.

A complete ocular examination is also performed, paying particular attention to the Bell's phenomenon, the ocular movements, the pupils and signs of myasthenia.

The treatment of most types of ptosis is surgical. Rarely, if the patient is unfit for surgery or if the risk of postoperative corneal exposure is great, one may have to resort to ptosis props attached to spectacles. These simply raise the eyelids mechanically. Alternatively, contact lens with ridges may be tried.

The type of surgical procedure undertaken depends very much on the degree of levator function.

If the levator function is fair to good (7–15 mm) a levator aponeurosis advancement procedure should be performed. In the case of adults, this should be performed under local anaesthesia with the patient's co-operation wherever possible. Where the levator function is between 4 and 7 mm a levator resection procedure is required.

If the levator function is poor (less than 4 mm) a frontalis sling will be required. Various materials can be used for this. Non-autogenous materials include supramid, polypropylene, mersilene mesh and preserved fascia lata. Alternatively, autogenous fascia lata may be used.

The main postoperative complication of ptosis surgery is corneal exposure.

Problem	Goal	Nursing intervention
Possible corneal damage from corneal exposure.	Maintenance of healthy cornea in the first days postoperatively.	1. Observe for corneal exposure during sleeping. 2. Consider the use of paraffin gauze under an eye pad if an eye pad is required. 3. Instil drops/ointment as prescribed. 4. If a Frost suture is used ensure it is firmly taped to the forehead, and firmly reattached after the instillation of prescribed medication.
Surgical wound at donor site if fascial lata graft used.	Healed surgical wound.	1. Maintain a firm dressing to the wound for 48 hours. 2. Advise the patient on the appointment for removal of sutures.

Other potential complications include under- or overcorrection, contour defects, conjunctival prolapse and skin crease defects.

Eyelid Retraction

There are a number of conditions that cause retraction of the upper eyelid, the most frequently encountered being thyroid eye disease. Additional non-neurological causes are the instillation of sympathomimetic drugs, the prolonged use of systemic corticosteroids, upper lid scarring and contracture or entrapment of the inferior rectus muscle.

Eyelid Tumours

Benign Eyelid Tumours

There are a number of benign eyelid tumours, many of which are easily recognizable by their characteristic features. The lesions most commonly encountered are chalazion, papilloma, seborrhoeic keratosis and xanthelasma.

Chalazion

A chalazion is the result of a reaction to retained meibomian gland secretions caused by an obstruction to the gland ducts. It presents as a firm, round, palpable swelling within the eyelid. There are usually no inflammatory signs unless the lesion becomes secondarily infected, in which case it may point and discharge through the conjunctiva or skin. Occasionally, excessive granulation tissue forms on the conjunctival surface, giving rise to a red fleshy mass.

There may be spontaneous resolution within a few weeks or months. This can be aided by the use of hot compresses, eyelid massage and the application of topical antibiotic ointment. If this does not occur, treatment is surgical by means of a vertical incision through the conjunctival surface of the lesion and curettage of the contents. The eyelid is held averted in a chalazion clamp which also helps to reduce haemorrhage. Antibiotic ointment is applied, together with a firm pressure dressing until the bleeding has stopped. The eyelids are then cleaned and a fresh eye pad is applied for 4–6 hours. The antibiotic ointment should be continued three times daily for a week. It is wise to warn the patient that there will be residual swelling for some weeks before complete resolution occurs.

A recurrence or atypical features raise the suspicion of a sebaceous gland carcinoma mimicking a chalazion. In these cases the lesion should be biopsied and submitted for histopathological examination.

Papilloma

This common eyelid lesion appears as a small fleshy growth attached by a thin pedicle. Treatment is by means of a simple excision. All specimens should be submitted for histopathological examination.

Seborrhoeic Keratosis

This is a very common cutaneous lesion of the elderly. It typically has a greasy, waxy 'stuck on' appearance. It is easily removed by a shave excision.

Xanthelasma

Xanthelasmata are slightly raised, often symmetrical, creamy-yellow deposits of lipid in the skin of the eyelids near the medial canthi. They may be associated with abnormalities of lipid metabolism. They are easily excised but recurrences are common.

Keratoacanthoma

A keratoacanthoma usually begins as a flesh-coloured papule which rapidly evolves into a dome-shaped nodule with a keratin-filled crater. It can involute spontaneously and disappear but excision is commonly undertaken for diagnosis, as it can be difficult to differentiate from squamous cell carcinoma of the eyelid, or for mechanical or cosmetic reasons.

It may be extremely difficult to make a correct diagnosis of an eyelid lesion without a biopsy. When a lesion thought to be benign shows growth, a biopsy should be performed. If a lesion is small an excisional biopsy should be performed with direct closure of the defect. If the lesion is too large to permit this, an incisional biopsy should be performed.

Malignant Eyelid Tumours

It is noteworthy that 25% of all malignancies involve the skin and 10% of cutaneous malignancies involve the eyelids. A total of 90–95% of malignant eyelid tumours are basal cell carcinomas (BCCs). It is important that a patient presenting with a malignant eyelid tumour undergoes a whole-body skin excamination to exclude additional cutaneous malignancies.

The clinical pattern of some eyelid malignancies can simulate other neoplasms; for example a pigmented eyelid neoplasm is much more frequently a basal cell carcinoma than a melanoma.

The lesions most commonly encountered are basal cell carcinoma, squamous cell carcinoma and sebaceous gland carcinoma. Other rarer tumours which are occasionally encountered are melanoma, Kaposi's sarcoma (most likely in AIDS) and lymphoma.

The management of all malignant eyelid tumours depends on a correct histological diagnosis, assessment of the tumour margins and an assessment of systemic tumour spread. Focal malignancy can be managed by surgery in conjunction with histological monitoring of tumour margins, radiation and cryotherapy. The choice of therapy depends on a number of factors, including the size of the tumours, its location, its histological type and the age and general health of the patient. The gold standard for the management of basal and squamous cell carcinomas is Mohs's micrographic excision (Mohs, 1986). Cryotherapy can be particularly useful for small BCCs in the region of the lacrimal drainage apparatus in patients who are unfit for surgery. Radiation treatment is effective but it is associated with ocular complications and recurrences can be extremely difficult to manage.

Basal Cell Carcinoma

This locally destructive tumour typically presents as a chronic, hard, non-tender, raised, pearly, well-circumscribed lesion with an elevated surround and a depressed, crater-like centre. In the periorbital region it is seen most frequently in the lower lid, followed by the medial canthus, the upper lid and lastly the lateral canthus. Orbital invasion by a BCC is manifest clinically as a fixed, non-mobile tumour and, in advanced cases, as a 'frozen globe'. Metastases are extremely rare.

BCCs that are particularly difficult to manage are tumours which are fixed, tumours located at the medial canthus, tumours showing orbital invasion and tumours that recur after radiotherapy.

Squamous Cell Carcinoma

This tends to appear as a thick, erythematous, elevated lesion with indurated borders and a scaly surface. Cutaneous horn formation or extensive keratinization are the most consistent features. The tumour can metastasize and tends to behave more aggressively than a BCC.

Sebaceous Gland Carcinoma

This is a particularly dangerous tumour as it tends to masquerade as a recurrent chalazion, hordeolum (stye) or chronic blepharoconjunctivitis ('masquerade syndrome'). It may metastasize before a correct diagnosis is established. The tumour has a predilection for the upper lid. It tends to affect older individuals and has a mortality rate of 20–30%.

EYELID RECONSTRUCTION

Reconstruction of eyelid defects must involve adequate replacement of both the anterior and posterior lamellae to achieve a good functional and cosmetic result. Defects of up to one third of the lid can usually be closed directly. Defects greater in size require the use of local tissue flaps or grafts of skin or cartilage. The use of these flaps or grafts is dictated by the precise nature of the lid defects and a detailed discussion is beyond the scope of this text.

EYELID TRAUMA

It is important to appreciate that apparently trivial eyelid trauma may be associated with serious, sight-threatening injury, which will go undetected unless a high index of suspicion is maintained during the patient's evaluation. The examination of such patients should be performed carefully and thoroughly to exclude associated trauma to the globe. Until proved otherwise, lacerations of the eyelid have an associated perforating injury of the globe and lacerations of the medial aspect of the eyelid involve the lacrimal drainage apparatus. An associated orbital fracture or retained foreign bodies should be suspected and appropriate radiological investigations performed.

All dirt and debris should be removed from the wounds and they should be thoroughly cleansed before undertaking any repair. The repair can be delayed up to 72 hours to await appropriate operating conditions. The blood supply of the eyelids and face is so good that apparently devitalized tissue frequently survives if left in place. Tissue should not therefore be discarded unnecessarily. Tissue should be replaced in its correct anatomical location to maintain normal eyelid integrity and to avoid the risk of trichiasis (see below), notching of the lid margin, entropion, inadequate closure (lagophthalmos) and epiphora.

Lacerations involving the lid margin require a meticulous repair. The lid margin should be reapposed using interrupted simple absorbable sutures to realign the tarsal plate and interrupted silk sutures placed in a vertical mattress fashion through the line of the meibomian gland orifices and through the lash line to realign the lid margin.

Lacerations involving the lacrimal drainage apparatus require a microscopic repair, using a bicanalicular stent wherever possible.

Miscellaneous Eyelid Disorders

Trichiasis

Trichiasis is a misdirection of the lashes toward the globe. It is frequently associated with chronic blepharitis but may follow opening of a poorly constructed lateral tarsorrhaphy. Trichiasis gives rise to an annoying foreign-body sensation and damage to the inferior corneal surface. Temporary relief is afforded by simple epilation or occasionally by the use of a soft bandage contact lens. Permanent relief is achieved with either electrolysis or laser for a few lashes, cryotherapy (freezing) for those not manageable with electrolysis, or surgical excision where the lashes are localized to a small area of the lid.

Distichiasis

This is a condition in which there is an accessory row of lashes arising from the meibomian gland orifices. This may be congenital or acquired. This is treated by splitting the lid along the grey line and applying cryotherapy to the posterior lamella.

Blepharospasm

Essential blepharospasm is characterized by an idiopathic bilateral involuntary contraction of the orbicularis oculi muscles. In the early stages of the disorder patients are frequently misdiagnosed and may even be dismissed as having a functional problem. Blepharospasm may also be seen in neurological conditions such as Parkinson's disease. The majority of patients respond very well to local injections of botulinum toxin. The neurotoxin interferes with the release of acetylcholine from the nerve terminals and relief from blepharospasm lasts 3–4 months following each injection. Frequent topical lubricants are required following the injection to avoid exposure keratopathy, as the blink is usually incomplete. Transient diplopia and ptosis are infrequent unwanted consequences of the injections.

Surgery in the form of orbicularis oculi excision and selective facial nerve avulsion for this condition is now only rarely required.

Coloboma

Coloboma is an embryological defect in the eyelid which may occur as an isolated anomaly or may be associated with other congenital defects.

Epicanthus

Epicanthus is a fold of skin which stretches from the upper to the lower eyelid and covers the medial canthal angle. In infants it can mimic a 'pseudosquint'.

Facial Palsy

A patient with a facial palsy may present with corneal exposure, paralytic ectropion, epiphora and poor cosmesis. The management depends on the underlying cause and the prognosis for recovery. If the palsy is acute, the immediate concern is protection of the cornea. This can usually be achieved by simple conservative measures such as topical lubricants, taping the lid closed at night or moist chamber goggles, or by means of a botulinum toxin-induced ptosis. If these measures are insufficient, a temporary lateral tarsorrhaphy will be required. This should be performed very carefully so as not to distort the lid margin should the tarsorrhaphy require opening at a later stage.

A lateral tarsorrhaphy is performed by splitting the grey line and excising the surface of the posterior lamella. The lids are then apposed using interrupted absorbable sutures passed through the depth of the grey line splits and tied together. The anterior lamellae are then sewn together using a continuous, fine absorbable suture. This method avoids the use of unsightly bolsters.

Established corneal exposure can be treated either by reducing the palpebral aperture or by improving eyelid closure. The palpebral aperture can be reduced vertically by lowering the upper lid and raising the lower lid, or horizontally by means of a lateral tarsal strip and a medial canthoplasty.

Herpes Zoster Ophthalmicus (HZO)

This is an infection of the ophthalmic division of the trigeminal nerve due to reactivation of the chicken pox (varicella-zoster) virus. It can occur at any age but is most commonly seen in patients over 50 years of age. It may be seen in immunocompromised patients. Symptoms begin with a severe unilateral neuralgia in the scalp and forehead corresponding to the involved dermatome. This is followed a few days later by the development of a vesicular eruption. The vesicles rupture, discharging serum and blood, forming extensive crusts which eventually heal leaving pitted scars. The often severe pain subsides in 2–3 weeks but postherpetic neuralgia persists in a number of patients, especially the elderly. Postherpetic neuralgia is notoriously difficult to control. Referral to a specialist pain clinic is indicated in resistant cases.

Impending ocular involvement may be suspected if vesicles develop on the tip of the nose, as this area, together with the cornea, is supplied by the nasociliary branch of the trigeminal nerve. Conjunctivitis is common, but more severe ocular involvement occurs in 50% of patients, including epithelial keratitis, corneal ulceration or uveitis. Other ocular complications include episcleritis, scleritis, secondary glaucoma, palsies of extraocular muscles and retinitis.

Recent studies have shown that acycloguanosine tablets reduce the duration of the rash if given within 3 days of onset. However, protection against ocular involvement and postherpetic neuralgia is limited. Povidone-iodine or steroid with antibiotic cream may be used to treat the ulcerative stage. The presence of ocular complications may require specific treatment, including acycloguanosine, steroid and cycloplegics.

Although not all patients with HZO have eye involvement they may still have been asked by their general practitioner to attend the ophthalmic unit for assessment. The decision to admit or not must take home and social circumstances into consideration in the assessment. As the rash develops, inflammatory oedema can encroach across the midline and involve the eyelids on the opposite side, giving the false impression of a bilateral condition. Nurses who have cared for patients with HZO know by experience that the patient's response can be highly individual and, by listening to these patients, the nurse can glean numerous points of helpful information to pass on.

Patients with HZO, again particularly the elderly, can be left feeling very depressed, especially in the early stages of general malaise, neuralgia and unsightly appearance. Should the general practitioner or district nurse not already be involved a referral should be made so that the patient can receive continued care at home in the knowledge that the consequences of his condition may be long-term.

References

Mohs F. E. (1986) Micrographic surgery for the microscopically controlled excision of eyelid cancers. *Archives of Ophthalmology*, **104**, 901–909.

Further Reading

Collin, J. R. O. (1982) *A Manual of Systematic Eyelid Surgery*, 2nd edn, Churchill Livingstone, Edinburgh.

Collin, J. R. O. and Leatherbarrow, B. (1990) Ophthalmic management of seventh nerve palsy. *Australian and New Zealand Journal of Ophthalmology*, **18**(3), 267–272.

14 THE LACRIMAL SYSTEM

Michael Raines, Tim Ossei Berkoh and Pat Lapworth

CHAPTER SUMMARY

FUNCTIONAL ANATOMY

The lacrimal apparatus has a secretory and drainage component, both of which are essential to the optical integrity and normal function of the eye.

The secretory component includes:

1. main lacrimal gland;
2. accessory lacrimal glands;
3. sebaceous glands of eyelids;
4. mucin-secreting cells of conjunctiva.

The main lacrimal gland is found in the superior temporal angle of the orbit. It is lodged beneath the orbital rim in the lacrimal fossa between the globe and lateral process of the frontal bone. The larger orbital portion and the small palpebral portion are separated in part by the aponeurosis of the levator palpebrae superioris muscle which elevates the upper lid.

The gland drains by a variable number of ducts. The ducts draining the orbital portion pass through the palpebral portion, before all ducts empty mainly into the outer part of the superior conjunctival fornix. It provides the aqueous component to the tear film.

The accessory lacrimal glands of Krause and Wolfring also contribute to the aqueous portion of tears. The former are found in the upper and lower conjunctival fornix and the latter in the conjunctiva surrounding the tarsal plates, mainly superiorly. The conjunctival goblet cells and the crypts of Henle secrete mucin to 'wet' the corneal epithelium. The oily layer of the tear film is derived from the meibomian glands and the sebaceous glands of Zeis, found in the lid margins.

Control of tear production is complex, but it is thought there are two methods of secretion.

1. Secretion comes at a steady rate from the accessory lacrimal glands of Krause and Wolfring (aqueous), from goblet cells (mucin) and from the meibomian glands and glands of Zeis (oily layer).
2. The 'reflex' secretion is derived from the main lacrimal gland. The stimuli for secretion can be peripheral (e.g. a foreign body on the cornea stimulating the Vth cranial nerve) or central in origin (i.e. emotion).

The precorneal tear film produced has three layers (Figure 14.1).

1. **The outer lipid layer** is derived from meibomian glands and glands of Zeis. This retards the evaporation of the aqueous layer and also helps maintain the surface tension, to prevent tears from overflowing the lid margins.
2. **The middle aqueous layer** is derived from the main lacrimal gland and accessory glands of Krause and Wolfring. It is 99% water. It supplies atmospheric oxygen to the corneal epithelium and also washes away debris on the ocular surface. It also maintains a smooth optical surface to the cornea.
3. **The inner mucin layer** is derived from conjunctival goblet cells and crypts of Henle.

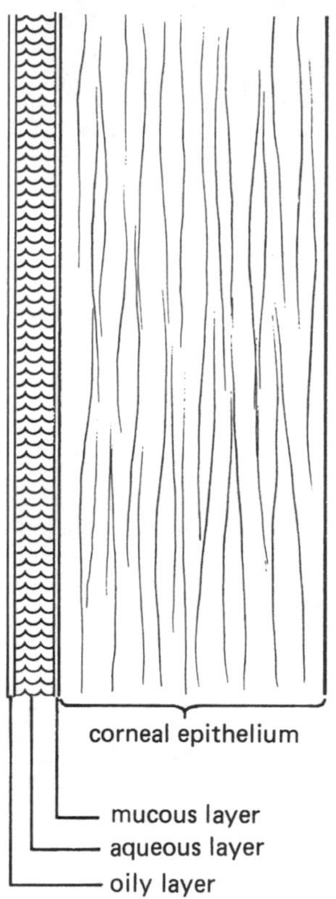

Figure 14.1 The tear film, showing the three layers.

Mucin, a glycoprotein, is absorbed on to the corneal epithelium and converts it from a hydrophobic to a hydrophilic surface. This allows the aqueous layer to maintain contact with the cornea.

Tears produced do evaporate, and blinking of the eyelids is an important manoeuvre which redistributes newly formed tears over the surface of the eye.

Tears contain most of the substances present in plasma but in slightly different concentrations. There is a high concentration of immunoglobulin 'secretory IgA', which may be locally produced and is active against external antigens such as bacteria and viruses. Lysozyme, a proteolytic enzyme, is also present, is able to dissolve bacterial walls and is an important factor in combating infection.

Generally there is a balance between tear production and tear elimination. If tear elimination is impaired, epiphora results. This should be differentiated from lacrimation, which is increased tear production.

Elimination of tears is through the drainage apparatus and comprises (Figure 14.2):

1. lacrimal puncta;
2. lacrimal canaliculi;

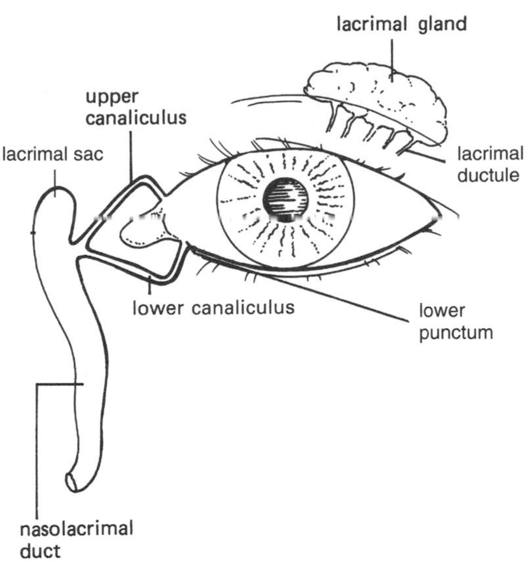

Figure 14.2 The lacrimal drainage apparatus.

3. lacrimal sac;
4. nasolacrimal duct.

Tears are attracted to the lacrimal puncta by gravity, capillary adhesion and eyelid blinking. A variable portion of the tears enters the puncta and further blinking compresses and shortens the canaliculus and propels the tears into the lacrimal sac. This sac is found in the lacrimal fossa, anteriorly on the medial wall of the orbit. A negative pressure in the lacrimal sac is produced on blinking, and this also draws tears into the sac. When blinking has ceased the sac collapses and forces the tears into the nasolacrimal duct. A series of mucosal folds in the duct may act as valves and prevent the upward passage of tears or air. The nasolacrimal duct opens into the interior meatus of the nose beneath the inferior nasal turbinate. The duct is an important site of blockage of tear flow.

Disorders of the Lacrimal Gland

Dacryoadenitis

Inflammation of the lacrimal gland is uncommon. It may be acute or chronic and usually results in some enlargement of the gland.

The palpebral portion of the gland is affected more commonly and often produces a mechanical ptosis. Pain is a common feature in acute infections and there may be redness of the overlying skin. Infection is usually viral and self-limiting, for example mumps.

Chronic dacryoadenitis occurs in a variety of diseases such as sarcoidosis, tuberculosis and leprosis and is most likely to result in slow, painless enlargement of the lacrimal gland. Treatment of dacryoadenitis is based on the underlying cause. Nursing problems can be as follows.

Problem	Goal	Nursing intervention
Pain	Pain-free	Administration of prescribed analgesia after discussion with the patient. Observation of the effectiveness of the analgesia. Application of heat after careful explanation, demonstration and supervised practice.
Swelling of the lacrimal gland and upper lid area.	Resolution of the swelling.	Application of heat (as above). Gentle handling of the lids at all times. Administration of prescribed antibiotics.

Problem	Goal	Nursing intervention
Temporary loss of visual acuity on the affected side due to lid oedema.	Safety of the patient until resolution of the oedema and normal binocular vision restored.	Assess visual acuity of unaffected eye. Establish with what activities of daily living patient requires assistance. Ensure patient does not bump into furniture, etc. by maintaining a safe environment.
Pyrexia – usually related to underlying disorder, e.g. mumps, infectious mononucleosis, sarcoidosis.	Reduction of pyrexia.	Administer prescribed antipyretics. 4–6-hourly TPR recorded and observed. Depending on degree of pyrexia, institute measures appropriate, e.g. maintain hydration – fluids at regular intervals, fluid balance chart to record intake and output. Tepid sponging if necessary. Initiate use of a cooling fan, etc. Administer prescribed treatment for underlying disorder, e.g. steroids for sarcoidosis, etc.
Underlying infection.	Freedom from infection.	Take conjunctival and lid swabs to determine causative organism. Report findings to medical staff. Administer prescribed topical and systemic antibiotics. Observe effectiveness of treatment.
Stickiness of the lids caused by mucopurulent discharge.	Clean, comfortable lids.	Institute lid toilet and hygiene as often as necessary to ensure patient comfort and the ability to open lids freely.
Anxiety due to illness.	Relaxed, co-operative patient.	Discussion with the patient to allow him time to ask questions about the cause of his illness and the treatments and investigations undertaken. Explanation that, as the treatment takes effect, the general malaise will improve and the oedema and inflammation will resolve.

Tumours

Tumours of the lacrimal gland may be divided into benign, malignant and secondary tumours. Benign mixed cell tumours are the most common. They are slow growing, usually in middle-aged individuals, and produce a painless swelling in the region of the lacrimal gland together with displacement of the globe downwards and medially.

Malignant tumours of the lacrimal gland can develop rarely from the benign mixed cell tumour or arise de novo. In these cases the growth is rapid; pain and diplopia may be present. Other types of tumour include adenocarcinoma, mucoepidermoid carcinoma, lymphoma and 'pseudotumour'. Plain skull X-rays, orbital CT scanning and ultrasonography are the most useful non-invasive investigations in diagnosing lacrimal lesions. Orbital biopsy is very helpful in carefully selected patients.

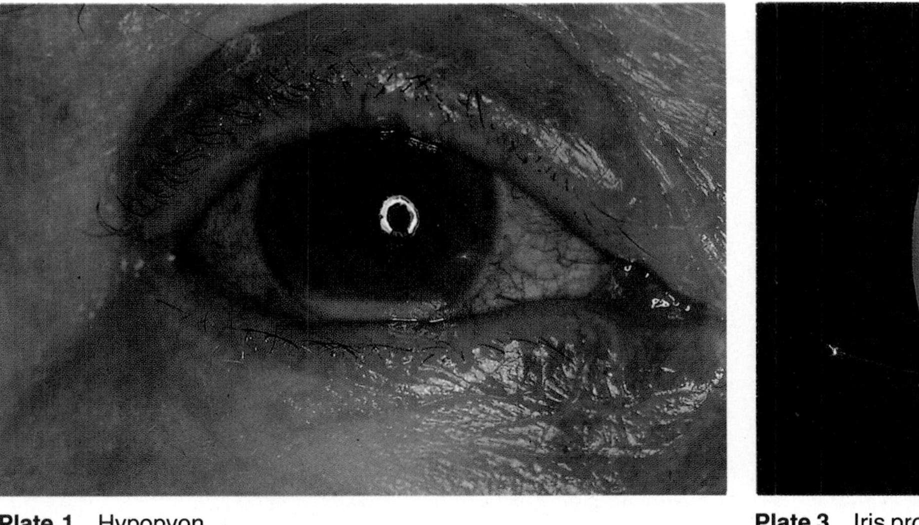

Plate 1 Hypopyon.

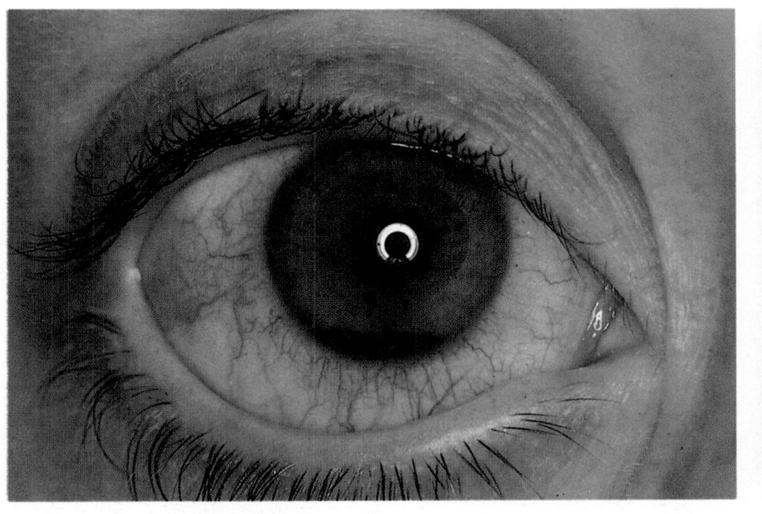

Plate 2 Hyphaema.

Plate 3 Iris prolapse following surgery. Note the distorted pupil.

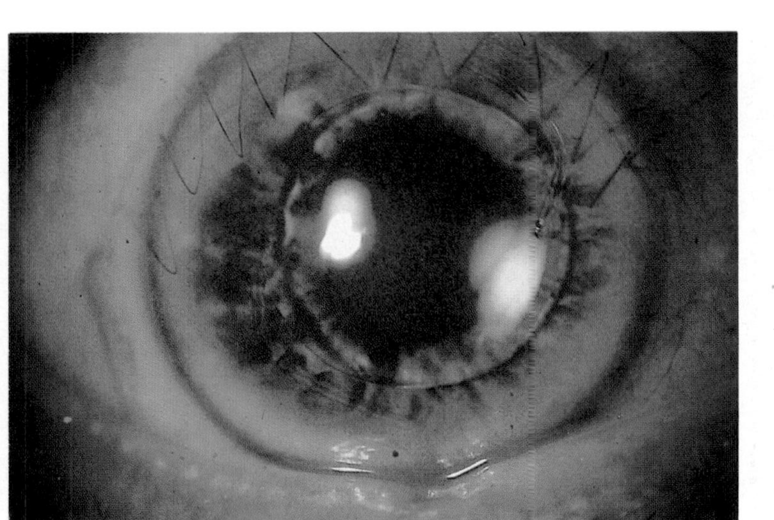

Plate 4 Anterior Chamber Lens Implant. A continuous suture can be seen at the corneal incision.

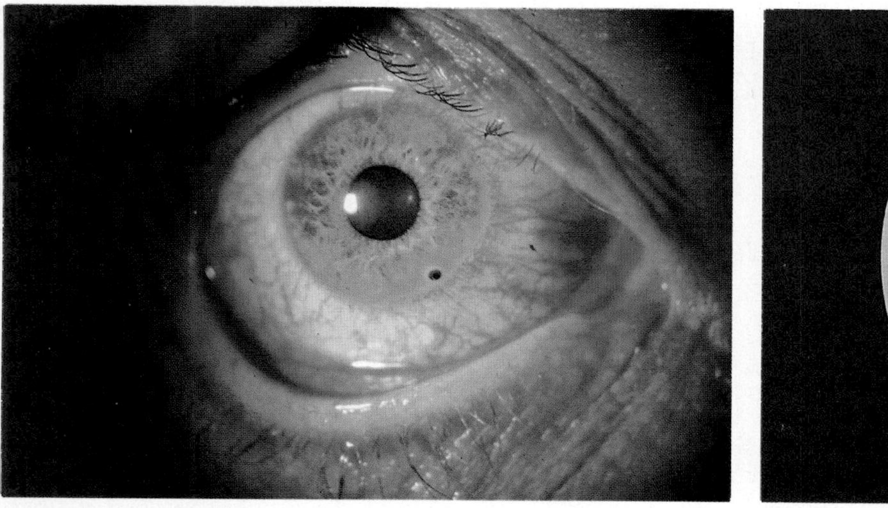

Plate 5 Typical appearance of a metallic foreign body located at the 5 o'clock position at the limbus.

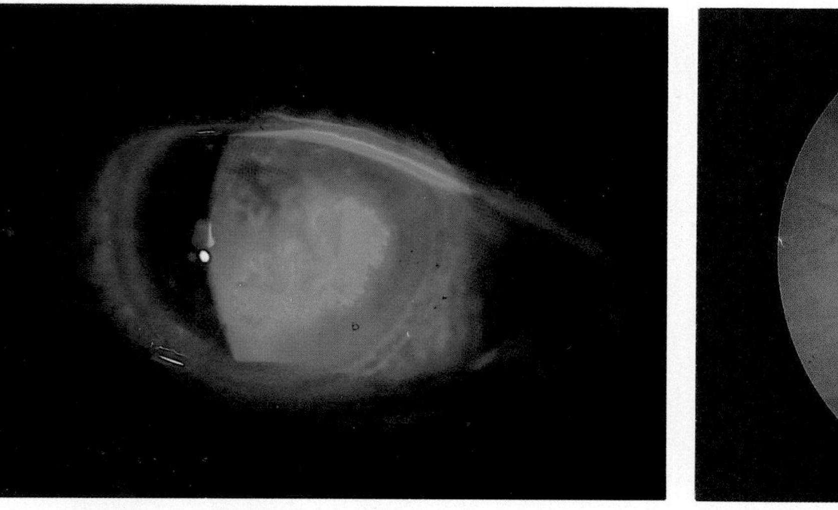

Plate 6 Geographic corneal ulcer due to herpes simplex virus (stained with fluorescein).

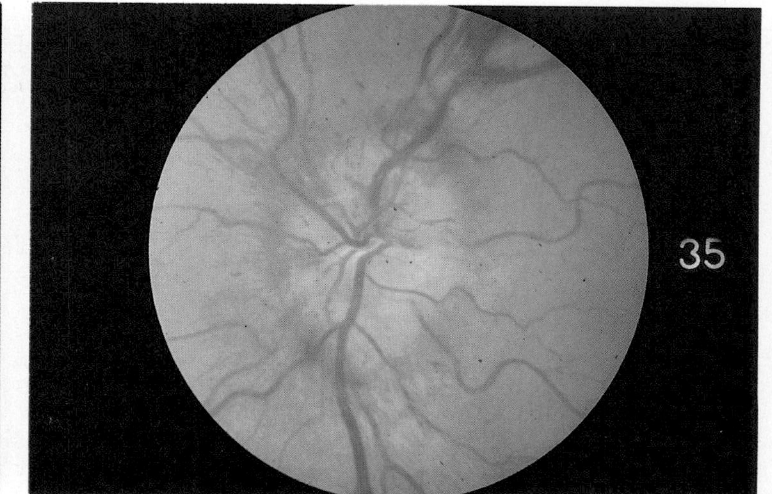

Plate 7 Papilloedema. Note the blurring of the disc margins, the congestion of the veins and flame-shaped haemorrhage.

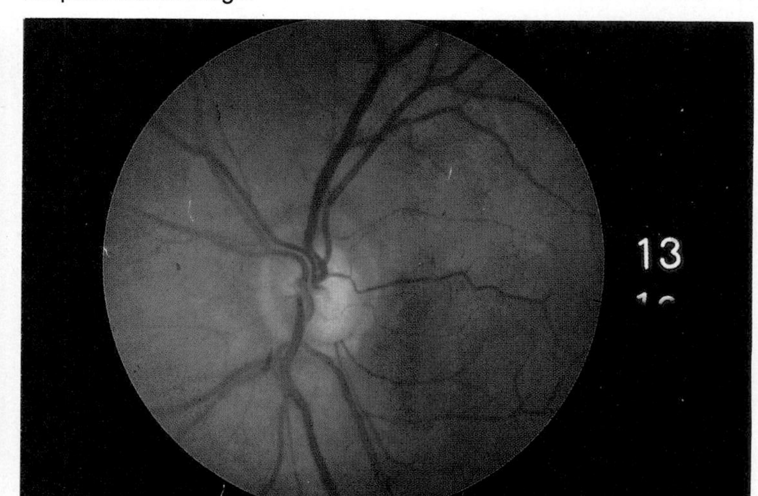

Plate 8 Optic nerve cupping, seen in a left eye. Note the 'disappearing' blood vessels at the infero-temporal margin.

Problem	Goal	Nursing intervention
Changes in normal appearance due to swelling of lacrimal gland involving upper eyelid.	To induce normalization of the anatomy of the upper eyelid.	Administer steroids or antibiotic drugs as prescribed and record same.
Visual disturbance caused by displacement of the globe arising from the tumour, e.g. diplopia.	Minimize visual disturbance.	Offer explanation and ensure patient understands. Relieve diplopia by patching or applying occlusive tape to glasses to cover the affected eye.
Discomfort/pain.	Promote pain-free state.	Administer prescribed analgesia and monitor the effects.
Anxiety due to pain and visual disturbance.	To promote anxiety-free state.	Encourage patient to verbalize fears and anxiety and offer support as necessary.

Treatment of lacrimal gland tumours depends on the type of tumour. Thus mixed cell tumours are treated by careful dissection of the tumour within its capsule. Adenocarcinoma is treated by radical excision, but still carries a poor prognosis. Lymphoma and pseudo-tumour may be treated by radiotherapy, systemic steroids or both.

The physical care of patients undergoing surgery is in principle the same as for patients undergoing major orbital surgery, as described in Chapter 21. Psychological problems are created by the stigma attached to the word 'tumour', and care should be planned according to the individual's response to this knowledge.

Patients requiring radiotherapy are usually referred for specialist treatment. Those patients undergoing conservative treatment may present with the following problems.

Dry Eyes

Dry eyes are a very common problem and can result from a deficiency of any of the tear film components: aqueous, mucin or lipid.

Keratoconjunctivitis sicca may occur as a result of atrophy and fibrosis of the main lacrimal gland with concomitant aqueous tear film deficiency. If the salivary glands are affected, causing a dry mouth, and other mucous membrane involvement is also present, the condition is known as primary Sjögren's syndrome. If there also exists a connective tissue disorder, for example rheumatoid arthritis, the condition may be called secondary Sjögren's syndrome.

Other causes of keratoconjunctivitis sicca include congenital alacrima, surgical removal of the gland and systemic diseases with lacrimal gland involvement, such as sarcoid.

Mucin deficiency may be caused by hypovitaminosis A (xerophthalmia), conjunctival scarring induced by chemical burns, Stevens-Johnson syndrome, ocular cicatricial pemphigoid and trachoma. The goblet cells that usually produce the mucin are destroyed in these conditions.

Deficiency of the superficial lipid layer of the tear film may result from chronic blepharitis, lid trauma or lid surgery with destruction of the meibomian glands, or alteration in their type of secretion.

Whichever type of deficiency or abnormality is present, the symptoms are universal – red, burning, itchy or gritty eyes. Paradoxically, intermittent reflex watering of the eyes may develop.

Signs on examination may be scanty. The marginal tear strip may be reduced in height and the bulbar conjunctiva loses its lustre and may appear thickened and hyperaemic. Mucus strands may be present and mucus filaments may appear attached to corneal epithelium. A fine punctate keratopathy may be present in the interpalpebral zone of the eyes. Rose Bengal 1% will stain the damaged corneal and epithelial cells mainly in the interpalpebral zone, and will highlight the mucous filaments. Note that rose Bengal application is extremely painful in patients with dry eyes and should be used judiciously.

Schirmer's test measures the aqueous components (Chapter 8). If performed without topical anaesthetic, the reflex function of the lacrimal gland is measured, together with the basic secretion. If performed with local anaesthetic in the eye, the basic secretion only is measured (e.g. accessory lacrimal gland function). Less than 5 mm wetting of the filter strip is considered a dry eye, but the test should be repeated on another occasion as it has false positives and negatives.

Severe dry eyes may result in recurrent corneal ulcers, corneal thinning and even perforation. Infections are more common and both corneal scarring and vascularization may result.

Treatment of the dry eye is by tear replacement. Artificial tears such as hypromellose are helpful in all forms. Mucin deficiency may be helped by mucomimetic polymers. If mucus filaments are present then mucolytic substances such as acetylcysteine 10% may be helpful. Avoidance of hot dry atmospheres is advisable and antibiotics to treat recurrent infections are necessary. Punctal occlusion with cautery preserves any natural tears that are present and is of benefit in some patients.

Nursing care is aimed at educating patients to be self-caring, so that they are able to administer their own treatment and to recognize potential complications should they occur.

Problem	Goal	Nursing intervention
Ocular discomfort. Grittiness. Burning. Itchiness.	Relief or prevention of discomfort.	Discuss with the patient the degree of discomfort and how this can be alleviated. Clean and bathe the lids whenever necessary to promote cleanliness and comfort. Instil prescribed drops, e.g. artificial tears, topical antibiotics and mucolytics, as prescribed. Discuss, demonstrate and supervise the patient in the instillation of these drops to encourage or maintain independence where appropriate.
Damage to cornea because of scanty tear film.	Healthy cornea.	Observe the cornea regularly at each dressing for signs of corneal damage – epithelial defect, haziness, ulceration. Ensure drops instilled on time and working effectively, i.e. moist, comfortable eye. Check to ensure adequate lid closure and no corneal exposure. Check to ensure no lashes rubbing and abrading cornea.
Ocular infection.	Normal flora present and no infection introduced.	Maintain moist corneal and conjunctival surfaces by drop instillation mentioned above and by instillation of prescribed topical antibiotics for prophylaxis. Teach patient good hygiene, particularly when he is responsible for self-administration of drops.
Dry mouth in Sjögren's syndrome.	Moist comfortable mouth and mucous membranes.	Discuss with the patient his normal fluid intake and his present requirement. Plan and record individual intake of fluids. Discuss with the patient choice of fluids. Frequent reassessment of the oral mucous membranes. Administer liquids for mastication and swallowing. Planned oral hygiene on an individual basis.
Poor or scanty tear film.	Preservation of tear film by punctal cautery.	Explain to the patient the reason for the procedure and the benefits for him. Explain the steps of the procedure and how the patient may help. Position patient comfortably, instil topical anaesthetic drops, e.g. guttae benoxinate. Comfort the patient during the procedure by holding his hand. Assist the doctor to carry out the procedure as smoothly and efficiently as possible. Check on patient's comfort at the end of the procedure and give prescribed analgesia if required. Observe the lids for bruising and swelling following the procedure.

Disorders of the Outflow Apparatus

Congenital

Congenital obstruction of the nasolacrimal duct usually becomes obvious a few weeks after birth when the formation of tears has started. The lower end of the nasolacrimal duct may not be patent at birth. It usually becomes canalized in the first few weeks of life but occasionally this may be retarded and epiphora results, often with secondary infection and a 'sticky eye'. As a result of stasis, the contents of the lacrimal passages accumulate and become purulent and may be regurgitated through the puncta by pressure over the lacrimal sac. Under these circumstances, massaging of the duct may help to expel the contents. Should the repeated massaging fail, then between 6 months and 1 year of age syringing and probing of the duct is indicated. This is performed under general anaesthesia with an appropriately sized metal probe and may have to be repeated on a further occasion if it fails to work the first time. Care must be taken to prevent the production of false passages with probes and to prevent damage to the lacrimal puncta.

If syringing and probing fails to resolve the epiphora, then intubation of the canaliculi and nasolacrimal duct with solid silicone tubes may be beneficial. This is performed under general anaesthesia and the tubes are left *in situ* for 4–6 months to keep the passages open. If this also fails, formal surgery may be required, particularly if there is persistent dacryocystitis.

Problem	Goal	Nursing intervention
Epiphora causing skin soreness and excoriation.	Relief of the epiphora. Dry and clean unexcoriated skin.	Teach the parents how to carry out massage of the lacrimal sac to express mucopurulent contents. *Technique*: Apply gentle but firm pressure on the skin of the most medial part of the lower lid, behind the most medial part of the anterior lacrimal crest. This may be performed once daily, providing the child is not too distressed. Teach the parents lid toilet and hygiene so that they are able to clean the lids whenever necessary.
Infection (caused by accumulation of lacrimal and conjunctival secretions within the sac) causing mucoid or mucopurulent discharge.	Freedom from infection.	Conjunctival swab taken for culture and sensitivity to determine the causative organism. Teach the parents to administer prescribed antibiotics. Lid toilet as above to remove discharge and sac massage as above.

Acquired

Acquired nasolacrimal obstruction is common in the elderly and may result directly from trauma and infection. The treatment is surgical.

Dacryocystography is very useful in investigating the lacrimal passages. Contrast medium is passed through the lacrimal passages via a small catheter and the passage is outlined by macrography. The site of blockage can be pinpointed accurately to aid the subsequent surgical approach.

Dacryocystorhinostomy entails producing a direct communication from the lacrimal sac into the nose and so bypassing any obstruction in the nasolacrimal duct or lacrimal sac. The operation may be combined with the use of silicone tubing to maintain the patency of the lacrimal passages in some circumstances, especially when the canaliculi are involved in the disease process. If silicone tubing is used it is left in place for 3–6 months before removal. The surgery is often performed under hypotensive anaesthesia to produce an almost bloodless site of operation and hence good visualization. Recently attempts have been made to produce this communication with minimally invasive techniques. Certain lasers are capable of cutting tissues including bone and can produce a communication between the lacrimal sac and the nose by endoscopic technique through the nose. A smaller passage is created but no skin scar is produced as the technique is performed through the nose. Long-term results of this technique are awaited to see if it is as successful as formal surgery.

Injuries to the Outflow Apparatus

Lacerations of the canaliculi are a serious problem because failure to repair them adequately is likely to lead to a lifetime of watering eye. With the use of an operating microscope, the severed end of the affected canaliculus can be identified and approximated over an internal splint of nylon or suture material or silicone tubing. Both canaliculi usually require to be intubated. Fortunately, the incidence of trauma to the lacrimal system has fallen since the introduction of the seat belt law in 1982. The following care plan can be utilized with injured patients.

Dacryocystitis

Infection of the sac is usually a result of obstruction of the nasolacrimal duct. Acute dacryocystitis presents with unilateral painful swelling and redness over the lacrimal sac

Problem	Goal	Nursing intervention
Potential infection following surgery.	Prevention of infection.	Nasal and conjunctival swabs taken for culture and sensitivity if appropriate. Results obtained and reported to doctor. Lid toilet and hygiene performed and patient teaching commenced by discussion, demonstration and supervised practice. Nasal cavities cleaned if appropriate by gentle swabbing with orange sticks and sodium bicarbonate lotion to remove crusts. Instillation of prescribed antibiotic drops.
Safety		
Inability to maintain normotensive state on account of hypotensive anaesthesia.	Safe postoperative course.	Observations of BP, pulse and respiration noted and recorded. (Patients may have been hypotensed during surgery so it is particularly important to observe for signs of bleeding as the blood pressure rises.)
Potential postoperative haemorrhage.	Prevent haemorrhage or detect the same as soon as possible in order to minimize the effects.	Check the wound dressing for signs of bleeding and report immediately. Reinforce dressing with extra gauze swabs if necessary. Check and report any swallowing of blood. Remind patient not to pull or disturb any tubes *in situ* from the canthus to the nostrils. Ensure blood has been sent for group and save preop if requested. Remind patient not to blow his nose as this can introduce infection and cause air to enter the tissues. Remind patient to sneeze with the mouth open to prevent similar problems to above.
Bruising and swelling of tissues around operative site.	Prevention and minimizing of bruising and swelling.	Ensure dressing remains *in situ* until first dressing completed. Once patient fully conscious, observations stable, and the patient feels well enough, allow to sit up.
Pain.	Prevention of pain.	Check and administer prescribed analgesia and record. Observe the effects.
Nausea and vomiting.	Prevention of nausea and vomiting.	Check and administer the prescribed antiemetic and record. Observe the effects.
Mobilization		
May feel slightly dizzy and unsteady; especially after hypotensive anaesthesia.	Return to normal mobility.	Discuss with patient how he is feeling. Sit up first either in bed or in a chair, then gradually mobilize, remaining with the patient while he is walking to ensure he is safe and that balance is normal.

Mobilization – ***continued***

Problem	Goal	Nursing intervention
Tubing may be malpositioned, causing damage to the cornea.	Tubing in correct position.	Note position of tubing at inner canthus and in the nostrils. If malpositioned notify the doctor.
Wound sutures may be loose or not intact.	Well-apposed wound.	Observe the wound edges and sutures and report and record any abnormalities to the medical staff.
	Sutures intact. Wound clean and dry.	Report and record any abnormal findings. Doctor may decide to remove loose suture or to resuture. No dressing required.
Nasal crusting from dried blood.	Clean, comfortable nasal cavities.	Using an orange stick moistened in sodium bicarbonate lotion, the crusts are gently removed from the lower part of the nostrils. If introduced too far up the nostril the orange sticks cause discomfort and will irritate.
Patient preparing for discharge home.	Relaxed, confident patient. Able to instil own topical medication safely. Able to carry out lid toilet and hygiene safely. Aware of abnormalities that may occur and understands when to return to hospital prior to appointment if necessary.	Full discussion and consultation with patient prior to discharge. Teach by demonstration and supervised practice like toilet and drop instillation. Discuss possible complications and explain reasons for return to hospital should they occur. Give time, date and place of next appointment on written card.

together with epiphora. There is often an overlying cellulitis and the patient may have malaise and fever. Staphylococci or streptococci are often the causative agents.

Treatment is with the appropriate systemic antibiotics and warm compresses. If a large abscess forms then incision and drainage may be carried out but there is a risk of fistula formation. Once the acute infection has settled down a dacryocystorhinostomy (DCR) should be performed to alleviate the offending blockage and so prevent further episodes.

Chronic dacryocystitis usually presents with unilateral epiphora, with or without regurgitation of the contents of the lacrimal sac (i.e. mucoid material or pus). Over a period of time the lacrimal sac may enlarge, producing a localized swelling of the sac full of mucoid material known as a mucocele. This is usually painless and some of the contents may be regurgitated through the canaliculi by pressure on the lacrimal sac.

Problem	Goal	Nursing intervention
Anxiety due to:		
– injury	Relieve anxiety.	Encourage patient to verbalize fears. Explain extent of injury to patient and need for hospitalization.
– bleeding;		Clean wound and apply dressing.
– hospitalization.		Inform relatives if necessary.
Potential secondary infection.	Prevent possible infection.	Clean wound and apply dressing.
	Protect from tetanus infection.	Give antibiotics prophylactically as prescribed and record. Give tetanus toxoid injection as prescribed and record.
Postoperative management of wound.	Ensure wound is clean and prevent any complications.	Ensure patient understands management. Clean wound as necessary. Instil antibiotic eye drops as necessary. If nasolacrimal tube is inserted, ensure that patient understands not to remove it. Instruct patient on management plan of care. Instruct patient not to manipulate eyelid when instilling eye drops to prevent breaking down of sutures.

Problem	Goal	Nursing intervention
Pain.	Relief of the pain.	Administration of prescribed analgesia 4–6 hourly as required after discussion with the patient. Application of heat by an appropriate method (i.e. hot spoon bathing) after careful explanation, demonstration and supervised practice.
Infection.	Control of infection.	Following the taking of swabs for culture and sensitivity, administer the prescribed systemic and topical antibiotics. Instruction and education of patient by friendly discussion to enable him to continue treatment at home. Lid toilet as required to ensure lid hygiene and patient comfort. Education of patient and instruction of how to continue lid toilet.
Pyrexia and general malaise due to infection.	Apyrexia.	4-hourly TPR to record changes in body temperature. Administration of prescribed antibiotics (as mentioned above) and antipyretics. Assistance with personal hygiene if required and assistance to change into clean dry clothes if perspiring profusely.
Anxiety due to pain and discomfort.	Relief of anxiety.	Enable patient privacy to discuss anxieties. Explain all treatments given. Explain the disorder and its outcome.

Treatment with topical antibiotics may prevent acute suppuration, but the treatment of choice is a DCR to relieve the obstruction. Probing is of minimal and short-lived success in adults.

Problem	Goal	Nursing intervention
Epiphora.	Relief of epiphora.	Punctal dilation and syringing of the lacrimal sac (Chapter 8). Recording of the findings. Explanation to the patient prior to dacryocystogram. Ensure patient comfort prior to, during and after this examination.
Excoriation and soreness of the skin, lids and cheek.	Dry, unblemished skin.	Lid and skin hygiene and toilet as appropriate. Advice to patient regarding conditions that could exacerbate the problem, e.g. cold winds.
Anxiety and social embarrassment.	Freedom from anxiety. No social embarrassment.	Explanation to the patient about the cause of his condition. Answer questions posed by the patient. Explanation of any treatment or investigation undertaken.

15

Conjunctiva

Andrew Tullo and Deirdre Donnelly

Chapter Summary

The conjunctiva is thought of by some as the 'poor relation' of the cornea. This is because minor conjunctival disturbances do not threaten sight; it is probably also because the conjunctiva is difficult to examine fully and therefore does not get the attention it deserves. However, the conjunctiva is a very important part of the ocular surface. When it is affected by chronic disease the patient may be severely affected and ultimately the cornea, and hence the vision, will suffer.

The majority of conjunctival conditions are treated on an outpatient basis. A patient's involvement in and understanding of care and treatment are, therefore, of the utmost importance, as it is the patient or his family who are going to carry out the treatment.

This chapter covers general guidelines of what nursing care is needed by patients in most common conjunctival conditions.

Functional Anatomy

The epithelium of the conjunctiva and cornea are continuous and together make up the ocular surface. The conjunctiva is composed of a stratified columnar epithelium which blends at the limbus with the corneal epithelium. If the corneal surface is lost through injury the limbus has the capacity to provide a source of replacement cells.

It is convenient to think of the conjunctiva as beginning at the eyelid margin where it forms a 'grey line' as it joins the skin. It lines the inside of the upper and lower lids, where it is tightly bound to the tarsal plates. It is then reflected at the fornices, lying more loosely over the eyeball as it comes forward to a point of insertion at the limbus. The tight binding of the tarsal conjunctiva (i.e. under the lid) is responsible for the characteristic changes that are seen there as a result of inflammation. Likewise the loose adherence over the globe is demonstrated when oedema lifts the conjunctiva to produce chemosis. This is the same space into which subconjunctival drugs are injected.

When the eyelids are closed a sac is effectively formed, lined by the epithelium of the ocular surface, of which 80% is conjunctiva. The function of the conjunctiva is to provide a moist lining to this sac, in order to maintain a clear cornea and a comfortable eye. As such, it is a thin but firm mucous membrane covered by a wear-and-tear epithelium.

At the medial corner (canthus) is a small area of modified skin called the caruncle which may become particularly inflamed in conjunctivitis. Next to it is the plica semilunaris, which is a curved fold. During squint and retinal detachment surgery it may be confused with the edge of the conjunctival incision, and must be avoided.

Numerous goblet cells are distributed in the conjunctiva, principally in the fornices that secrete mucin into the tear film. Mucin is essential to allow the tear film to sit comfortably on the conjunctival surface. Accessory lacrimal glands (of Krause) are also present in the fornices.

The nerve supply to the conjunctiva is from the first division of the trigeminal nerve. If it is defective (e.g. after neurosurgery), such that both the cornea and the conjunctiva are insensitive, there is a considerable risk of corneal ulceration and even perforation. This is particularly likely if a facial palsy is also present, because the protective role of the lids is compromised.

Blood is supplied both externally from the lids and internally from the anterior ciliary arteries, which anastomose at the limbus. The superficial vessels are congested in conjunctivitis and appear bright red. Disease of the eyeball itself, such as acute glaucoma or iritis, results in congestion of the deeper vessels producing a duller purple red.

Unlike the globe, the conjunctiva does have a lymph supply which drains to the preauricular gland. Conjunctivitis associated with a swollen gland in front of the ear should be assumed to be infectious.

CONJUNCTIVITIS

Inflammation of the conjunctiva is the most common eye condition of all and makes up a large proportion of cases of 'red eye' (Figure 15.1). The symptoms of conjunctivitis are soreness, watering, discharge and foreign body sensation.

In several ways the conjunctiva is like the throat. It is a mucous membrane generously supplied by lymphoid tissue designed to deal with organisms that pass that way. When inflamed this tissue enlarges, forming lumps, just visible to the naked eye, called follicles. The same

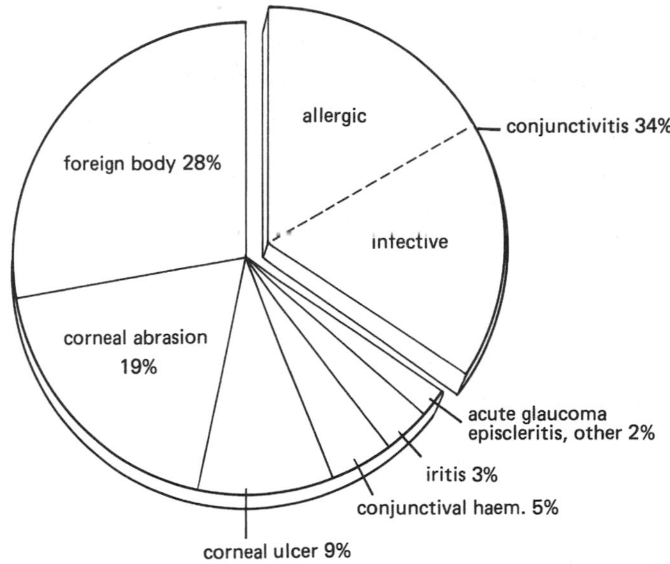

Figure 15.1 The cause of 'red eye' in a series of 500 consecutive new cases.

organisms infect the throat and conjunctiva, sometimes simultaneously.

The principal agents are the adenoviruses, which are notorious for spreading to other patients in eye departments, sometimes in epidemic proportions. Thus hand-washing and careful hygienic practice are of utmost importance for all staff. Adult patients should also be advised to use their own towel, flannel and pillow case; they should if possible administer their own treatment, and always wash their hands before and after touching the eye. If they follow this advice they pose little threat to other members of the family or those at work. If a child is thought to have an infectious conjunctivitis they should be off school until symptoms and signs have 'peaked'. After this stage organisms become very difficult to isolate.

Although the precise organism in conjunctivitis will remain unknown in most cases, the experienced observer can often make the correct diagnosis from the history and slit-lamp findings. This is important because the results of laboratory investigations often take days to come through (see below).

Conjunctivitis is treated primarily with the instillation of topical medication in the form of eye drops. Most patients present in the Accident and Emergency Department and so the nurse is in contact with the patient for only a short time. During this time she has to ensure that the patient is able and willing to carry out his treatment at home.

Problem	Goal	Nursing intervention
Patient unaware how to instil eyedrops because of insufficient knowledge and/ or skill.	To ensure patient is able and willing to comply with treatment regime.	1. Explain purpose and frequency of treatment to patient. 2. Advise patient (or parent, etc.) always to wash hands before and after procedure (to prevent spread of infection). 3. Explain how drop instillation is carried out – tip head back, pull down lower lid with one hand while holding the drop bottle in the other like a pen, positioning hand with bottle so that drop falls into lower fornix without bottle touching eye, lids or lashes. 4. Demonstrate procedure and then allow patient to instil the drops under supervision. 5. Ensure patient is happy with this technique and is aware of the frequency and purpose of the drops. 6. Remind patient to wash hands after the procedure.

Although not painful, conjunctivitis is nevertheless fairly uncomfortable for the sufferer. Unpleasant symptoms will resolve once the condition has been successfully treated, but it is much appreciated by the patient if the nurse can suggest means of providing symptomatic relief in the meantime.

Some of the symptoms experienced with conjunctivitis and how these can be dealt with are covered below.

Problem	Goal	Nursing intervention
Patient is unable to open eyes properly due to discomfort from bright lights.	To relieve photophobia.	1. Advise patient to avoid brightly lit rooms and sunny places while conjunctivitis persists. 2. Suggest wearing of dark glasses. 3. Explain that photophobia will disappear as condition improves.
Eyelids crusted and stuck together, particularly in the morning, due to accumulation of discharge.	To relieve problems of crusting.	1. Teach patient how to carry out lid hygiene. 2. Instruct him to boil one pint of water with one teaspoon of salt, allow to cool and then bathe eye using cotton wool balls or clean tissues until crusting has cleared. 3. Repeat for other eye, using different tissues/cotton wool. Renew solution daily.
Eyes watering due to reflex lacrimation arising from irritation.	To relieve discomfort without spreading infection.	1. Explain that watering will ease as condition improves. 2. Advise use of tissues and not hankies. 3. Use separate tissues for each eye to prevent spread of infection.
Patient complaining of gritty sensation in eyes due to actual condition.	To ease discomfort.	1. Explain that the grittiness is to be expected and will ease as condition improves. 2. If it is extremely irritating, advise patient to take mild analgesia, e.g. paracetamol.

The importance of avoiding the further spread of the infection has already been pointed out. Advice on preventing the spread of infection to, for example, other members of the family is therefore an essential part of patient education in the treatment of conjunctivitis.

Problem	Goal	Nursing Intervention
Potential risk of infection spreading to another person because of lack of knowledge on the patient's behalf.	To enable the patient to prevent further spread of infection.	1. Explain to patient that conjunctivitis can easily be spread to those with whom he is in close contact. 2. Outline importance of careful hygiene, always washing hands after touching eyes or instilling drops. 3. Advise the use of separate towels, flannels, etc. from other family members until the infection is cured. 4. Do not allow anyone else to use the same drop bottle. 5. Avoid close contact with others while infection is present; avoid picking up and hugging children as infection is easily spread.

Infectious Agents

Adenoviruses

These are the most important cause of conjunctivitis. They are both the commonest identifiable agent and highly infectious. There are a number of different serotypes, some of which cause a particularly severe keratoconjunctivitis and on occasion lasting visual disturbance due to characteristic round corneal lesions. Antibiotic drops are normally given for this usually self-limiting condition, even though it is a viral infection. It is important to keep follow-up appointments to a minimum to prevent cross-infection.

Herpes Simplex Virus

This virus is best known for recurrent keratitis (Chapter 16). However, it may also cause an acute follicular conjunctivitis when encountered by a non-immune individual, in other words someone who is meeting the virus for the first time. Vesicles on the lid margin are a clue to the diagnosis. Treatment is with an antiviral agent such as acyclovir, and complete recovery is the rule.

Bacteria

True bacterial conjunctivitis in the otherwise healthy individual is less common than generally supposed. Normal commensal organisms may be blamed and antibiotic drops are commonly prescribed on entirely speculative grounds. When present it is most likely to be due to *Staphylococcus aureus*.

There are, however, two particular bacteria that deserve particular consideration.

Chlamydia is the cause of a common sexually transmitted disease. In the West, at least, ocular infection is uncommon (see also Chapter 23). However, it occasionally causes conjunctivitis in the young adult. Treatment is with tetracycline 1% drops and ointment. Tablets are also required to eradicate the genitourinary tract infection that is the source of the infection. *Neisseria gonorrhoeae* is an unusual cause of eye infection in the adult but, like *Chlamydia*, originates from the genital tract.

The most important feature is that a baby born to a woman whose genital tract is infected by either of these two organisms is likely to develop ophthalmia neonatorum (conjunctivitis within 30 days of birth). This condition may require hospitalization and intensive treatment. *Chlamydia* responds to intensive topical tetracycline and systemic erythromycin (systemic tetracycline stains the future teeth and must not be prescribed). Infection with the gonococcus is potentially more serious as the cornea can become involved, causing blindness. The treatment of choice is intensive penicillin drops, though some strains are now resistant.

This situation requires delicate handling by the nurse, as the mother will need to have treatment as well as the baby. The mother may well feel guilty and responsible for having caused the infection and thereby harming her baby. At this stage it is vital that the baby's care is not taken out of her hands and that she does not feel pushed to one side; the nurse should encourage her to be fully involved in both the baby's general care and its eye treatment.

Sticky eye is, in fact, common in the newborn and is mostly due to staphylococcal infection which generally responds well to chloramphenicol 1% ointment or fucidic acid and does not come to the attention of the eye unit.

ALLERGY

Conjunctivitis is commonly of an allergic nature. It may occur in association with other allergic reactions such as hay fever or asthma, or it may be localized in the eye.

The common features of allergic conjunctivitis are follicles and chemosis (jelly-like oedema). The condition may be seasonal and is usually self-limiting.

Problem	Goal	Nursing intervention
Mother feels responsible for baby's condition and may feel that she is not a good mother. Both mother and baby require treatment to eradicate infection.	To promote maternal bonding by encouraging mother to be involved in baby's care and to eradicate infection.	1. Explain to mother the probable means by which her baby acquired the infection and the need for both to have further treatment. 2. Ensure mother is allowed and encouraged to be involved in baby's general care so that she does not feel inadequate. 3. Encourage mother to seek treatment for herself and try to make her feel less responsible for the situation. 4. Involve mother in the care of her baby's eye infection by teaching her how to instil drops, clean baby's eyes and, if only one eye is affected, explain the importance of lying baby on her affected side to prevent the infection from spreading to the other eye.

The cause of the allergy is usually hard to identify but there are a number of possible causes that the patient may already be aware of. Both nurse and patient can then work together to cope with the allergen (e.g. pollen, animals) responsible in his particular case.

Problem	Goal	Nursing intervention
Patient is unaware of cause of allergy so there is a risk of the symptoms continuing unabated or of them recurring at a later date.	To identify cause of allergy and to ensure the patient has the necessary knowledge regarding avoidance of the specific allergen.	1. Explain the nature of an allergic response to the patient. 2. Suggest potential allergens and determine by discussion with the patient whether there is any possibility of one of these being responsible in his case. 3. Discuss the course of the allergic reaction with the patient: its duration; whether it is seasonal or worse at any particular time, e.g. after meals; specific foods eaten; drops used; make-up worn; contact lens fluids used; and also other factors that give rise to general allergic reactions, such as house dust, feathers, animals, etc. 4. Eliminate possible causes one by one until, if possible, a single allergen is identified. Advise patient to avoid this.

The patient with an allergy may be prescribed drops if the condition caused is severe, in which case he will need tuition about drop instillation as given to patients with infective conjunctivitis.

Dealing with an allergy can be a protracted affair, and indeed the allergen may never be identified. It can be worrying for the patient not to know what is causing the condition, particularly if it recurs frequently. Should this happen the nurse should play a supportive role and provide encouragement to help him during this period.

A minority of individuals are seriously affected by allergic eye disease. They are children and young adults who are often highly atopic (i.e. have eczema and/or asthma). Chronic severe conjunctivitis requires careful supervision by both the hospital and the parents, especially if steroid drops are needed. Some patients develop a 'cobblestone'-like appearance under the upper lid, which may be associated with corneal ulceration. This is a sight-threatening complication which occasionally requires scraping under general anaesthesia to help resolution. Black patients appear to be particularly prone to involvement of the limbus in allergic disease.

Some contact lens wearers develop a 'giant papillary conjunctivitis' under the upper lid. This may be improved by a change in contact lens solution, although it is sometimes so troublesome that the lenses have to be abandoned.

Laboratory Investigation

The surface of the eye is readily accessible and a number of different investigations are possible and often helpful in diagnosis. These apply equally to the investigation of corneal disease.

Culture

A conjunctival swab is taken by rolling a cotton-tip applicator firmly across the length of the lower fornix. In the case of a corneal ulcer, including dendritic ulcers, the lesion itself is swabbed, preferably at the slit-lamp. For suspected chlamydial infection the result is more likely to be positive if the applicator is rolled firmly up under the upper lid.

The swab is then placed directly on to a culture plate or into transport medium. Such media are different for bacteria, *Chlamydia* and viruses. It is obviously important that specimens reach the laboratory as soon as possible, with as much information for the laboratory as possible.

The result of a bacterial swab may be available the next day. Herpes virus takes 3 days to appear in culture and adenoviruses and *Chlamydia* take several days or longer. In the meantime the diagnosis and hence the treatment are based on clinical impression.

Cytology

A scraping can be used to provide a quick answer by staining and microscopic examination.

Gram staining gives an immediate answer as to whether bacteria are present in large numbers. It may provide a clue but does not tell precisely which organism is responsible. On the very rare occasion when fungi are present branching hyphae may be seen.

Using Giemsa stain the presence of large numbers of particular cells may give a clue to the diagnosis; for example, lymphocytes suggest viral infection.

Electron Microscopy

Although not routine, electron microscopy of tear samples can on occasion demonstrate the presence of viral particles within a matter of hours.

Serology

In suspected viral infection the taking of blood samples separated by an interval of 10 days can show a diagnostic rise in antibody levels to the causative organism. By the time these results are available the condition may have resolved and therefore the usefulness of this test is limited. Single serum samples are usually a waste of laboratory time.

The use of more sophisticated methods such as those based on the polymerase chain reaction (PCR) is likely to become more commonplace in the future and may allow diagnosis to be made in the clinic or casualty department.

Problem	Goal	Nursing intervention
Patient unaware of what taking a conjunctival swab will require of him because of lack of specific knowledge.	To prepare patient for test prior to its being carried out.	1. Explain purpose of test to patient, how it is done and what he will be expected to do during it. Ensure he understands. 2. Ask him to sit back in a chair (or to lie down) with head well supported, open eyes and look up. 3. Pull down lower lid gently and explain that patient will feel slight discomfort as swab is rolled along the length of the lower fornix from the inner to the outer canthus. 4. Once taken, place swab in appropriate transport medium and wash hands. 5. Tell patient that the test is over. Ensure he is all right and that eye feels comfortable. Inform him of when results will be known.

Spontaneous Conjunctival Haemorrhage

The sudden appearance of a bright red patch on the white of the eye will often bring an alarmed patient to the Accident Department. While there is occasionally some sensation associated with the onset, such haemorrhages are usually silent. Consequently they are often noticed first by someone else, thus adding to the worry. In the vast majority of cases this is an innocent condition and requires no treatment. The patient may be hypertensive, so the blood pressure should be checked. Systemic steroids seem to be the cause in some instances. Occasionally it is brought on by a coughing or sneezing bout.

Problem	Goal	Nursing intervention
Patient anxious due to the sudden appearance of his red eye.	To reassure patient that his red eye is harmless.	1. Explain that this redness is caused by a tiny burst blood vessel in the eye and will resolve within 2–3 weeks. 2. Ask patient if he had coughed or sneezed or been doing any marked physical activity shortly before he noticed it, as this could have caused it. 3. Measure and record patient's blood pressure and report any abnormality to the medical staff. 4. Reassure patient that it will not do him any harm.

Trauma

Laceration

A small laceration to the conjunctiva will heal of its own accord, but a larger laceration, especially if dirty, requires cleaning and suturing if the edges of the wound are not properly apposed. This is normally done under local anaesthetic. In the case of a child, a general anaesthetic will be needed, which has the advantage of allowing a full examination of the eye. It is the responsibility of the nurse to ease any anxiety by explaining what the procedure involves (and by assisting the doctor in the performance of the procedure). A drop of topical anaesthetic will often allow a further examination.

Problem	Goal	Nursing intervention
Patient is apprehensive due to prospect of having to have stitches in his eye.	To relieve anxiety by making the patient aware of what will happen to him. To ensure patient is comfortable during and after procedure.	1. Explain procedure to patient by telling him what he will be expected to do during it, how long it will take and what it will feel like. 2. Point out that he will be asked to lie flat, with his head on a hard pillow (and that his head and other eye will be covered by a sterile sheet), that local anaesthetic drops will be put in his eye, which will sting at first but which will soon feel numb, and that he will be asked to lie very still for 10–30 minutes. Emphasize the fact that, although the procedure is disconcerting and uncomfortable, he will feel no actual pain although he will be aware of someone touching his eye/eyelids. 3. Warn patient that if he should feel that he wants to cough or sneeze, he should indicate this rather than try to prevent it from happening. 4. After procedure, if shaken, allow the patient to stay lying down until he feels better. Offer him a cup of tea and the chance to sit and rest quietly for a while before going home.

The risk of infection following injury is covered by the use of antibiotic drugs and ointment. The patient who will be responsible for carrying out the treatment must know when and how to instil the medication.

Problem	Goal	Nursing intervention
Risk of infection developing in the conjunctiva following laceration. Patient unaware of this potential problem.	To prevent/reduce the risk of infection developing.	1. Explain to patient that there is a risk of infection developing in the eye because of the wound. 2. Discuss the recommended treatment with him and explain how it is carried out. 3. Allow the patient to instil any prescribed antibiotics drops/ointment under supervision, emphasizing the importance of washing hands before and after doing this. 4. Tell him how long the course should last and outline the symptoms that might occur should infection develop: increased reddening of the eye, irritation, discharge, crusting and stickiness, and to return to the hospital if this occurs. 5. Reassure patient that the wound will probably heal quickly and that infection is unlikely to develop if the treatment is carried out correctly.

Foreign Bodies

Patients frequently attend the Accident and Emergency Department with 'something in their eye'. The foreign body in question can be anything from a fly to a speck of metal. Treatment is by removal using the same approach as for a subtarsal foreign body (Chapter 6).

It is important, however, that a proper nursing history is taken before any attempt is made to remove the foreign body. If, for example, the object was a piece of metal travelling at high speed into the eye there is a risk of it penetrating the globe, in which case a different course of action is required.

Exposure of the Conjunctiva

Exposure of the conjunctiva may develop for a variety of reasons: proptosis, burns, injury to the lid resulting in inadequate coverage of the conjunctiva, or chemosis of the conjunctiva following surgery or direct injury to the conjunctiva.

Problem	Goal	Nursing intervention
Patient unable to close his eyes fully due to exposed conjunctiva preventing lid closure.	To relieve patient's discomfort and to prevent permanent damage to conjunctiva by keeping it moist.	1. Explain to patient what you are about to do and why. 2. Moisten/lubricate exposed conjunctiva with prescribed ointment, cover with Bactigras or Vaseline gauze if ordered. Cover with eyepad. 3. Try to close eyelids as much as possible. Ensure eye remains moist and is not in direct contact with the pad. 4. Assess degree of proptosis, chemosis, etc. daily and treat underlying cause as appropriate. 5. Ensure patient's eye feels comfortable to him.

Systemic Disease

Severe conjunctival damage may result from involvement in two generalized conditions.

Stevens–Johnson Syndrome

This is an acute condition, usually occurring in the first three decades, which may be brought on by drugs such as sulphonamides, or infection by some viruses. Often, however, the cause is not known. Multiple skin lesions, called **erythema multiforme**, are associated with ulceration of both the mouth and conjunctiva, which may be very severe. In young children involvement of the lungs may be life-threatening. The condition is self-limiting, but may leave the conjunctiva so damaged that the patient is left with chronically sore eyes and poor vision for the rest of his life. The damage can be limited by the use of intensive steroid drops in the very early stages.

Cicatrizing Pemphigoid

This is another condition of the mucous membranes, this time affecting the elderly. It is often slow in onset, but at its worst can result in chronically inflamed eyes and eventually corneal vascularization and blindness. Early intervention with steroids and tear supplements improves the prognosis. Nursing care in these cases must depend on the underlying cause of the conjunctival problem, the treatment being given for this and the effect the disorder is having on the patient.

Conjunctival Degenerations and Tumours

Pingueculum

This is a common benign change resulting in a yellow-white lesion close to the nasal limbus. No treatment is required.

Pterygium

In this disorder a tongue-shaped sheet of tissue grows on to the cornea from the nasal limbus. It is very common in tropical regions but rarely develops in temperate climates. Surgery may be indicated for cosmetic reasons or because the lesion has encroached on the pupillary area and affects the vision. Surgery may be followed by recurrence, in which case irradiation becomes necessary.

Dermoid

This is a congenital lesion, usually found at the limbus, which may contain hair! Excision is possible for cosmetic reasons; a partial-thickness corneal graft is used. Reassurance as to the non-malignant nature of the above lesions should be given.

Pigmented Lesions

Benign patches of pigment are common in the conjunctiva of black patients and occasionally occur in caucasians. Any such lesion which undergoes a change in size or colour requires excision to achieve a histological diagnosis. Any new pigmented lesion of the conjunctiva should be considered as possibly malignant and excised with the aid of the operating microscope.

Conjunctival tumours are rare but when they occur they produce the same response in the patient as any other tumour – fear, anxiety and apprehension. In order to deal with these reactions it is first of all important to determine whether the tumour is benign or malignant.

Malignant tumours are generally characterized by fairly rapid change in size and possibly in pigmentation. Action needs to be taken rapidly to prevent spread, and wide excision of the tumour with postoperative irradiation may be indicated. The nurse can do a lot to help the patient to come to terms with the problem.

Problem	Goal	Nursing intervention
Anxiety and fear caused by knowledge of a malignant tumour in the conjunctiva.	To alleviate anxiety and provide reassurance and support.	1. Discuss situation with patient. Allow him to express his feelings; anger, horror, fear, resentment, etc. 2. Try to answer any question he may have. 3. Provide emotional support and reassurance both pre- and postoperatively. 4. Discuss situation with relatives, if the patient wishes this. Help them to express how they feel and try to suggest ways in which they can help by involving them in both the physical and psychological care of the patient.
Patient unprepared for surgery to remove tumour as he does not know what this involves.	To prepare patient mentally and physically for theatre by explaining situation to him.	1. Outline procedure and preparation, explaining what the patient is expected to do. Ensure he understands this. 2. Discuss physical preparation for theatre and carry it out as appropriate. 3. Talk over any particular worries he may have regarding surgery. 4. Give a brief description of aftercare and what he can expect to feel like.

Long-term follow-up will be needed for the patient following the removal of a malignant conjunctival tumour and if possible the nursing staff with whom he has become familiar during this early stage should be involved.

16

Cornea and Sclera

Andrew Elliott and Gail Thomas

Chapter Summary

Cornea

Sclera

Cornea

The cornea is the transparent anterior part of the structural coat of the eye. Its interface with air is the principal site of refraction of light in the eye. As such, its clarity and uniformity must be maintained, and if it is damaged by scarring or disease, there is a significant loss in visual acuity.

Any loss or disturbance of vision is very distressing to the patient. The nurse should be aware that these psychological problems may form a major aspect of her nursing care when looking after patients with corneal scarring or disease. Many such conditions are treated in the Accident and Emergency Department, so the nurse is in contact with the patient for only a short time. Certain corneal conditions, such as severe keratitis and injury, that need intensive therapy necessitate admission to hospital. The nurse is then involved with all aspects of inpatient care.

Functional Anatomy

The cornea has an ordered, five-layered structure on which its clarity depends (Figure 16.1). It has a diameter of approximately 11 mm and is a mere 0.5 mm thick in the centre. Not only must light pass through the cornea but it must also be refracted. Slight differences in the radius of curvature result in astigmatism (Chapter 12).

Layers 1 & 2: The Epithelium and Basement Membrane

To ensure an even surface the superficial cells of the epithelium have tiny projections (microvilli) holding a fine layer of mucus, which is the inner layer of the tear film (Chapter 14) and which makes the cornea 'wettable'. The epithelium is a highly active tissue. Thus, when the cornea is abraded, cells slide in to fill the gap and multiply to replenish its several layers. The cornea derives most of its oxygen supply from the atmosphere. If it is deprived of this by overwear of a contact lens, swelling of the cornea occurs, particularly of the epithelium.

The stability of the epithelium depends on its fixation to its basement membrane. If this is damaged by injury or disease recurrent spontaneous ulceration is a possible future consequence.

The cornea is richly innervated exclusively by sensory nerves belonging to division I of the trigeminal nerve. The nerve endings lie in the epithelium, making the corneal surface a highly sensitive area.

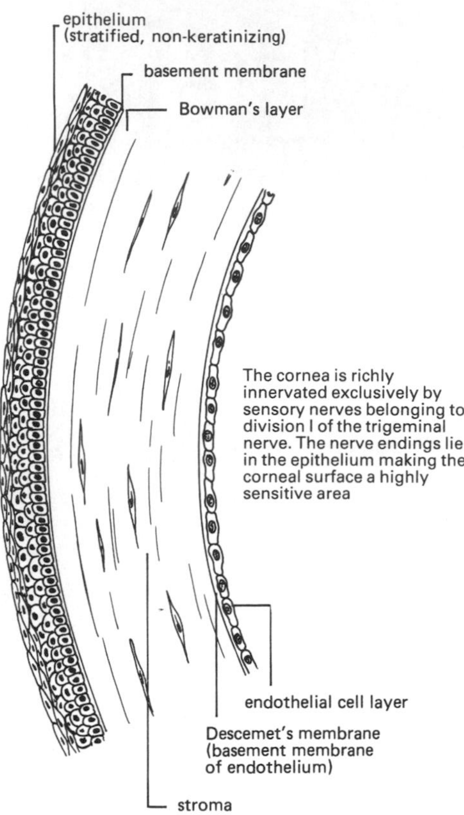

Figure 16.1 The cornea, showing its five layers.

Layer 3: Bowman's Membrane and the Stroma

Beneath the basement membrane lies a compressed part of the stroma called Bowman's 'membrane'. If this is damaged by injury or disease lasting opacification is inevitable and if it occurs in the visual axis vision will suffer.

In the stroma proper there are highly organized collagen fibrils through which light can pass. Disruption of the regular design causes corneal opacification. The few cells scattered within the stroma are called keratocytes. They are normally quiescent, but after injury or corneal surgery they become active. They then lay down and arrange new collagen, which is responsible for wound healing.

Layers 4 & 5: Descemet's Membrane and Endothelium

The innermost layers of the cornea are endothelium lying upon Descemet's membrane.It is a single layer of cells with no capacity to regenerate. It is responsible for pumping water out of the cornea in order to keep it 'dehydrated' and thereby regular and transparent. Once the endothelium is damaged the cornea becomes swollen, opaque and painful.

Foreign Bodies and Injuries

The commonest corneal problem is the foreign body, often in industrial workers and DIY enthusiasts. There is usually a history of 'something going into the eye' but the patient may complain of a gritty, watery and photophobic eye without this background. Most foreign bodies are metallic

(Plate 4) and if ferrous, cause a surrounding rust ring in the superficial stroma.

Surface fragments can be removed with a moistened cotton bud but for the embedded foreign body less damage to the cornea is caused by using a hypodermic needle point under slit-lamp magnification. The rust ring is removed, causing as little damage to the stroma as possible. This is surprisingly pain-free if a few drops of anaesthetic are used (e.g. amethocaine). The risk of corneal infection is reduced by using antibiotic drops for a few days and the eye can be kept comfortable with cycloplegic drops (e.g. mydrilate). A small residual stromal scar and depression often result but this is only a problem if the central cornea is involved, when blurring and glare ensue. Foundry workers and sandblasters are at particular risk and should wear eye protection.

Foreign bodies lodged under the upper eyelid (subtarsal foreign body) cause similar symptoms and the cornea may be abraded as the lid moves up and down. Nurses should know how to evert the eyelid (Chapter 10) in order to remove such a foreign body.

Corneal abrasions, caused by garden twigs, toddlers' fingers or contact lenses, for example, can be extremely painful and the eye is intensely photophobic and waters copiously. Abrasions stain brightly with fluorescein drops which are then usually visible to the naked eye. Relief is obtained by dilating the pupil and firmly padding the eye closed until the epithelium is healed. It may take two or three days for the epithelium to slide and replicate to fill the gap, but healing is often surprisingly rapid.

In some patients the new epithelium does not adhere very well to the basement membrane and can easily be disturbed, giving rise to the recurrent abrasion syndrome, in which symptoms can recur spontaneously or after trivial trauma like rubbing the eye. Ointment to lubricate the surface, especially at night, is helpful but recurrences are possible even years after the original trauma.

Lacerations of the cornea are commonly due to broken glass and are now much less frequent since car seat-belt legislation. Pain is not a good guide to severity and signs such as distortion of the pupil, visible aqueous leak and a soft eye are important indications of ocular perforation. Radiography is essential as fragments of metal or glass may be inside the eye and should be removed.

Small, high-speed fragments of metal can penetrate the eye, classically when a heavy hammer hits a metal chisel, causing a splinter of metal to fly off; collision of metal on metal in other industrial settings can produce the same result. The entry wound may not be obvious so it is important to suspect the injury. Penetration of the eye may subsequently be complicated by cataract and retinal detachment.

The nurse is one of the first people the patient sees. There is a need to identify the cause and extent of the injury. The nurse usually takes a history and the eye is examined.

Problem	Goal	Nursing intervention
Injury to the eye of unknown extent.	To ensure correct action is taken.	1. Take a history from the patient, finding out how and where the injury took place. Explain reasons for questions in order to identify foreign body if present, or extent of injury – whether X-rays are needed or if surgery may need to be performed. 2. Examine the eye. It may be necessary to instil fluorescein; asking the patient to look up, one drop is instilled into lower fornix. 3. Explain reason for instilling the eye drops to the patient. Explain that a bright light may be shone into the eye and the patient will be asked to look in different directions. 4. Identify the extent of the injury and take appropriate action.

As corneal foreign bodies and superficial injuries, e.g. abrasion, cause the patient to have pain, it may be impossible for the nurse to examine the eye without first relieving the pain.

Problem	Goal	Nursing intervention
Pain due to abrasion or foreign body irritating the eye.	To ease pain and allow examination of the eye.	1. Sit patient in a chair with his head on head rest. 2. Explain the reason for instilling the anaesthetic drops into the eye, that they will ease the pain and allow patient to open the eye. 3. Warn patient that the drops may sting, but that this will quickly wear off. 4. Ensure patient is comfortable and able to open the eye after the instillation of the drops.

After examination of the eye, if a foreign body is present and it is superficial, it can be removed with the aid of magnification. If a superficial abrasion is present following foreign body removal, there is a need to promote healing and prevent secondary infection.

It may be necessary for the patient to return to the Accident and Emergency Department in 48 hours for removal of the rust ring from a ferrous foreign body.

Problem	Goal	Nursing intervention
Irritation of the eye due to foreign body.	Patient will be relieved of discomfort following removal of the foreign body.	1. The procedure for removing the foreign body should be explained to patient, ensuring he understands what he has been told. 2. Instil anaesthetic drops into the eye if they have not already been instilled – explaining reason for the drops. 3. The patient should be seated at the slit-lamp with head forward and chin on rest. 4. Ensure patient understands to keep very still and does exactly as requested. 5. Inform patient that slight pressure may be felt, but no pain. 6. The nurse, if specially trained, or doctor gently removes the foreign body with aid of a 21G disposable hypodermic needle or moistened cotton bud, being careful to avoid damage to surrounding corneal epithelium. 7. The nurse may assist the doctor if necessary by holding the patient's upper lid and steadying patient's head. 8. Ensure patient's comfort on completion of the procedure.
Risk of secondary infection following removal of foreign body.	Patient to understand the reasons for complying with treatment.	1. Antibiotic ointment should be instilled into the eye and an eye pad applied. 2. The patient should be told the reason for the eye ointment and the pad. Instruct patient to keep the pad on the eye for at least 24 hours to allow the epithelium to heal. 3. If ointment or drops are prescribed for use at home, the frequency and reason for the drops should be explained to the patient. 4. Advise patient to return for check if requested by doctor, or if eye does not settle after a few days.
Pain due to corneal abrasion and potential problem of secondary infection due to break in corneal integrity.	To relieve irritation, prevent infection and promote healing. Patient to report pain levels at acceptable limit to him and understand the reasons for compliance with treatment.	1. Instil antibiotic ointment or drops as prescribed and show patient how to do this. 2. Pad the eye for 24 hours to promote healing. 3. Ensure the patient understands the importance of keeping the eyelids closed underneath the pad. 4. Ensure the patient can comply with treatment and that he is made aware of potential complications, e.g. risk of infection, delayed healing, recurrent abrasion. 5. Give patient sufficient eye pads for use at home and give date and time for review in Accident Department. 6. Give the patient advice on suitable analgesics.

If the eye is padded to help healing, this leads to a visual limitation and the nurse should ensure that the patient is aware of the dangers (Chapter 6).

Problem	Goal	Nursing intervention
Visual disturbance caused by pad that could lead to physical injury.	Patient to understand the need for increased awareness of ensuring his own safety.	1. Explain the effect of visual field loss that padding the eye causes. 2. Giving reasons, instruct the patient not to drive a car or operate machinery while the eye is padded. 3. Advise the patient to take extra care when crossing the road. 4. Ensure patient understands the information given. 5. Give reassurance that this is only a temporary measure to aid healing.

Corneal injuries vary greatly in extent, from a small laceration to actual penetration. These injuries require surgical intervention, which necessitates admission to hospital. The nurse is then involved in all aspects of inpatient care.

If there is a penetrating injury it may be necessary to reform the anterior chamber, abscise an iris prolapse if present and suture the wound. The patient would be admitted as an urgency and would need to be prepared for theatre soon afterwards.

This can be a frightening experience for patients, particularly young adults. The nurse needs to give reassurance and psychological support during this preoperative period and, following surgery, should ensure the patient understands any precautions that need to be taken to promote healing and prevent complications.

A traumatic cataract may be forming and the patient may have noticed a deterioration in vision. The patient should be told that this will be dealt with at a later date.

The patient is usually followed up in the Outpatient Department until the wound is completely healed. It should be explained to the patient that any sutures in the eye may have to be removed at a later date and that when the eye has settled his vision will be fully assessed. This may remain blurred during the healing period while drops are being instilled, and especially if further surgery is going to be necessary.

Problem	Goal	Nursing intervention
Patient unprepared for emergency surgery and anxious over what is going to happen because of lack of knowledge.	Patient to be mentally and physically prepared for emergency surgery by the time of operation.	1. Establish patient's knowledge base. 2. Outline preoperative procedure and preparation, explaining what the patient will have to do. Make sure he understands what he has been told. 3. Allow patient to ask questions about surgery and voice any fears. 4. If the patient is young, ensure parents are able to talk to the doctor about any worries they may have. 5. Give supportive reassurance to family. 6. Discuss physical preparation for theatre and carry this out accordingly. 7. Give a brief outline of postoperative care, what patient should expect and feel. 8. Giving reasons, inform the patient that the eye may be covered for 24 hours with a pad or shield and that he may be expected to stay on bed rest during this period. 9. Advise the patient that eye drops will be instilled after surgery to prevent infection and it will be necessary for the patient or patient's family to continue this treatment at home. 10. Systemic antibiotics may be recommended. Explain reason for this medication to patient and administer as prescribed.
Risk of infection or wound rupture due to patient not being aware of postoperative precautions.	Patient to be fully educated regarding the prevention of postoperative complications.	1. Teach patient or relative to instil eye drops as prescribed and provide supervised practice to develop and consolidate the skill, giving reasons. 2. Advise patient to avoid putting hankies near the eye and never to rub the eye. If eye waters, wipe cheek with clean tissue. 3. Giving reasons, advise the patient to wear protective eye shield at night for 2 weeks. 4. Advise patient to avoid heavy lifting and to stay away from work or school until medical staff say it is safe to restart. 5. Ensure patient understands information and is aware of early signs of problems: if there is pain, if vision deteriorates or eye becomes sticky to seek medical attention immediately.

Burns

The three types of burn affecting the ocular surface are chemical, thermal and radiation. In all cases it is important that first aid treatment is given rapidly in order to minimize any damage to the eye.

Chemical Injury

A variety of chemicals can damage the cornea; some can render the cornea permanently opaque, whereas others may damage only the epithelium. Alkalis such as ammonia and sodium hydroxide have a justifiably terrible reputation as they break down tissue barriers in the cornea and penetrate deeply.

It is vitally important to irrigate the eye at once with copious amounts of water. Fancy eye washes and eye baths may be available but putting the victim's head under the nearest cold tap is likely to be quicker and speed is more important than technique. In hospital the eye is anaesthetized with drops and the irrigation is repeated. An i.v. giving set with normal saline is a convenient way but more specific solutions may be used depending on the pH of the chemical. Prolonged irrigation – up to half-an-hour – is necessary for alkaline burns. In addition, solid matter (such as cement particles) should be removed from the conjunctival sac after everting the lids (Chapter 6).

Any patient with severe chemical injury to the ocular surface (i.e. cornea, conjunctiva or both) will be admitted. Topical steroids up to 2-hourly are often used in the first 48 hours. Evidence suggests that topical ascorbic acid (vitamin C) may also be helpful.

One potential problem with both chemical and thermal burns is symblepharon – adhesions forming between palpebral and bulbar conjunctiva under the lids. If these

Problem	Goal	Nursing intervention
Risk of adhesions forming between layers of conjunctiva following a burn to the eyes.	Patient will understand reasons for rodding to be carried out prior to the procedure.	1. Explain to patient that what you are about to do will prevent further damage to his eye(s). Ensure understanding. 2. Ask him to sit or lie still, with his head well supported and to move his eyes as directed. Point out that it will feel uncomfortable but is nevertheless very important. 3. Apply sterile lubricant to sterile glass rod and, asking patient to look up, roll the rod backwards and forwards horizontally along the lower fornix. Note whether or not there are any signs of adhesions. Repeat procedure for upper fornix after asking patient to look down and everting upper lid. 4. Repeat 4-hourly or more frequently if necessary. 5. Ensure patient is comfortable on completion of the procedure.

develop then the fornices are lost and the total area of conjunctiva is drastically reduced. The formation of symblepharon can be prevented by rodding or the insertion of a symblepharon ring.

In severe cases later treatment may involve corneal grafting but the success rate is very poor and this emphasizes how important those first few minutes after injury are. The amount of damage done depends on the amount of time elapsing between the injury and irrigation, and also on the concentration of the chemical involved.

Psychological problems experienced by patients with burns to their eyes include anxiety and fear, which are both compounded by the considerable pain likely to have been caused by the injury.

Problem	Goal	Nursing intervention
Pain caused by burns to the eye(s).	To relieve pain or reduce to an acceptable level to the patient within 24 hours.	1. Ask the patient how often he has pain and how severe it is. 2. Give analgesia as prescribed. Ensure the patient is comfortable. 3. Monitor effect of analgesia about 30 minutes after administration. 4. Observe for further signs and/or symptoms of pain and give analgesia as necessary. Report to medical staff if pain relief is not being achieved.

Anxiety and fear are prevalent whenever the prospect of losing one's sight is present.

Problem	Goal	Nursing intervention
Patient anxious/ frightened about how the burn to his eye will affect his sight because of lack of information.	Patient will understand the effects of the burn and feel informed about his progress.	1. Encourage the patient to voice any particular worries he has. 2. Keep him informed of the progress of treatment and of his condition. 3. Try to give him realistic expectations regarding his sight and reassure whenever possible/appropriate. 4. Ensure patient understands the information given.

Some burns will be serious enough to warrant hospitalization and nursing care needed by a patient being admitted to hospital in an emergency should be given as appropriate. However, if the patient is being treated as an outpatient, he will need to be taught how to instil drops himself and to be made aware of what treatment will involve. As in any case where the integrity of the ocular surface has been damaged, there is a risk of infection and the patient needs to know how to minimize the chance of this occurring.

Problem	Goal	Nursing intervention
Risk of infection developing following burns to the conjunctiva.	Patient will understand the problems that can occur following a burn to the eye and the importance of compliance with treatment.	1. Instil antibiotic drops and show patient how to do this. Allow the patient to practise under supervision. 2. Pad the eye to promote healing. 3. Ensure patient is aware of how to carry out his own treatment/care and is also aware of the potential complications of a burn, e.g. infection, and that he should seek further help should they develop.

A severe burn can also have long-term consequences for the patient if there has been any disfiguration as a result. He may need further surgery to replace scar tissue or to release adhesions. If coupled with a visual impairment this can lead to a marked loss of body image.

Problem	Goal	Nursing intervention
Patient suffering from a change of body image following scarring to the eye and surrounding tissue.	To help patient to come to terms with his deformity.	1. Talk to the patient about his worries, fears, feelings and what upsets him particularly about his injury. 2. Try to help him deal with these problems, talking them through individually and suggesting possible ways of overcoming them. 3. Discuss what further surgery would involve (if this is needed) and how he feels about this. 4. Try to build up his self-esteem and help him adapt to cope with any visual loss.

The majority of chemical burns take place at work and many could be avoided if proper precautions were taken at the time. It is also important that workers are aware of first aid treatment required and are able to carry it out, as this can be of the greatest importance in minimizing the damage done. By talking to the patient about preventive measures, the nurse can do much to reduce the risk of similar accidents recurring.

Thermal

Thermal injury ranges from a superficial abrasion due to a lighted cigarette to deep burns caused by molten metal. The former is treated as an abrasion, the latter may be as severe as a lime burn.

Radiation

Ultraviolet radiation is absorbed by the cornea and causes epithelial damage. Typically, a painful photophobic eye follows the use of a sun lamp or arc welding equipment ('arc-eye') without eye protection. Affected individuals may be alarmed by the onset of symptoms several hours after exposure to ultraviolet light. Treatment is symptomatic and padding the eye(s) closed helps the discomfort. The nursing care involved is similar to that of a corneal abrasion, already covered, with appropriate health education.

The prevention of industrial eye injuries is governed by the Statutory Instrument 1974 No. 1681 Factories *The Protection of Eye Regulations* and occupational health nurses play a big role in advising and educating employers and employees in their implementation.

The hospital nurse in an Accident and Emergency Department can use the opportunity of an eye injury to reinforce the safety and prevention aspects. This can apply equally to DIY accidents in the home.

The education of parents concerning the prevention of eye injuries in children is also an important aspect in which the ophthalmic nurse plays a role with other professionals such as health visitors, teachers and health educationalists.

Corneal Infection

The patient usually presents with watering, photophobia and severe pain, which is a marked feature because of the irritation of the many sensory nerve endings in the corneal epithelium. The patient may be distressed by the pain and irritation. The nurse should explain that the pain and other symptoms will gradually ease as the condition responds to treatment.

Corneal infection may be of bacterial, viral, amoebic or fungal origin. The type of treatment and nursing care depends upon the causative organism and the severity of the condition. The main aim of the treatment is to combat infection and limit corneal scarring and loss of vision.

Most patients present at the Accident and Emergency Department, so the nurse only sees them for a short period of time. As the patients will have to carry out the treatment at home, the nurse should ensure that they are able and willing to comply. If the condition is severe, and in particular if there is evidence that infection is spreading within the eye, admission to hospital is necessary. The nurse is then involved with inpatient care of a patient with ulceration, which usually consists of intensive drop therapy or injections of concentrated antibiotics. Deep, severely infected ulcers are sometimes very slow to heal and cause quite extensive corneal scarring. The patient may have to spend a long time in hospital and this slow healing problem makes him very anxious about his condition.

Bacterial Keratitis

It is unusual for bacterial corneal ulcers to develop in a normal eye; a predisposing factor is often present, such as a corneal abrasion, contact lenses, dry eyes, bullous keratopathy or even malnutrition.

A bacterial ulcer has an underlying dense stromal infiltrate of leucocytes and often a hypopyon, which is an accumulation of white cells in the inferior anterior chamber (Plate 1). Causative organisms include *Streptococcus pneumoniae*, *Staphylococcus aureus*, *Pseudomonas aeruginosa* and *Moraxella*.

Vigorous bacteriological investigation must be undertaken and admission is often indicated. Initial treatment is frequent concentrated broad-spectrum antbiotic drops, such as gentamicin and cefuroxime. Subconjunctival antibiotic injections may also be used. The antibiotics may be changed later once the causative organism has been cultured and sensitivities to antibiotics are known.

Progression to perforation is possible when treatment is late or ineffective. This is heralded by formation of a descemetocele, where Descemet's membrane bulges through an area of extreme corneal thinning. Even when treatment is rapidly effective there may be residual stromal scarring and thinning, causing faceting of the corneal surface which produces lasting visual disturbances if central.

The condition and the medical intervention may produce the following problems for the patient that require nursing care.

When a corneal ulcer is present it is necessary to take a corneal scrape to identify the causative organism. The nurse should explain the reason for this investigation to the patient. Likewise a dendritic ulcer (Plate 6) is sometimes

Problem	Goal	Nursing intervention
Painful eye due to corneal ulceration and exposure of sensitive nerve endings; this depends on the depth of ulceration.	Pain reduced to a level acceptable to the patient within 24 hours.	1. Talk to the patient about the pain, its type and severity. 2. Give the patient a mild analgesic to take 4–6 hourly. If inpatient, monitor, to see effect. 3. If the pain is not relieved by mild analgesia, inform the medical staff and ask for a review of the patient's condition and treatment. 4. If the patient is at home and the pain is very severe, advise him to return to hospital.
Photophobia preventing patient from opening his eye.	Patient will be relieved of discomfort caused by the light within 6 hours.	1. Explain to the patient that this will improve as condition improves and infection clears. 2. Suggest wearing dark glasses. 3. Advise the patient to avoid brightly lit rooms or bright sunshine during this active period.
Blurred vision creating anxiety about visual prognosis.	Levels of anxiety reduced to a level acceptable to the patient within 24 hours.	1. Discuss with the patient his worries and fears about his condition. 2. Keep the patient informed of his condition. 3. Try and give realistic expectations regarding duration of treatment and sight, giving reassurance when possible.
Eye sticky, discharging pus or mucus, causing eyelids to stick together.	To enable the patient to open his eyes.	1. If the patient is at home, teach him how to carry out lid hygiene. 2. Instruct him to boil water with a teaspoon of salt, allow to cool and then gently bathe the eye with cotton wool or tissues. 3. Remind the patient to wash his hands before and after procedure. 4. Ensure the patient understands the information given. If inpatient, note amount and type of discharge and keep medical staff informed of this.
Eye watering as a result of its condition.	Patient to be relieved of the discomfort and annoyance of his eye watering.	1. Explain to the patient that watering will ease as condition improves. 2. Give reasons, advise the patient to wipe the cheek with a clean tissue, but to avoid hankies and not to rub the eye. 3. Explain that if the eye is rubbed this can cause further damage and spread of infection. 4. Advise the patient to use a separate tissue for each eye to prevent spread of infection. 5. Ensure the patient understands the information given.

debrided to remove infected cells for diagnosis and to facilitate healing. Both procedures require the patient to sit at the slit-lamp to have the lesion swabbed or scraped.

As the specimen is taken directly from the corneal lesion, it is usually performed by the medical staff, while the patient is examined at the slit-lamp. The nurse would assist

Problem	Goal	Nursing intervention
Patient unaware of what taking a corneal scrape involves because of lack of knowledge.	Patient is prepared for the test prior to it being carried out.	1. Explain the purpose of test to the patient, how it is carried out and what he is expected to do during the procedure, and ensure he understands. 2. Patient is asked to sit at the slit-lamp with his head well forward with open and still eyes. 3. Explain that the patient will feel slight pressure as the cornea is swabbed or scraped. 4. The specimen should be placed in the correct medium and hands should be washed. 5. Tell the patient the test is finished and ensure he is comfortable. 6. Inform the patient when the results will be ready.

the doctor by instilling anaesthetic drops and giving support and explanations.

It may also be necessary for the patient to have a subconjunctival injection of concentrated antibiotic. As this can be a frightening experience, the nurse should ensure that the patient is well prepared for the procedure.

(For an outpatient, the nurse should ensure that transport home is available and instructions on when to restart the eye drops are given to the patient or relative.)

During hospitalization

Problem	Goal	Nursing intervention
Frequent disturbances due to the instillation of intensive treatments.	Patient to feel adequately rested.	1. Explain to the patient the need for frequent instillations of medication. 2. Accommodate the patient in a quiet area of the ward so as to encourage rest between treatments. 3. Arrange for uninterrupted meals between treatments. 4. Instil medications as efficiently as possible to keep disturbances to a minimum. 5. Encourage rest and sleep between treatments, which may be 24-hour. 6. Encourage the patient to be involved in his own treatment. 7. If disturbed sleep patterns are adversely affecting the patient, negotiate with the medical staff for a reduction in treatment frequency during the night.

As an outpatient

Problem	Goal	Nursing intervention
Difficulty with frequent instillation of intensive treatments.	Patient is willing and able to comply with treatment.	1. Explain purpose and frequency of treatment to the patient. 2. Advise patient or family always to wash hands before and after procedure to prevent spread of infection. 3. Explain how drops instillation is carried out. Tip head back, pull down lower lid with the hand while handling the drop bottle in other hand like a pen, positioning the bottle so that a drop falls into the lower fornix, without the bottle touching the eye. 4. Demonstrate the procedure and then allow the patient to instil the drops himself under supervision. 5. Ensure patient is happy and understands frequency and purpose of the drops. Advise on keeping a check list of times of instillation. 6. Remind patient to wash hands after procedure.
Patient unaware of what a subconjunctival injection involves, and what he is expected to do, because of lack of knowledge.	The patient is well prepared for the injection prior to it being carried out.	1. Explain purpose for the test to the patient, ensuring that he understands what is expected. 2. The patient is asked to lie down on the couch or bed or sit in a chair with his head supported.

As an outpatient – *continued*

Problem	Goal	Nursing intervention
		3. Inform the patient that it is necessary to instil anaesthetic drops, e.g. amethocaine, into the eye and that (a) they sting but this soon wears off and (b) they enable the procedure to be carried out without it being painful. 4. Tell the patient that he may feel pressure and some discomfort during the injection but it only lasts for a short time. 5. The nurse should advise the patient to keep very still during the procedure. 6. Explain to the patient that a speculum may be inserted into the eye or the eyelids may be held open by the nurse. 7. Tell the patient he may be asked to look in different directions during the procedure. 8. The nurse should hold the patient's hand and give reassurance. 9. The injection already prepared should be given under the conjunctiva slowly, avoiding blood vessels and areas close to the limbus. 10. After the injection is given the nurse should apply a pad to the patient's eye. 11. Analgesic can be given and the patient should be advised to rest. 12. Explain to the patient that the pad should stay on for 2–4 hours and then intensive drops should recommence as prescribed. 13. Ensure the patient is comfortable on completion of the procedure. 14. Clear away all equipment used and wash hands.

Marginal Ulcers

Marginal ulcers, a different problem altogether, are relatively common. They cause discomfort, watering and photophobia. Infiltrates are seen at the limbus and there may be a clear zone between the infiltrates and the limbus. The overlying epithelium breaks down as a secondary event. The lesions themselves contain no bacteria but are thought to represent an immune reaction to staphylococcal toxins from infected lid margins. The ulcers rapidly resolve with topical steroids but recurrences occur unless the underlying cause is treated.

Herpes Simplex Keratitis

An important corneal infectious agent is the herpes simplex virus (type I), because of its ability to cause recurrent disease. The patient should be made aware of this so that he understands to attend early for treatment of any flare-ups, as this prevents further damage and limits corneal scarring.

The classic lesion is the dendritic ulcer, which results from virus that has remained dormant in the trigeminal nerve ganglion after the primary infection. Cold sores on the lips develop in a similar way. Trigger factors include stress, sunlight and intercurrent illness, but usually there is no obvious precipitating event in the case of eye disease.

Dendrites stain brightly with fluorescein and the virus-infected cells at the edge stain with rose Bengal. Injudicious steroid drops can cause the ulcer to enlarge to geographic shape (Plate 5) and the eye may even perforate. This is why steroid drops should never be used for the undiagnosed red eye.

Topical antivirals include idoxuridine and acyclovir; they shorten the natural healing time of these ulcers, as does wiping off the infected corneal cells (debridement).

The corneal stroma can also become involved, either by viral invasion or by an immune hypersensitivity reaction, giving stromal oedema and adjacent keratitic precipitates (disciform keratitis). Because an immune mechanism is implicated, weak topical steroids are often used (with antivirals) in stromal disease.

Repeated epithelial and stromal keratitis gives rise to corneal scarring and facets (excavations which disrupt the smooth surface contour), which reduce the vision and for which corneal grafting may be considered. Unfortunately, recurrences still occur after grafting and associated vascularization makes corneal graft rejection more likely.

Herpes Zoster

Herpes zoster (shingles), which is caused by a recrudescence of the chicken pox virus, is a devastating disease that can affect the eye when the ophthalmic branch of the trigeminal nerve is involved. Epithelial disturbance, stromal keratitis and uveitis are some of the many acute manifestations. Ocular inflammation, especially of the cornea, may continue for months and even years after the skin rash. It may also undergo exacerbation. The skin may be scarred in an unsightly fashion and a few patients will suffer seriously from postherpetic neuralgia.

Problem	Goal	Nursing intervention
Patient unaware that herpetic infection may recur and that there is a need to attend early for treatment.	Patient understands the need for returning promptly if problems develop.	1. Inform the patient that this type of infection can recur. Ensure that he understands the importance of seeking early medical treatment to minimize further scarring. 2. Make the patient aware of early signs and symptoms: irritation in the eye (i.e. foreign body sensation), watering eye, reddening of the conjunctiva and pain.

Fungal Infection

This is very rare in the UK. Diagnosis can be delayed unless the condition is suspected and corneal scrapes are inoculated into the appropriate media. There may be a history of a corneal abrasion, for example with a twig, when vegetable matter may have entered, or the infection may be suspected when an apparently bacterial ulcer is not healing with antibiotics. Projections from the edge of the infiltrate and satellite lesions are suggestive. Treatment includes topical drops and occasionally systemic antifungals and the choice depends on whether the infection is due to a filamentous organism (e.g. *Aspergillus, Fusarium*) or a yeast (e.g. *Candida albicans*).

Contact Lenses and Infection

Some corneal infections are caused by contact lenses, particularly soft lenses worn for extended periods. *Pseudomonas*

Problem	Goal	Nursing intervention
Patient is unaware of risk of infection if contact lenses are not cleaned properly or checked regularly, because of lack of knowledge.	Patient will correctly care for his lenses and attend for regular check-ups.	1. Giving reasons, advise patient to have contact lenses regularly checked by his optician. 2. Ensure that lenses are not worn during an infection. 3. Advise the patient always to follow correct cleaning techniques as instructed by the optician, using sterile solutions. 4. Recommend the patient to throw away old cleaning solutions and lens cases. 5. Make the patient aware of early signs of problems: red eye, lens irritating the eye, excessive watering – ensure he understands to seek medical attention. 6. If lenses are not worn for long periods or the patient has had an infection, lenses should be sterilized and wearing time should be built up slowly.

and *Acanthamoeba* are notorious in this context. As many people wear contact lenses today, they should always be taught and encouraged to use correct cleaning techniques. Any contact lens wearer should be advised that it is important to have lenses checked regularly as scratches or excessive protein build-up on lenses can lead to corneal problems.

It is applicable to use the same principles when advising patients who are wearing a bandage lens as to the care required.

Corneal Oedema

The cornea is maintained in its transparent and relatively dehydrated state by the endothelial cell layer, which actively pumps water from the cornea into the aqueous. Corneal oedema or waterlogging of the cornea occurs when this mechanism fails. This can occur if endothelial cells are damaged during cataract extraction or corneal surgery or if the cell numbers progressively decrease, as in Fuchs's dystrophy (see below). Intraocular lens implantation may increase the risk of corneal injury because a single touch by the Perspex on the endothelium can kill many cells. There would be no problem if the cells could replicate but this does not occur in man and the complement of cells present at birth declines throughout life. Cataract extraction is being undertaken at much earlier stages and corneal decompensation after surgery is now a major indication for corneal grafting. Corneal oedema can also be produced by very high intraocular pressure such as in rubeotic glaucoma, which may follow central retinal vein occlusion, or severe diabetic eye disease and angle closure glaucoma.

Oedema fluid collects in between and under the epithelium, causing blebs or bullae which blur the vision and cause acute pain when they burst. In addition, the broken epithelium can easily become infected, giving rise to bacterial ulcers.

Soft bandages lenses protect the cornea and ease the pain but increase the infection risk. Clearly, lowering an abnormally high intraocular pressure will help, but when the condition is due to endothelial cell failure the only long-term solution is corneal transplantation.

Hypertonic saline drops are sometimes used to make the cornea less swollen.

Keratoconus

Keratoconus ('conical cornea') describes well this gradually progressive disease that alters the shape of the cornea

(Figure 16.2). Thinning and protrusion of the apex of the cornea often starts at around puberty and progresses over the next 10 to 15 years. Both eyes are usually affected unequally. Later the protrusion may be easily seen by looking at the eye from the side or by observing the distortion of the lower lid in downgaze (Munson's sign). As the cornea has a major rọle in refracting light the irregular distortion causes blurring of vision which cannot be corrected by spectacles.

The basic cause is unknown but keratoconus is often seen in atopic individuals, in other words those with eczema and/or asthma. It also occurs in Down's syndrome. The condition may generate anxiety, not only in the patient, who is often introspective, but also in parents who may be worried about schooling and career.

Sudden corneal oedema with associated pain and photophobia can follow breaks in Descemet's membrane and the endothelium. Surprisingly, corneal perforation is an extreme rarity.

The myopia and astigmatism caused by the structural change are initially helped by spectacles. Hard contact lenses can dramatically improve vision by making the refracting surface of the eye more spherical, but may become difficult to retain as the disease progresses. At this stage corneal transplantation is justified and is necessary in approximately 15% of keratoconic individuals. Fortunately most cases stabilize before such surgery is necessary.

The nursing care involves outpatient preparation for the surgery, inpatient, pre- and postoperative care and aftercare. A brief account will be given of this.

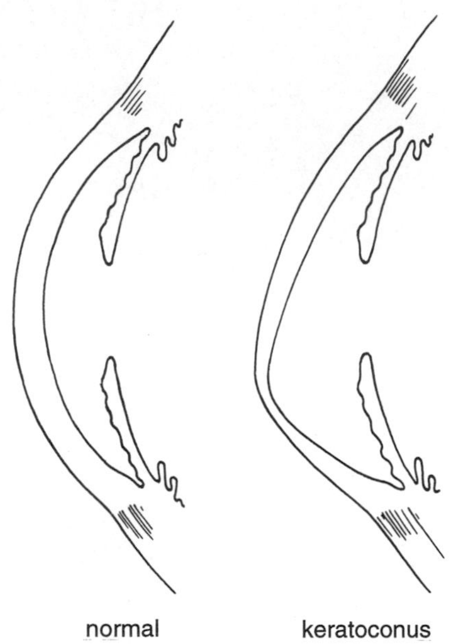

Figure 16.2 Comparison between a normal and a keratoconic cornea.

Outpatient Preparation for a Patient Listed for Corneal Graft Surgery

This section applies not only to keratoconus but also to other indications such as bullous keratopathy, herpes simplex keratitis and dystrophies.

It is important to identify and deal with any problems that may jeopardize the success of the corneal graft. At the time a graft is first considered the suitability of both the eye and the patient are considered.

The tear film must be adequate and a Schirmer's test will be requested. If the cornea is vascularized, and especially if a previous graft has failed, tissue typing may be undertaken in order to identify a matched donor, which will reduce the chance of graft rejection.

Patients must understand that admission to hospital may be rapid when a donor becomes available. They will require numerous follow-up appointments and drops for many months.

Problem	Goal	Nursing intervention
Patient unaware of what will happen pre-admission to hospital because of lack of knowledge.	Patient will be aware of preoperative preparation prior to his admission.	1. Reinforce the surgeon's explanation of the surgery, allow the patient to ask questions, voice any fears. 2. Discuss what being on the waiting list means: the patient will have to wait for donor eye material to be available. This period can vary and it is kinder not to give approximate time periods. 3. The nurse should also explain that the admission date will probably be notified by telephone. The surgeon will already have informed the patient of this, but patients do not always remember what they have been told. 4. Carry out any investigation ordered by surgeon, e.g. tissue typing – explain the reason for and importance of this to the patient. This test helps the surgeon obtain a good tissue match. 5. Check that the patient understands what he has been told and that his name, address and telephone number(s) are written in his notes.

The prospect of being able to store donor tissue is now being realized, and already most corneal grafts are a planned rather than an emergency procedure.

Corneal grafts may be full thickness (penetrating) or lamellar (partial thickness). The latter is only undertaken occasionally and is indicated for a superficial corneal problem. Despite preparation for admission, the emergency nature of the surgery still produces extra problems for the patient.

Epikeratoplasty is a form of lamellar transplantation in which a lathed disc of stroma is sutured firmly on to the surface of a keratonic eye to flatten the steep cornea and, less commonly, to treat aphakia. Such partial-thickness forms of transplantation are not threatened by immunological rejection. Emergency admission for surgery remains a possibility, for example if a corneal perforation has occurred. In such circumstances access to stored corneas in an eye bank is clearly very helpful.

PREOPERATIVE NURSING CARE COMMENCED ON ADMISSION

Problem	Goal	Nursing intervention
Anxiety over emergency admission and impending surgery because of the suddenness of the event.	Patient will achieve anxiety level acceptable to him within 24 hours of admission.	1. Orientate the patient to the ward surroundings. 2. Explain the routine and introduce the patient to fellow patients and staff. 3. Allow the patient to ask questions about his impending surgery. 4. Inform the patient that he will be going to theatre for the operation later in the day. 5. Give any instructions and information to the patient's relatives/friends regarding approximate time of surgery and visiting times. 6. Ensure all information given has been understood. 7. Explain to the patient the preoperative preparation and carry out this preparation accordingly.

Problem	Goal	Nursing intervention
Patient unaware of the potential ophthalmic problems which may follow surgery, through lack of knowledge.	Patient will understand the need for restriction in activities by his first postoperative day.	1. Remind the patient that bed rest for up to 24 hours may be required. 2. Explain the reason for rest: to recover from anaesthetic and to prevent pressure on the corneal wound. 3. Reinforce the advice about not leaning over the bedside and not rubbing or touching the eye dressing. 4. Perform the first dressing aseptically the day after surgery. 5. Examine the eye at each dressing and ensure any abnormalities are reported to the medical staff, e.g. broken sutures, shallow or flat anterior chamber, hazy donor tissue. 6. Instil eye drops as prescribed. 7. Explain to the patient the need and importance for these drops. 8. The eye may be covered with an eye shield or pad until epithelialization has taken place. After approximately 48 hours the shield is just worn at night to protect the eye from injury during sleep. 9. Assist the patient with hygiene and allow gentle mobilization to commence during the early healing stage. 10. Remind the patient not to touch the eye, if it waters, but to wipe the cheek only with a clean tissue.

Problem	Goal	Nursing intervention
		11. Observe the eye at each dressing and report any abnormalities to the medical staff. 12. Allow the patient to ask about his care. 13. The nurse should reassure the patient that vision may be blurred while healing is taking place. Irritation will ease also as the eye begins to heal. 14. Ensure all information given is understood.

POSTOPERATIVE NURSING CARE

The patient is usually in hospital for 3–5 days, if no complications occur. This period will vary depending upon the surgeon and the condition of the eye. The patient should be advised about aftercare. Vision may be blurred during the healing phase and while drops are being instilled. The sutures will usually remain *in situ* for at least 6 months, but this also varies depending upon the healing of the eye and the surgeon's strategy. It should be explained that the vision will be assessed at a later date when the eye has settled and healed. Good aftercare is important with graft patients, so that any signs of ocular complications, for example rejection, can be prevented or treated early.

Problem	Goal	Nursing intervention
Patient not aware of importance of good aftercare because of lack of knowledge.	Patient understands the importance of aftercare, and the need to seek medical attention if problems develop, by the time he is discharged home.	1. Good assessment of the patient on admission will indicate any likely postoperative problems. 2. Discuss the aftercare with the patient, asking him whether any help is available at home and informing him of services that can be arranged to help him. 3. Arrange for the district nurse to supervise drop instillation and hygiene if required. 4. Contact the Social Services to assess the patient's home circumstances and provide help if required. 5. Remind the patient of precautions, i.e. to avoid rubbing or wiping the eye, heavy lifting and to stay away from school/college/work until the medical staff say it is safe to return. 6. Make the patient aware of any problems that might occur: pain, red eye, watering or increased blurring of vision; ensure he understands to seek medical attention as soon as possible should these occur.

Refractive Surgery

A number of procedures for manipulating the shape of clear corneas are being actively developed. These include surgical relaxing incisions for astigmatism after corneal transplantation. Surgical incisions and now the excimer laser are being used to treat moderate degress of myopia. Most of these procedures are performed on outpatients.

Corneal Dystrophies

There are many different corneal dystrophies, most being quite rare. They are bilateral and familial, e.g. lattice dystrophy, macular dystrophy. Recurrent erosion may occur if the superficial layers of the cornea are involved. The condition usually progresses slowly so reasonable vision is often maintained until middle age. No treatment is usually needed until vision has been severely affected, when a lamellar or penetrating keratoplasty will be necessary.

Fuchs's endothelial dystrophy may be familial but often has no clear pattern of inheritance. A progressive depletion of endothelial cells eventually gives way to stromal and epithelial oedema due to insufficient water pumping by this important cell layer. Concentrated sodium chloride or sucrose drops dehydrate the cornea by osmosis and improve sight in early cases. When a graft is undertaken it may be combined with a cataract extraction and lens implantation.

In general, corneal transplantation is the best treatment for most dystrophies if and when vision is significantly affected. Success rates are high although some dystrophies can eventually recur in the transplanted cornea.

Nursing care for graft surgery has already been outlined. As some of these dystrophies are hereditary, it is important that all family members are screened. The surgeon usually screens the family as a matter of course, but the nurse should give additional encouragement to patient and family to ensure that all the family are seen by the medical staff.

Arcus

A whitish-yellow ring of cholesterol and triglyceride deposits in the corneal stroma, usually separated from the limbus by a clear margin of cornea, is termed arcus. Over the age of 60 it is a common ageing change of no particular significance, often referred to as arcus senilis. However in younger patients there may be an underlying disorder of fat metabolism which should be investigated. Arcus does not affect sight. Patients, and those with an untrained eye, do not usually notice this phenomenon. The condition may be observed in outpatients when the patient attends with another complaint. On discovering this condition, the nurse should advise the patient to seek medical advice.

Problem	Goal	Nursing intervention
Patient unaware that unknown fatty deposits may exist elsewhere in the body, because of lack of knowledge.	Patient is aware of the problem and seeks advice as soon as possible.	1. Giving reasons, urge the patient to seek medical advice. 2. Inform the patient that medical staff may order blood test, e.g. serum cholesterol levels – explain reason for this test. 3. Any systemic condition found will be treated to prevent complications. 4. Give assurance to the patient that early identification and treatment will prevent complications. 5. Ensure the patient understands the information given.

Band Keratopathy

Band-shaped keratopathy is caused by depositions of calcium carbonate in Bowman's layer and the superficial stroma of the cornea in the palpebral fissure. This grey-white band is not uniform and is punctuated by small translucent holes.

It can be produced in conditions associated with high blood calcium, such as hyperparathyroidism and multiple myeloma, but also occurs in chronic ocular disease, including uveitis in juvenile chronic arthritis and conditions causing degeneration of the eye. There is sometimes no apparent cause.

Gradual visual loss can be reversed by removing the deposits either with EDTA solution, which binds calcium, or directly by superficial keratectomy. This also helps the discomfort which, in advanced cases, arises from epithelial disturbance over the layer of calcium deposits but if the rest of the eye is already severely diseased, it may be of no visual value to carry out this procedure.

Sclera

The sclera is the tough white outer coat of the eye, which is continuous with the cornea. It is made of irregularly arranged collagen bundles with perforations to allow the transmission of blood vessels and nerves, the most important being the optic nerve which leaves via the cribriform plate – a sieve-like modification of the sclera.

The loose connective tissue rich in blood vessels that covers the sclera is called the episclera.

Episcleritis

Episcleritis is a fairly harmless condition which may be asymptomatic or can cause mild discomfort. The episcleral vessels dilate, resulting in redness of the eye which may be localized or diffuse and is often unsightly. Sometimes, swelling and injection is noticeable as a distinct lump which is tender. Topical steroids are occasionally used but often no treatment is required. Recurrences are common and the patient should be aware of this. It is not a sight-affecting condition.

Scleritis

Scleritis is a rare but much more important diagnosis as it may result in loss of the eye. It is commonly associated with such conditions as rheumatoid arthritis, systemic lupus erythematosus and polyarteritis nodosa. It is also a chronic feature of herpes zoster ophthalmicus.

The inflammation causes vessel dilation deep in the episclera and gives a bluish appearance in daylight. Inflammation can be localized or widespread and may occasionally affect only the posterior sclera, which clearly makes diagnosis difficult. Sometimes the sclera is destroyed so much that the choroid becomes visible and perforation of the eye is possible. Scleritis is extremely painful. High doses of systemic steroids and other immunosuppressive drugs are often necessary to control the inflammation.

Scleral Injury

Scleral injuries can be of various types, caused by blunt, sharp or flying particles. They often go hand in hand with penetrating corneal wounds. Flying particle injuries are common in industry, particularly if the patient has not been wearing protective goggles. Important causes of scleral laceration are air gun pellets, dart injury, pub fights and road accidents. Seat-belt legislation has resulted in a dramatic decline in severe injury to both cornea and sclera.

The need to identify the nature and extent of the injury is very important as this determines the treatment needed. Most of these patients would be admitted to hospital for surgical repair. If the injury is very extensive and deep, the integrity of the globe is at risk and visual function may be permanently destroyed.

The nursing care depends upon the nature and extent of the injury and the treatment ordered. In cases where visual function is at risk a considerable amount of psychological support is needed. The patients are usually young, so parents also will be distressed and they appreciate this support. Young adults are often drunk at the time of the accident and may be devastated by the implications of what has happened when they are sober.

As mentioned previously, identifying the nature and extent of the injury is important to determine treatment. If the injury is very deep and extensive, and the integrity of the globe and visual function is at risk, the patient and/or parents will be very anxious.

The nurse plays an important role in reassuring and supporting the patient and/or parents, during this period.

Problem	Goal	Nursing intervention
Patient has a scleral injury which is causing some distress.	Patient will understand the need for treatment prior to it being carried out.	1. Take a history from the patient, finding out where and how the injury occurred. 2. If an object hit the eye, ask about the type of object, whether blunt or sharp, or a flying particle. 3. Instruct the patient that the eye will be examined by the surgeon and that the size and extent of the injury will be noted. 4. Inform the patient that further investigations, e.g. X-ray, may be ordered to identify a foreign body, if present. 5. Explain the reasons and importance of the investigations to the patient. 6. Give reassurance as necessary. 7. Inform the patient that treatment is ordered accordingly. 8. Ensure the patient understands the information given.
Patient or parents anxious about extent of injury and visual outcome, because of lack of knowledge.	Anxiety levels will be reduced to a level acceptable to the patient/parent within 24 hours of the injury occurring.	1. Allow the patient to voice any fears and ask questions about condition. 2. Keep the patient informed of his condition. 3. Give the patient realistic expectations concerning the expected visual outcome. 4. Ensure consultation with medical staff.

17

Uveal Tract

Joscphinc Duvall-Young and Efty Joannadu

Chapter Summary

Functional Anatomy

The uvea lies in the middle of the three coats of the eyeball between the sclera and the retina.

The uvea is a vascular structure and is divided into three parts: the iris anteriorly, the ciliary body, and the choroid posteriorly (Figure 17.1). Each part has in common a highly vascularized stroma as well as unique anatomical characteristics reflecting specialized functions. The iris forms the

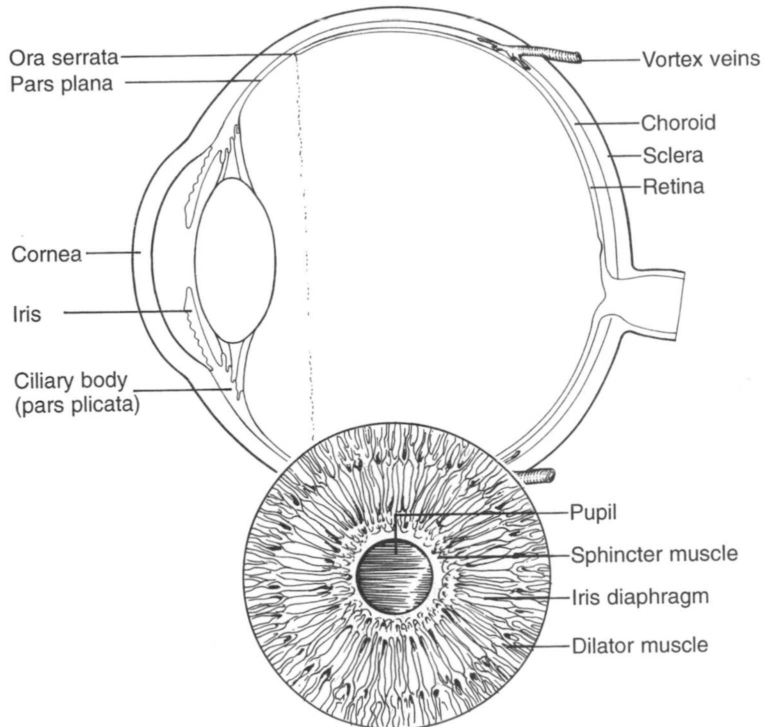

Figure 17.1 The uveal tract, showing its component parts and the iris in greater detail.

diaphragm controlling the amount of light entering the eye, in a fashion similar to the aperture setting on a camera. The size of the pupil is controlled by two muscles in the iris: the sphincter muscle around the pupil and the dilator muscles at the periphery. These two muscles are under the control of the autonomic nervous system, constriction being mediated by the parasympathetic nerves and dilation by the sympathetic. (Think of the sympathetic activity as a fear response. A frightened person has widely open eyes and dilated pupils, a relaxed person has small pupils.) To work as a diaphragm, the iris itself must not allow transmission of light through the stroma. On the deep surface is a layer of heavily pigmented epithelium. In the dark, the pupil dilates to allow as much light as possible to enter the eye, whereas in bright light it constricts, eliminating the dazzling effect of excessive light. Part of the accommodative response, which is the mechanism brought into play when reading, is constriction of the pupil, which increases depth of focus. The other components of accommodation are convergence of the eyes and an increase in power of the lens due to contraction of the ciliary muscle.

The anterior part of the ciliary body is thrown into radial folds, called ciliary processes. The folds give origin to the term pars plicata (folded part) for the anterior part of the ciliary body, to which are attached the zonular fibres that support the lens. Alteration in the tension of the zonular fibres changes the shape of the lens and is mediated by the ciliary muscle, which contracts, pulling the ciliary processes forward, relaxing the zonular fibres and making the lens rounder and able to focus images of near objects on the retina. Behind the pars plicata is the pars plana, which has little functional significance although it has considerable surgical importance as a frequently used 'safe' access to the interior of the eye during vitrectomy, as it lies between the pars plicata and the peripheral extent of the retina.

The ciliary body epithelium, which is the source of aqueous, circulates in the anterior segment of the eye nourishing the lens and cornea, both of which are avascular.

The choroid provides a rich blood supply to the outer retina for its high metabolic demand. The capillary bed which lines the choroid, the choriocapillaris, is the richest in the body.

Symptoms of uveal disease may be due to loss of clarity of the intraocular fluids because of exudation or haemorrhage, both causing blurring of vision. Blood or exudate in the aqueous may block the mechanism for draining aqueous, leading to secondary glaucoma, which may produce blurring of vision because of corneal oedema, or pain if the pressure is very high. Pain in uveitis is due to spasm of the ciliary muscle and is often associated with photophobia due to multiple reflections of light within the aqueous from suspended inflammatory cells. Ciliary body disease may present similar problems and in addition may result in the loss of aqueous production, with a fall in intraocular pressure and ultimate degeneration and shrinkage of the globe, termed phthisis bulbi. Choroidal disease may cause visual disturbance by interfering with the blood supply of the retina or by spreading of inflammation into the retina. Choroidal tumours interfere with the adhesion of the retina and may result in retinal detachment. In the long term, cataract and corneal opacification may result from interference with nourishment of the lens and cornea by the aqueous.

Inflammation

Inflammation of the uveal tract is termed uveitis. Broadly, uveitis can be divided into anterior uveitis (also termed iritis and iridocyclitis), involving the iris, ciliary body or both, and posterior uveitis (also termed choroiditis). If all parts are involved, the diagnosis is panuveitis.

Anterior Uveitis

Anterior uveitis is common and acute. The pathological response is characterized by vascular congestion, exudation of proteinaceous fluid and white blood cells into the aqueous and subsequent resolution. The signs and symptoms of acute uveitis can all be explained on the basis of knowledge of the pathology of inflammation. The patient complains of pain and redness. Vascular congestion can be seen in the conjunctival vessels at the limbus of the cornea and sometimes on the iris. The patient complains of blurred vision because of the presence of exudate in the aqueous increasing turbidity, and sometimes also because the exudate may obstruct aqueous flow, causing an acute secondary glaucoma with corneal oedema. The exudate can be seen in the aqueous on slit-lamp examination as 'flare' and 'cells', often likened to the beam of a cinema projector seen in a dark room. If the cellular exudate is extensive it may deposit on the posterior surface of the cornea (keratic precipitates) or settle as a fluid level (hypopyon). Loss of function may occur if the ciliary body is involved, when aqueous production may be lost and the intraocular pressure falls. Acute uveitis sometimes resolves without any residual scarring. However, adhesions commonly occur between the iris and lens, when they are called posterior synechiae. When the pupil is dilated distortion of the pupil margin is seen at the

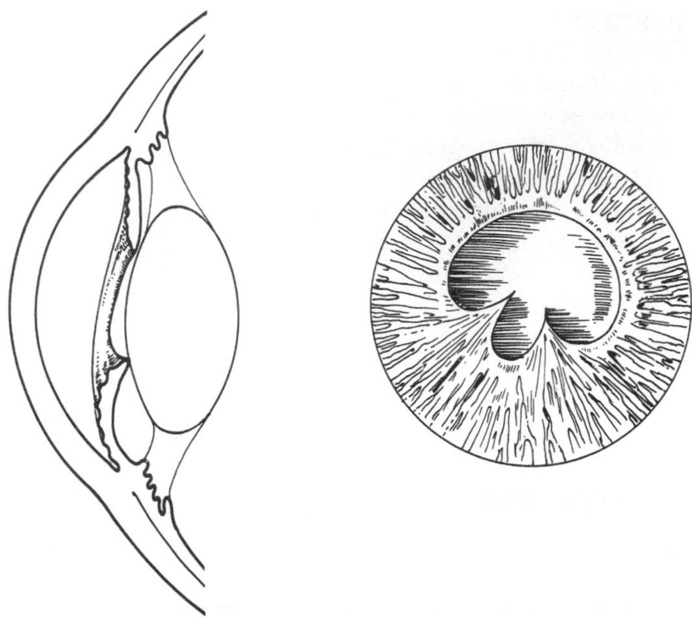

Figure 17.2 Posterior synechiae, where the iris is adherent to the front of the lens.

site of the adhesion (Figure 17.2). Extensive posterior synechiae can cause secondary glaucoma if they are extensive enough to completely block the pupil (iris bombé).

The majority of cases of acute anterior uveitis are idiopathic, that is, no cause is identified, although they are presumed to have an immune aetiology. Infective anterior uveitis is very rare, although in the past syphilis and tuberculosis were implicated. A number of conditions are associated with anterior uveitis, such as ankylosing spondylitis, Reiter's syndrome and sarcoidosis. In severe recurrent or bilateral cases investigation for associated disease is undertaken.

Chronic anterior uveitis is associated with less pain, redness and visual disturbance, but is complicated by the development of cataract and corneal opacities as a consequence of the disturbance of the normal aqueous composition. Organization of exudate with fibrous adhesion formation is common, with secondary glaucoma. A mass of organized tissue may occur behind the lens (cyclitis membrane). By the time this occurs, the ciliary body has usually ceased to produce aqueous, the lens and cornea are opaque and the eye blind. A very low-grade inflammation occurs in Fuchs's heterochromic cyclitis, which causes only a mild visual disturbance until late when cataract and secondary glaucoma develop. Chronic uveitis in children may be associated with juvenile arthritis.

Management

Steroids are usually administered in drop form at a frequency which varies, with severity, between half-hourly and 2-hourly. In very severe cases, a subconjunctival injection of steroid ensures a continued high dose to the eye. Cycloplegics such as homatropine (1% or 2%) are used to enlarge the pupil and draw it away from the lens, reducing the risk of fibrous adhesion formation. Pain originating from spasm in the ciliary muscle is also relieved by cycloplegics by paralysing the muscle.

Problem	Goal	Nursing intervention
Fear and anxiety because of reduced vision and red eye.	Awareness and acceptance of condition and possible course of the disease.	1. Explain to the patient the condition and treatment and possible course of the disease. 2. Advise on coping strategies, reduced vision from the condition and effects of treatment, e.g. effects of mydriatics. 3. Advise on safety aspects related to reduced vision, e.g. during work.
Pain and photophobia.	Alleviation of pain.	1. Explain the cause of the pain. 2. Encourage compliance with topical treatment. 3. Advise on the use of analgesics. 4. Advise on the wearing of dark glasses. 5. Explain the use of topical heat treatment to relieve pain and enhance the effects of topical treatment.
Anxiety about the need for many investigations.	Acceptance of the need for investigations.	1. Explain the types of investigation and the reasons for them. 2. Where possible, have all investigations performed at the same time. 3. Ensure the patient is aware of when the results will be available.
Potential complications of acute secondary glaucoma.	The early recognition and treatment of complications.	1. Ensure the patient is aware that increased pain, further reduction in vision or an increase in conjunctival injection requires further medical consultation. 2. Advise patient to seek urgent medical consultation if any signs of complications appear.
Possibility of recurrence.	The recognition and early treatment of a recurrence.	1. Ensure the patient is aware of the signs of recurrence and the need for early commencement of treatment. 2. Advise on the means of seeking urgent medical consultation should recurrence be suspected. 3. Advise not to use old medication prior to seeking medical consultation.

The treatment is continued until an improvement is seen, and then slowly reduced. Treatment is usually continued for between 2 and 6 weeks. At follow-up visits, the intraocular pressure must be measured, as a side effect of steroid treatment is secondary glaucoma.

Patients with acute uveitis are usually first seen in the Accident and Emergency Department and following investigation the patient usually returns home to continue self-care, although a severe bilateral episode may need intensive inpatient treatment.

Chronic uveitis is treated similarly, with particular attention to the intraocular pressure. Fuchs's heterochromic chronic cyclitis is notoriously unresponsive to topical treatment, but the prognosis is much better following cataract extraction than it is in other types of chronic uveitis such as Still's disease.

POSTERIOR UVEITIS

Posterior uveitis is less common than anterior uveitis. It may present with dull pain and loss of vision due to inflammatory exudate clouding the vitreous, but tends to run a more protracted course than anterior uveitis. As in anterior uveitis most cases are idiopathic, but some are caused by sarcoidosis and tuberculosis. Histoplasmosis is endemic in the USA and causes a type of chorioretinitis. In toxoplasmosis the protozoon may infect the individual *in utero* and can cause widespread central nervous system disease, or may affect the choroid, often bilaterally. *Toxoplasma* infection acquired later in life causes similar ocular effects but is milder and is usually unilateral. *Toxocara* infection causes a uveitis, principally in children. The ova of parasitic worms in the intestines of dogs and cats are ingested by children and hatch in the intestine. An alarming 25% of random soil samples taken from parks contain toxocaral ova. The parasite burrows into the circulation and is carried round the body to several sites, including the eye. Mild cases present with a focal area of choroiditis, but the most florid involve the retina extensively and result in permanent visual damage. This is, however, a rare infection.

Appropriate health education should be given to the patient and family in relation to hygiene, especially handwashing after playing with pets and the control of *Toxocara* infection in pet dogs by routine worming.

The treatment for idiopathic posterior uveitis is systemic steroid administration only if the focus of inflammation threatens to encroach on the macula or is in the vicinity of the optic nerve head. At these two sites progressive inflammation and scarring may cause severe and permanent visual loss. Elsewhere, the inflammation subsides in time, with the formation of a scar that does not significantly interfere with visual function. Topical steroids are valueless as they do not reach the choroid in sufficiently high doses to suppress inflammation. Systemic steroids are avoided in mild cases because the side effects are usually worse than the risk of long-term visual impairment.

Somc of the patient's problems may be similar to that of anterior uveitis, such as fear and anxiety from reduced vision, anxiety about the need for many investigations and the possibility of recurrence.

Problem	Goal	Nursing intervention
Patient unaware of need for systemic steroid therapy because of insufficient knowledge.	The effective use of steroids with a minimum risk of complications.	1. Ensure the patient understands the importance of steroid therapy, the prescribed dose and the frequency. 2. Ensure the patient understands the need to carry a steroid treatment card. 3. Monitor weight, urinalysis and blood pressure at frequent intervals.

Non-infective endophthalmitis may occur as an immune response to ruptured lens (lens-induced endophthalmitis), following necrosis of an intraocular tumour or in sympathetic ophthalmitis, which is discussed below in the section on trauma.

Infective endophthalmitis may follow intraocular surgery and penetration; non-traumatic cases occur following perforation of corneal ulcers with the introduction of infection or may be caused by the spread of infection elsewhere in the body, when it is termed endogenous endophthalmitis. This occurs, for example, in patients with septicaemia and intravenous drug addicts.

In managing endophthalmitis the infective agent, if any, requires to be identified. If an ulcer is present in the cornea, swabs and scrapings must be taken for culture. Otherwise the best source of material for culture is the vitreous. The organism may be bacterial or fungal.

The treatment of infective endophthalmitis is an antibiotic to which the organism identified is sensitive, or a cocktail of antibiotics to cover Gram-positive and Gram-negative organisms. The antibiotic may be administered intravenously, subconjunctivally or into the vitreous with care since some antibiotics are toxic to the retina. In addition steroids may be given, topically or preferably systemically. In other circumstances, the rule is that steroids must not be given in the face of infection since they promote bacterial growth, but in endophthalmitis the risk to vision is from scarring, not the infection itself. Scarring within the vitreous forms bands which are adherent to the retina and which contract as they mature, producing traction retinal detachment. Steroids limit the amount of scarring and therefore improve the prognosis for vision. If the infection is fungal, appropriate antifungal medication is prescribed.

The prognosis in endophthalmitis is poor and some eyes have no residual useful vision following treatment. They may fail to settle on treatment and remain actively inflamed and painful. In these cases surgery is usually advised. The two possible operations are evisceration and enucleation. Evisceration involves removal of the cornea and intraocular content, leaving a variable amount of sclera and the optic nerve undisturbed. In an enucleation the extraocular muscles are cut from the eye, the optic nerve is severed and the entire globe is removed. Evisceration has the theoretical advantage of leaving the optic nerve undisturbed and minimizing the risk of spreading the infection along the nerve, but has the disadvantage that there is the possibility of leaving small amounts of uveal tissue behind, which could excite a sympathetic ophthalmitis in the fellow eye (Chapter 21).

Patients with endophthalmitis are treated intensively as inpatients, the aim being to preserve as much useful vision as possible. Medication administered by subconjunctival injection may be repeated frequently (e.g. daily) and the care required during this procedure is outlined in Chapter 6. Intravenous antibiotics may be administered by infusion or by bolus injections into an indwelling cannula, local policy dictating the method and the grade of a person administering the same. Intravitreal injection may be performed in the ward or the operating theatre, as a minor surgical procedure. There may be some residual pain following the procedure, which is controlled by mild analgesics. In instances when intensive topical treatment is prescribed this can create the following problem for the patient.

Tumours

The commonest primary intraocular tumour is malignant melanoma, but the commonest intraocular tumour overall is a metastasis secondary to carcinoma of the breast, lung or gastrointestinal tract. Metastatic tumours deposit in the uveal tract, usually in the choroid, and may be the first indication of malignant disease in the patient or may be a manifestation of carcinomatosis. The patient complains of loss of part or all of the visual field in one eye, and on examination has a retinal detachment with an underlying mass.

Problem	Goal	Nursing intervention
Frequency of medication instillation, causing lack of sleep and interruptions to routine.	To maintain feeling of well-being while continuing prescribed medical treatment.	1. Explain to the patient the need for frequency of drops. 2. Reduce other interruptions as far as possible. 3. Plan so that all care is given at the same time. 4. Encourage rest between administrations. 5. Serve meals after a drop instillation so that meals are uninterrupted. 6. Discuss with the medical staff the possibility of reducing the frequency of instillations between 12 midnight and 6 am as the patient responds to treatment.

Malignant melanoma of the uveal tract may affect the iris, ciliary body or choroid (Figure 17.3). It is increasingly common with age but may affect any age from young adulthood onwards. If the tumour is in the iris, the patient may notice a darkly pigmented spot when he looks in the mirror. If it is more posterior, he may present with visual disturbance. This occurs early in tumours of the posterior pole and later in more peripherally placed tumours. The symptoms are those of retinal detachment, since that is what accounts for the visual loss. In very large or necrotic tumours the patient may present with glaucoma or endophthalmitis. The diagnosis is based on fundus examination,

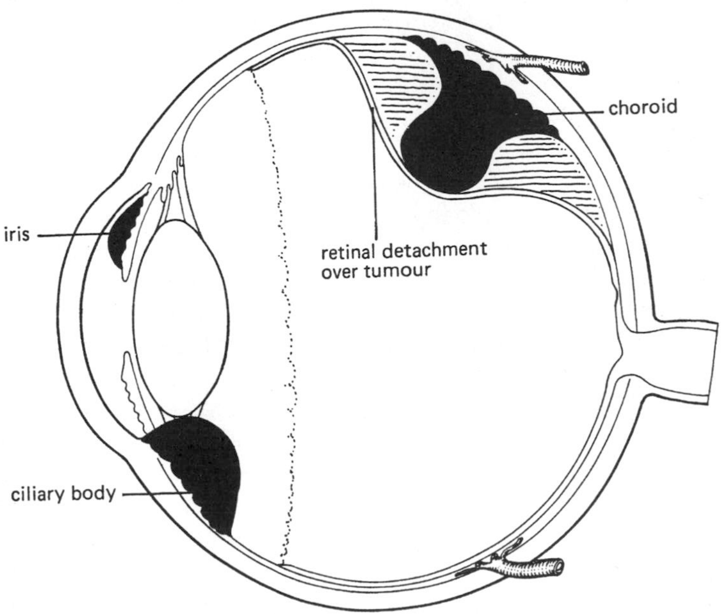

Figure 17.3 Sites of tumour within the uveal tract.

with gonioscopy in tumours of the ciliary body and iris root. Additional investigations include fluorescein angiography, ultrasonography and looking for evidence of spread to the liver.

The treatment of intraocular melanoma is a subject of controversy. Until relatively recently most eyes harbouring tumours were enucleated. An implant may be inserted into the orbit, on to which the muscles are fixed, which will move with the fellow eye. The prosthetic eye is moulded to fit over the implant and will have a certain amount of movement and an improved cosmetic result.

It has been reported that the prognosis for life for patients with malignant melanoma is not improved by enucleation and may even be reduced theoretically because of vascular spreading of the tumour when the eye is handled during surgery. Malignant melanomas spread out of the eye through the choroidal circulation and the vortex veins and deposit locally in the orbit or at distant sites, most commonly the liver. The other options available are close observation to ascertain whether or not the tumour is growing, and if so to intervene either with local excision with preservation of the globe or irradiation by a plaque placed surgically. With large tumours in which nothing is to be gained visually, enucleation is advised. The prognosis for life for anteriorly placed tumours is good.

The care of a patient having an eye removed is covered in Chapter 20 for children and Chapter 21 for adults. In the cases of malignant melanoma, consideration must also be given to the psychological effects of a malignant condition and possible long-term problems that may ensue.

TRAUMA

Trauma to the uveal tract is common and may be caused by either a blunt or sharp injury. Sharp injury to the eye causes perforation, in which case the uveal tract is frequently involved. Perforating injuries of the cornea are usually plugged by a knuckle of iris, which may allow the anterior chamber to remain formed. In very small perforations of the cornea the only sign of injury may be a slight distortion of the pupil as a result of iris entrapment in the wound. Sometimes perforating injury is associated with a foreign body which may be retained in the eye. This is obvious in, for example, gunshot wounds, but may be missed in other circumstances. It is very important to recognize an intraocular foreign body which, if there is extensive intraocular haemorrhage, may not be visible. Intraocular foreign bodies left in the eye for any length of time usually cause a very severe inflammation and loss of vision, especially if they contain iron or copper. An exception is a fragment of glass which causes very little inflammation. Hammer and chisel injuries are notorious for causing a tiny perforation when a fragment of chisel flies into the eye. An X-ray will reveal the present of metallic foreign body, which should be removed surgically.

The management of corneal perforation is nearly always surgical. If surgery is undertaken within hours of the injury, the entrapped iris may be pushed back into the eye but if there is a delay the iris begins to undergo necrosis and if it is replaced within the eye there is a danger of bacterial endophthalmitis. In such cases the part which has been exposed to the outside is excised. Similarly, anterior scleral ruptures are repaired surgically, often with excision of exposed uveal tissue.

Blunt injury most commonly causes bleeding into the anterior chamber (hyphaema: Plate 2). Blood cells floating in the aqueous are seen as floaters by the patient unless the bleeding is profuse, in which case vision may be severely affected. Common causes of such injury are blows to the face with a fist or squash ball. The blood comes from torn vessels in the region of the iris root. A tear in the iris root may involve the drainage angle, in which case aqueous drainage may be affected and glaucoma may later ensue. Patients with hyphaemas are usually admitted to hospital for bed rest to allow the blood to resorb and the clot in the blood vessel to organize. If the patient remains active the clot will be dislodged and the iris mass will bleed again, often more profusely than before. After a few days, the risk of rebleeding is very small. If the anterior chamber fills with blood the blood clot cannot leave the eye through the drainage system and a severe rise in intraocular pressure may follow. Rarely, blood has to be removed surgically.

Blunt injury often causes anterior scleral rupture, especially in eyes that have had previous surgical procedures, in which case the site of the surgical scar gives way. Elderly patients may fall and catch the eye on an item of furniture. In such cases the ciliary body prolapses through the wound and appears under the conjunctiva as a dark mass.

Another pattern of injury seen in severe blunt trauma to the eye is posterior choroidal rupture. Linear or crescentric white areas appear in the fundus in the posterior pole and if involving the macula, cause lasting visual loss.

In eyes which have had injuries, including surgery, involving the uveal tract there is a risk of developing sympathetic ophthalmitis, a chronic panuveitis affecting both eyes that can occur at any time after 2 weeks following injury. The precise cause of this condition remains unknown but it is considered to be an immune response to uveal tissue which, when damaged, reveals antigens that are not recognized by the body's defence mechanism and are attacked as foreign. The same antigens are present in the fellow eye and are also attacked by the immune system. The incidence of sympathetic ophthalmitis has fallen as surgical techniques improve, and it is now rare. To minimize the risk of the condition open injuries affecting the uvea must be carefully repaired and steroids must be used liberally. If the condition occurs the prolonged use of high doses of steroid topically and systemically improves the prognosis. If inadequately treated, substantial visual impairment is suffered following severe protracted inflammation. Severely damaged eyes with no hope of useful vision should be enucleated early, as with the extensive uveal injury they are more likely to excite sympathetic ophthalmitis. The eye should be enucleated within 10–12 days of the injury, since sympathetic ophthalmitis does not occur until after that time.

The nursing care of patients with trauma involving the uveal tract follows basic principles. In cases where the trauma has opened the eye surgical repair is indicated. The physical care of the patient in this instance is similar to any intraocular pre- and postoperative care. The psychological and socioeconomic problems for the patient are different. The urgency of the surgery and the nature of the injury will increase the anxiety of the patient as to the impending surgery and the possible visual outcome. In many instances, vision may be considerably reduced by scarring and loss of tissue after treatment or the eye may ultimately have to be removed. Not only may this be psychologically traumatic for the patient, but it may affect his social status and his earning capacity. The full team may be involved with the care of this patient, depending on the individual problems that manifest themselves.

Congenital Abnormalities

Defects in the uveal tract are called colobomata. During development of the eye the optic cup forms and fuses inferonasally. The closure may fail anywhere along its length from the iris to the optic nerve giving rise to a coloboma. In the iris the defect is seen inferonasally and in the choroid a white patch of sclera is seen through the choroidal defect anywhere along a line corresponding to the site of the fetal fissure, ending at the optic disc. An iris coloboma is largely a cosmetic defect with a minor optical defect and may be corrected with a painted contact lens. A field defect corresponding to the affected area is present in coloboma of the choroid.

A number of other malformations in the iris occur. There may be distortion of the pupil (corectopia), or multiple pupils (polycoria). The iris may be almost completely absent (aniridia), which has an autosomal dominant pattern of inheritance and is frequently associated with glaucoma. Albinism is a hereditary absence of pigmentation that may affect the eye, skin and hair, or the eyes only. It is associated with macular hypoplasia and nystagmus. Affected individuals often have very poor vision and marked photophobia.

18

AQUEOUS DYNAMICS

Gordon Dutton and Meg Johnson

FUNCTIONAL ANATOMY

The eye maintains its spherical shape because it is 'inflated' to above atmospheric pressure. The normal range of intraocular pressure is between 12 and 20 mmHg, the average being 14 mmHg. Aqueous humour (often abbreviated to aqueous) is formed by the ciliary epithelium. Its formation can be divided into two components, ultrafiltration and secretion. Ultrafiltration describes the process whereby aqueous humour is 'filtered' out of the bloodstream as a result of the blood pressure in the ciliary capillaries being higher than the intraocular pressure. Secretion is an active metabolic process and is not dependent on pressure; it is diminished by drugs (e.g. acetazolamide) which inhibit the formation of aqueous, and ischaemia.

The flow of aqueous is illustrated in Figure 18.1. Aqueous initially passes into the posterior chamber between the iris and the lens; it then flows into the anterior chamber through the pupil. Aqueous leaves the anterior chamber through the trabecular meshwork, whose structure is akin to that of a miniature sponge, and passes into the canal of Schlemm from where it flows through collector channels which join up with veins on the surface of the eye. Most of the aqueous passes through the face of the ciliary body in the chamber angle and drains into the venous system of the uvea. This is known as the uveoscleral outflow. Some of the aqueous also permeates into the vitreous humour from whence passage of water is known to take place across the retina into the choroid. The exact mechanisms which control and maintain the intraocular pressure within the normal range are unknown.

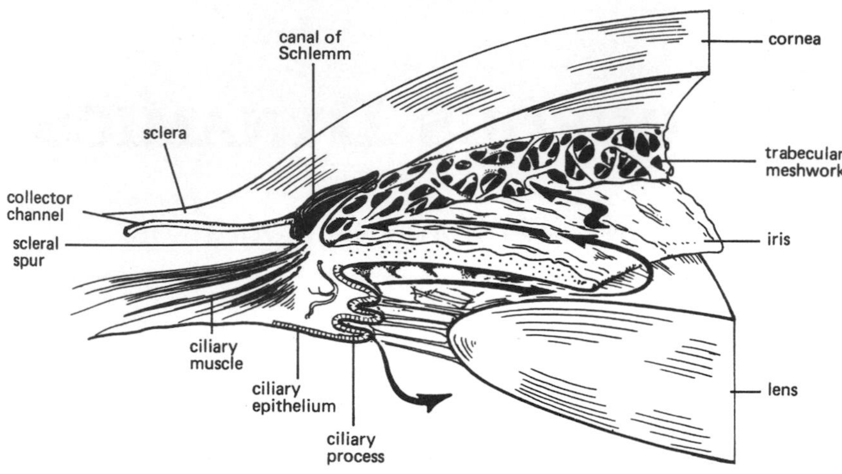

Figure 18.1 Schematic diagram of a wedge-shaped section taken from the anterior segment of an eye. This diagram illustrates the site of formation and the direction of flow and drainage of the aqueous humour.

Assessment of Patients

Measurement of Intraocular Pressure

Applanation tonometry is the most commonly used accurate method of measuring the intraocular pressure. To understand the principles of this technique, four forces must be considered (Figure 18.2(a)): the pressure exerted by the tonometer head (1) is equal to the intraocular pressure (2) when the surface being applanated (i.e. flattened) is just over 3 mm in diameter. At this diameter the resistance of the cornea to flattening (3) is equal to the surface tension forces of the tear film (4), which pull the tonometer head on to the cornea.

In order to know what force is required to produce a circle of contact 3 mm in diameter the principle of a split prism is employed. Fluorescein and local anaesthetic are instilled into the eye. A blue light is shone on to the tonometer head, through which the observer focuses upon the fluorescent tear film. If the tonometer head were to have no prisms, then as the tonometer was pressed harder against the eye one would see an enlarging green fluorescent circle. However, in order to know when the circle has reached the 'end point' of 3 mm in diameter there are two prisms incorporated into the tonometer head, one above the

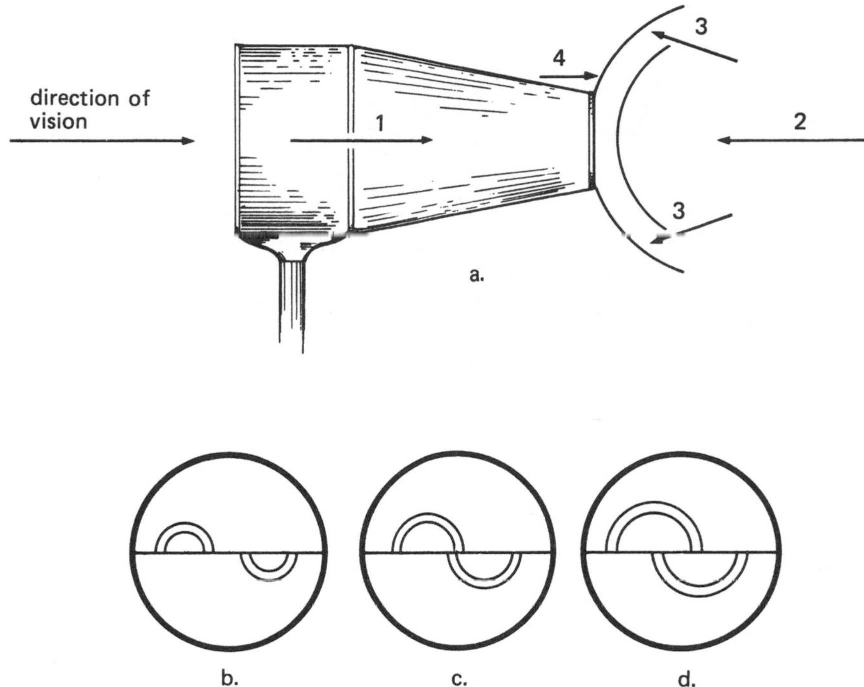

Figure 18.2 **(a)** Schematic diagram illustrating the principles of applanation tonometry. The tonometer is pressed on to the cornea to produce flattening. The forces (1–4) which are considered are described in the text. **(b, c, d)** These three diagrams illustrate the appearance seen when looking through the applanation tonometer. The force being exerted by the tonometer is gradually increased until the appearance shown in **(c)** is seen. At this point the force being exerted (1) is equal to the intraocular pressure (2); **(b)** and **(d)** illustrate the appearances when the tonometer head is pressing too lightly **(b)** or too heavily **(d)** upon the cornea.

other. This means that the enlarging circle is seen as enlarging half circles which are above each other and are displaced laterally (Figure 18.2 (b)–(d)). The diameter of contact equals 3 mm when the two halves just overlap (Figure 18.2 (c)). The pressure being exerted upon the eye, which is then equal to the intraocular pressure, is read from the calibrated dial.

The Perkins tonometer is a portable applanation tonometer. It is very useful for examination of the bedbound and the anaesthetized patient.

The monitoring of intraocular pressure is a function undertaken by the specialist nurse and the following care plan can be utilized.

Problem	Goal	Nursing intervention
Patient uncomfortable and tense, causing lack of co-operation due to fear from lack of awareness and understanding.	The patient is comfortable, relaxed and co-operative throughout the procedure.	Explain the reason for the test and the importance of monitoring the intraocular pressure in order to see how successful the treatment is and whether the patient needs to commence treatment. Explain that the drops you will instil are local anaesthetic drops, so the test should not be painful. Explain to the patient where you want him to position his head and the importance of trying not to blink, again assuring him that it will not hurt. Explain that the test will only take a couple of minutes. Move the slit-lamp as close to the patient as possible. Ensure patient is at the correct height; use cushions or a lower chair if necessary. Adjust the slit-lamp height so that the patient can rest his chin comfortably on the chin rest. Position the chin rest so that the patient's eye is level with the marker line. Ensure patient comfort and that he is not stretching at all prior to commencing the test. Instil local anaesthetic drops (lignocaine and fluorescein) prior to commencing the test.
Potential damage to corneal epithelium during the test.	The patient has an intact corneal epithelium at the end of the procedure.	Recheck the patient's comfort and understanding. Ensure the tonometer is attached securely to the slit-lamp. Ensure prism has been soaking in Milton solution for 10 minutes and dry carefully before using. Fix prism into tonometer securely and ensure prism holder is in the correct position. Make yourself as comfortable as possible. Remind the patient to keep his eyes wide open and not to blink. Move the slit-lamp slowly forward until the prism is in contact with the cornea. Looking through the eye pieces measure the intraocular pressure as accurately and as quickly as possible. Pull the tonometer away from the eye as soon as you have measured the intraocular pressure. Ensure the measurement is recorded immediately to prevent the test having to be repeated. (If the patient is unable to co-operate, use one hand to open the lids, ensuring that no pressure is put on the eyeball, and follow the procedure as above.)

Indentation Tonometry

The indentation or Schiotz tonometer is now rarely used because it is not as accurate as applanation tonometry. The amount of indentation produced by the instrument when it is placed upon the cornea of a recumbent patient is read from a scale. This is proportional to the intraocular pressure, which is determined from calibration tables.

Automatic Tonometers

The air-puff tonometer is used by many optometrists because the eye is not touched by the instrument. A fine beam of light is shone by the instrument upon the cornea, which acts as a mirror. A jet of air of rapidly increasing force is played upon the central cornea, transiently deforming it. The angle of reflection of the incident beam of light thus rapidly changes and the reflected beam is thereby transiently reflected into a light detector when the cornea has been flattened by the air jet. A computer in the instrument determines the intraocular pressure by ascertaining the force of the air jet required to flatten the cornea and thus reflect the light into the detector.

Gonioscopy

In glaucoma, a wide range of abnormalities may be seen in the iridocorneal angle by gonioscopy, which is an essential basic technique for the evaluation of any patient with the disease.

Gonioscopy (Figure 18.3) is an assessment of the drainage angle to identify any abnormal structures, and to estimate the width of the angle and therefore the likelihood of closure in the future. As the angle cannot be visualized directly through the cornea, it involves placing a contact lens with a mirror on to the cornea to eliminate total internal reflection of light emerging from the angle. It is performed by medical staff but, as it involves full patient co-operation, an explanation by the nurse may help to prepare the patient for the examination.

GLAUCOMA

Glaucoma may be defined as raised intraocular pressure, which, if maintained, will lead to pathological changes in the eye. There are a number of different types of glaucoma and these may be classified as shown in Figure 18.4.

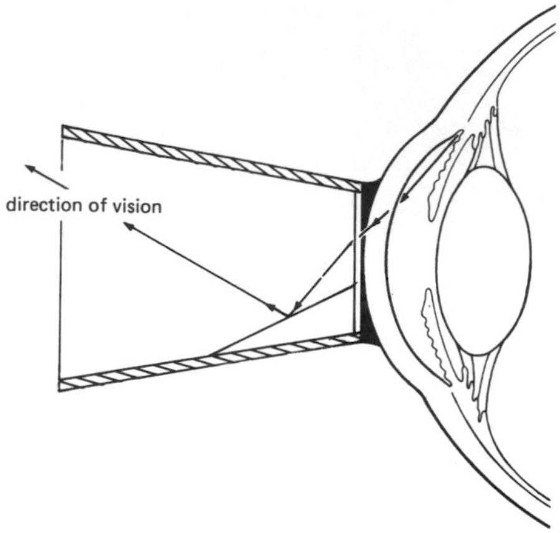

direction of vision

Figure 18.3 Diagram illustrating the principle of gonioscopy. A contact lens enclosing a mirror is placed on the eye and the mirror is positioned in such a way that the observer is able to see into the angle between the iris and the cornea.

ACQUIRED GLAUCOMA

PRIMARY OPEN-ANGLE GLAUCOMA (POAG)

Apart from those patients in whom severe disease has resulted in loss of vision, primary open-angle glaucoma (also known as chronic simple glaucoma) is a symptomless and therefore insidious disease which is most often detected when a patient visits his optician for spectacles. The patient will then be referred to an ophthalmologist, who will assess the patient and often organize further tests to clarify the diagnosis, to stabilize the condition and for patient education.

If admission is not planned, then patient education, treatment and observation of the ability to instil drops should take place in the Outpatient Department. It is therefore the responsibility of the nurse in the department to assess and satisfy herself as to the patient's competence. The same tests are likely to be carried out whether the patient is admitted or not, and therefore the same care can be applied to each individual situation.

DIAGNOSIS

There are three diagnostic criteria:

1. raised intraocular pressure;
2. cupping of the optic disc;
3. visual field loss.

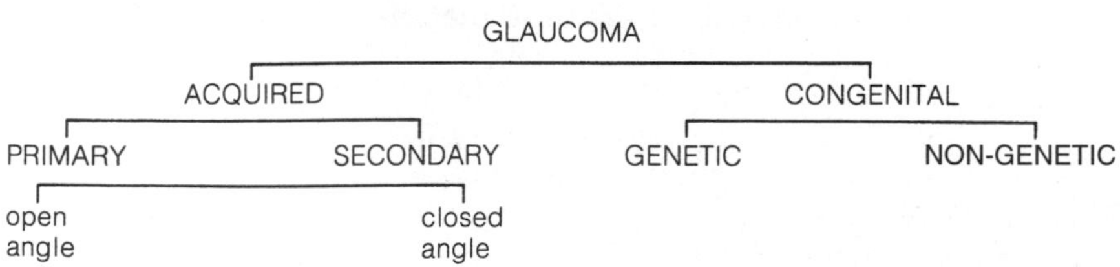

Figure 18.4 Classification of glaucoma.

Raised Intraocular Pressure

The normal range of intraocular pressure is 12–20 mmHg. The pressure varies during a 24-hour period, being lower during the day than at night. In POAG the intraocular pressure is persistently elevated and the diurnal variation in pressure may be greater. In addition, in the normal eye the intraocular pressure is greater when lying than when standing; this phenomenon may be accentuated in patients with POAG.

Cupping of the Optic Disc

The optic disc is supplied by capillaries derived from branches of the posterior ciliary arteries. A raised intraocular pressure decreases the blood pressure in the optic disc capillaries and thereby diminishes the flow of blood. Excavation and atrophy of the optic nerve head (Plate 6) is the result of local impairment in the capillary circulation, with subsequent loss of the nerve fibres passing into the optic nerve. The normal optic disc has a small central depression (the physiological cup). The vertical diameter of the physiological cup should not exceed half the vertical diameter of the whole optic disc (cup to disc ratio of 0.5). When the cup to disc ratio is greater than 0.6 open-angle glaucoma must be suspected.

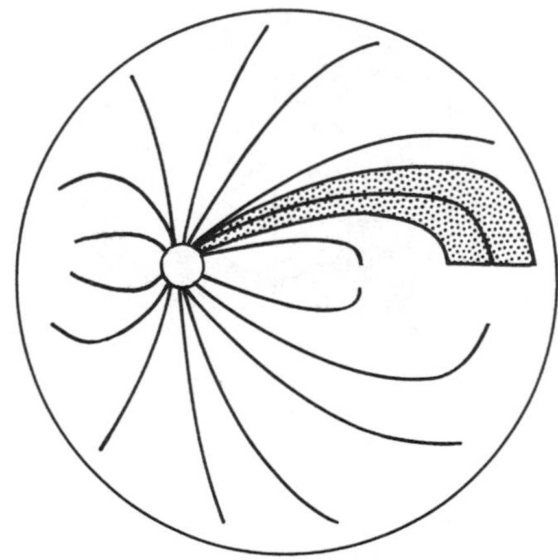

Figure 18.5 Diagram illustrating the distribution of nerve fibres over the surface of the retina. The small circle represents the position of the optic nerve and the curved lines the positions of the nerve fibres. The shaded area illustrates the position of a nerve fibre bundle which is characteristically damaged in primary open-angle glaucoma and which results in the type of visual field loss defect seen in Figure 18.6.

Visual Feld Loss

Loss of visual field results from damage to nerve fibre bundles as they enter the optic disc. The distribution of the nerve fibres in the retina resembles the pattern produced by iron filings when placed upon paper overlying a bar magnet (Figure 18.5). When a bundle of nerve fibres is damaged and lost, arcuate areas of retina lose their innervation, with resultant visual field loss in the upper or lower half of the field. Typically, the pattern of visual field loss is arcuate in character and may extend to the blind spot or out to the periphery (Figure 18.6(a) and (b)). Peripheral visual field loss of this nature results in a nasal step (Figure 18.6(a)). Such visual field loss is initially only minimal but is gradually progressive and may eventually result in total blindness if the disease is not treated.

Many of the tests that are routinely and regularly carried out on patients with primary open-angle glaucoma are in themselves likely to create concern for him and his ability to co-operate fully with the nurse or the doctor. A full explanation of each, as well as reassurance, are required to allow the patient to be more relaxed and to co-operate fully with the investigators.

If the patient is admitted to hospital he can expect to have tonometry performed at least four times a day in order to assess correctly the diurnal variation. Additional late night and early morning readings may be taken. He will probably have a visual field test performed every 3–6 months and gonioscopy at least once, so again a careful explanation at the beginning of his treatment will help to allay anxiety during the period of his care.

If the reason for the rise in pressure is uncertain it may be necessary for the patient to undergo one or more provocative tests. These are tests devised to establish whether the eye is developing an abnormally high rise in intraocular pressure under certain conditions.

They include:

1. the water drinking test. The patient drinks one litre of tap water on an empty stomach and the intraocular pressure is measured over 15 minute intervals for one hour. An intraocular pressure rise occurs in POAG;
2. tests to produce a rise in intraocular pressure by pupil block:

   (a) sitting in a dark room for one hour;
   (b) lying prone in a dark room for one hour;
   (c) one drop of mydrilate (0.5%);
   (d) one drop of phenylephrine (10%) followed by one drop of pilocarpine (2%) once the pupil has begun to dilate.

In all these tests a rise of 8 mmHg between the beginning and end of the test is usually taken as a positive result.

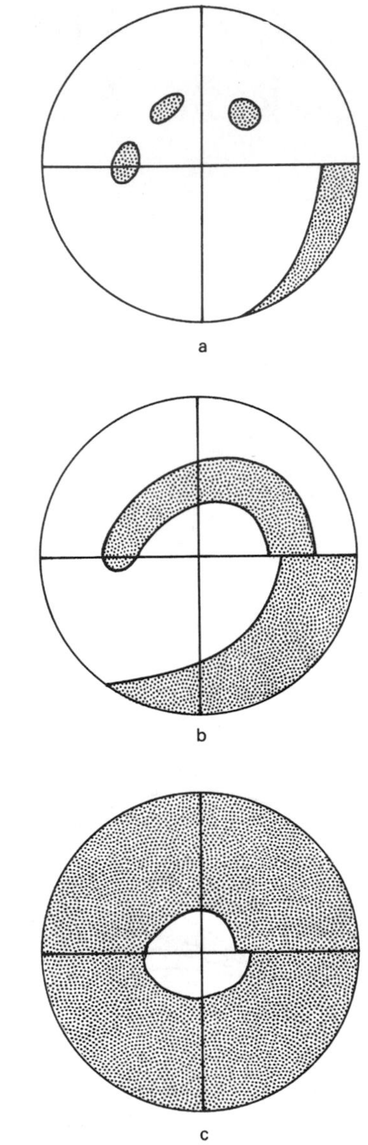

Figure 18.6 Characteristics of typical progressive visual field loss in glaucoma. The outer circle indicates the field of vision of the left eye and the centre of the cross indicates the position of fixation of vision.

Epidemiology

The commonest causes of blindness in the UK are senile macular degeneration, cataract and glaucoma. The main factors which place someone at risk of developing POAG are a family history of the disease, involvement of the other eye by the disease, and old age. For this reason, first-degree relatives of a patient with POAG who are over the age of 40 should be advised to be screened for it.

Treatment

The principal aim of treatment is to reduce the intraocular pressure and thereby to improve capillary perfusion at the optic nerve head.

Such treatment must provide permanent reduction in intraocular pressure, and the efficacy of treatment must be regularly assessed for the remainder of the patient's life. It is therefore important that the patient understands his disease and is aware that medical treatment, at least, must be continued indefinitely; moreover, the patient must understand that treatment is designed to prevent further loss of vision and is unlikely to give rise to any significant improvement in visual function. Three methods are currently employed :

1. medical treatment;
2. laser treatment;
3. surgery.

Medical treatment is currently the mainstay of therapy in most cases. However, laser treatment and surgery may also be considered as primary therapeutic modalities in certain cases.

Medical Treatment

A number of drugs may be used alone or in combination.

1. Parasympathomimetic eye drops (e.g. pilocarpine 1–4% three to four times a day) are commonly used.
2. Anticholinesterase eye drops (e.g. eserine 0.5–1% three to four times a day) are now rarely used.

   Both groups of drugs act on the ciliary muscle by stimulating the parasympathetic system. This muscle inserts into the scleral spur (Figure 18.1). When this muscle contracts the pores of the trabecular meshwork are opened and the outflow of aqueous humour is facilitated.
3. Beta-blocking drugs reduce the intraocular pressure by inhibiting the formation of aqueous. Currently the most commonly used drug is timolol in a concentration of 0.25% or 0.5%. This is usually instilled into the eye twice a day. Other such drugs include betaxolol, metipranolol and carteolol.
4. Adrenaline is a sympathomimetic drug and dilates the pupils. It is thought to reduce the formation of aqueous by causing vasoconstriction in the ciliary body and increasing the outflow of aqueous. Propine is a pro-drug and releases adrenaline into the aqueous after it has been absorbed. Mixtures of adrenaline and guanethidine are also sometimes employed and are more effective in lowering intraocular pressure than is either drug alone.

If the above drugs separately or in combination fail to control the intraocular pressure, oral treatment may be given. The most commonly used drugs are acetazolamide and dichlorphenamide. These drugs are carbonic anhydrase inhibitors and act by decreasing the secretion of aqueous. Side effects include paraesthesia (tingling) of the fingers, reduction in plasma potassium levels and renal stone formation. These drugs must not be given to patients who are acidotic or who have chronic pulmonary disease.

The patient's understanding of his newly diagnosed condition may vary considerably, depending upon his previous knowledge, from hopes of a complete cure to fear of inevitable gradual blindness. Therefore, as soon after diagnosis as possible a teaching session should be arranged. Ideally this should take place in a small group of four or five patients because feedback, as questions from patients, can be more readily expressed in that environment. This is obviously easier if the patient has been admitted, but the important thing is to ensure that the patient has a basic understanding of his condition and is thus motivated to comply with the prescribed treatment.

Problem	Goal	Nursing intervention
Poor knowledge of condition and its causes and treatment.	Patient has basic knowledge of open-angle glaucoma and the reason for his prescribed treatment.	1. Always make yourself available to answer patient's questions during his stay. 2. Prepare teaching plan covering: (a) basic anatomy and physiology related to glaucoma; (b) the tests likely to be performed and the reasons behind them; (c) treatment that may be or has been prescribed; (d) the importance of compliance. 3. Introduce literature from agencies such as the International Glaucoma Association and answer any further questions. 4. Evaluate patient's response during and after the session and adjust information given accordingly.

A major problem is compliance with treatment. There may be several reasons for non-compliance. The main reason is a lack of understanding of the treatment and its effect upon the eye. This hopefully will be diminished as the patient is made aware that the treatment is required to prevent blindness and will not improve vision. Another reason is that many patients with primary open-angle glaucoma are elderly. They may be forgetful, and many who live alone do not have the support and encouragement of a partner or family. Patients often have reduced manual dexterity due to, for instance, arthritis. They may have reduced visual acuity because of cataract formation or senile macular degeneration. All these factors will affect their compliance with treatment and may diminish their ability to instil drops.

Problem	Goal	Nursing intervention
Patient unaware of how to instil his own drops.	To ensure patient is able and willing to comply with prescribed medication safely himself.	1. Explain the effect of the treatment and the reason for it. 2. Advise patient always to wash hands before instillation of drops. 3. Explain what the patient is to do: pull down lower lid with one hand; hold drop bottle like a pen in the other hand. Position bottle over lower fornix, squeeze the bottle without touching the eye. 4. Demonstrate the procedure and then under supervision allow patient to instil his own drops. 5. Repeat the instruction and demonstration until patient and nurse are confident he is competent. 6. If necessary investigate positions in which patient may feel happier.
Lack of motivation to comply to treatment of open-angle glaucoma.	Patient motivated to comply based on adequate knowledge of the effect of the treatment.	1. Assess patient's understanding of his condition. 2. Go over again any points not understood. 3. Explain the effect of the treatment that the patient has been prescribed. 4. Ensure patient understands the necessity to control intraocular pressure over 24 hours. 5. Enquire as to any adverse side effects the patient may be experiencing – reducing motivation. 6. Assess any difficulties patient may be experiencing due to his personal circumstances, job, etc.

These factors and the patient's general physical and social condition need to be taken into account when assessing drop technique and in seeking to help the patient become fully motivated and able to comply.

When teaching a patient to instil drops it is important to have an open mind as to the way in which the procedure is to be performed. It is important to ensure hygiene and safety. The patient may wish to stand, to sit or even to lie on his bed to put in the drops, any of which are perfectly acceptable. It is worthwhile teaching the patient to instil the drops without using a mirror as this aids independence.

The care and teaching given to the patient to assist safe instillation of drops also involves assessing and ensuring that he is physically able and motivated to comply with treatment.

When the nurse is satisfied that the patient fully understands treatment and is able to instil the drops she should go on to teach punctal occlusion following instillation. This reduces the systemic absorption and therefore the risk of side effects from the drop.

Problem	Goal	Nursing intervention
Patient unaware of value of punctal occlusion	Patient competent at punctal occlusion, and motivated to do so, based on his understanding.	1. Explain the reason for punctal occlusion. 2. Teach patient how to occlude the punctum following drop instillation. 3. Teach the patient to occlude for about one minute following drop instillation.

If drop technique and motivation to comply are in question when the patient visits the Outpatient Department then he should be admitted for education and observation. If during admission it is decided that the patient is unable to put in his own drops it should be the job of the nurse to include and educate the family to do so. If the patient has no family support, district nurse services should be introduced.

It may be that a patient is not complying with treatment because of side effects (e.g. blurring of vision) or simply because of his job (e.g. shift work). This can be tactfully assessed by the nurse during interview and suggestions then made to help the patient feel able to comply despite his present lifestyle.

Laser Treatment

The application of between 50 and 100 argon laser burns, each 50 μm in diameter, to the trabecular meshwork gives rise to a significant reduction in intraocular pressure. This treatment, which is known as **argon laser trabeculoplasty,** may be used in selected patients as a first-line or second-line form of treatment for primary open-angle glaucoma. It is thought that the scarring engendered by the laser treatment stretches the tissue between the burns, opens the spaces of the trabecular meshwork and thus facilitates the drainage of aqueous from the eye.

Should the patient fail to be adequately controlled on medical treatment then laser treatment may be advised. The patient may have preconceived ideas about laser treatment and a careful explanation should be given explaining the aim of the treatment, what will be expected of him during the procedure and what the expected outcome will be.

Problem	Goal	Nursing intervention
Anxiety, caused by a lack of understanding of laser treatment and its long-term effect on vision, and fear of pain and discomfort during the procedure.	Patient fully aware of what is expected of him during the procedure, the reasons for the treatment and expected outcome.	1. Explain carefully that the patient will be required to sit, as for gonioscopy, and that a lens such as the goniolens will be applied to the eye. 2. Explain, by referring back to the basic anatomy that the patient knows, the reasons for laser treatment and the expected outcome. 3. Ensure that the patient is confident that careful observation will be made of the eye following the procedure. 4. Explain that the procedure may be uncomfortable but should be pain-free. 5. Explain that the patient may experience a slight headache following the procedure.

Following a laser trabeculoplasty it is important to monitor the intraocular pressure regularly as there may be a significant rise in pressure due to resulting inflammation and it may be necessary for the patient to be given acetazolamide as a prophylactic measure.

Surgical Treatment

Surgical treatment for primary open-angle glaucoma is usually employed when medical treatment has failed to control the intraocular pressure or prevent loss of visual field. Non-compliance with medical treatment is also an indication for surgery. In some centres surgery is regarded as a first-line form of treatment, especially if a patient is thought to be unlikely to use topical treatment. The principle of surgery is to create a fistula between the anterior chamber and the subconjunctival space. It is thus known as drainage surgery. There are a number of operations based on this principle: trabeculectomy, Scheie's procedure, the trephine procedure and iridencleisis, in which a 'wick' of iris is incorporated into the fistula. By far the most commonly performed procedure is trabeculectomy.

The principles of trabeculectomy are illustrated in Figure 18.7. The conjunctiva is divided and retracted to allow access to the proposed drainage site. A small, rectangular, half-thickness flap of sclera is elevated and a deep piece of sclera is removed, making a hole into the anterior chamber. A peripheral iridectomy is performed. The scleral flap and conjunctiva are then resutured in place. The fistula which has been created gives rise to a permanent reduction in intraocular pressure in the majority of cases. The complications of this procedure include 1) overdrainage of aqueous

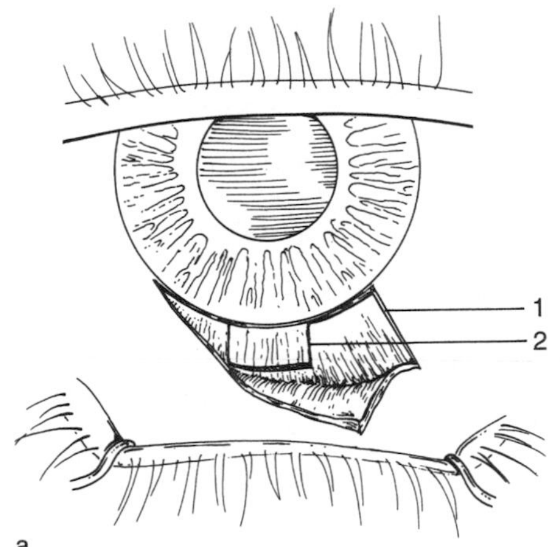

Figure 18.7 First stage in the procedure of trabeculectomy as seen by the surgeon from above. **(a)** An incision is made into the conjunctiva (1) and the conjunctiva is reflected. A rectangular half-thickness cut is made in the sclera (2).

with a flat anterior chamber, 2) infection and 3) cataract formation.

Postoperative care of a patient following trabeculectomy is similar to that of a patient who has had anterior segment surgery (Chapter 7). Special note should be made at first and subsequent dressings of the depth of the anterior chamber and the presence of a drainage bleb. If the ocular condition is satisfactory the patient can be progressively self-caring and mobile from the first day postoperatively until discharge.

The intraocular pressure is monitored during the postoperative period and a significant drop is expected following surgery. Successful surgery may mean eventual control of the intraocular pressure with no medical treatment following the initial postoperative period.

In some cases in which trabeculectomy has not worked, a plastic drainage tube may be implanted to reduce intraocular pressure. This is sometimes carried out as a two-stage procedure.

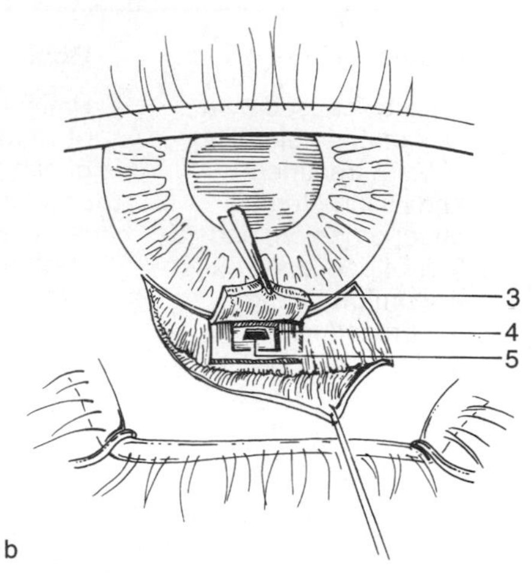

Figure 18.7 Second stage in the procedure of trabeculectomy as seen by the surgeon from above. **(b)** A flap of sclera (3) is then dissected free. A smaller rectangular hole (4) is then cut into the anterior chamber. A hole is then made in the peripheral iris (peripheral iridectomy) (5) so that the iris cannot balloon forwards and block the hole after the operation is complete. Finally the scleral and conjunctival flaps are sutured back into place. A fistula is thus created between the anterior chamber and the subconjunctival space.

Primary Closed-Angle Glaucoma (Acute Closed-Angle Glaucoma)

This condition is most common in middle to old age. It occurs about twice as frequently in females. An eye in which the anterior chamber is shallow is susceptible to the disease. The two commonest causes for a shallow anterior chamber are 1) hypermetropia and 2) enlargement of the lens. A hypermetropic eye has a short axial length and the anterior chamber depth is thus foreshortened. Throughout life the lens continues to grow. As it enlarges the anterior chamber becomes shallower.

When the pupil is in the mid-dilated position the combined actions of the sphincter and dilator muscles tend to push the pupillary margin up against the lens (Figure 18.8). Aqueous is formed in the posterior chamber of the eye, flows through the pupil and drains into the canal of Schlemm through the trabecular meshwork. When the flow of aqueous through the pupil is impaired in any way, the peripheral iris bows forward (Figure 18.8) and, in eyes in which the anterior chamber is shallow, the peripheral iris comes into contact with the adjacent cornea, blocking off the trabecular meshwork. In this situation the aqueous cannot escape from the eye and the intraocular pressure rises to levels as high as 70 mmHg. At such a high level of intraocular pressure the amount of blood which can enter the eye (the perfusion) is reduced and all the intraocular structures, especially the optic nerve, may be severely damaged by ischaemia. Acute closed-angle glaucoma thus constitutes an ophthalmic emergency and must be treated immediately as

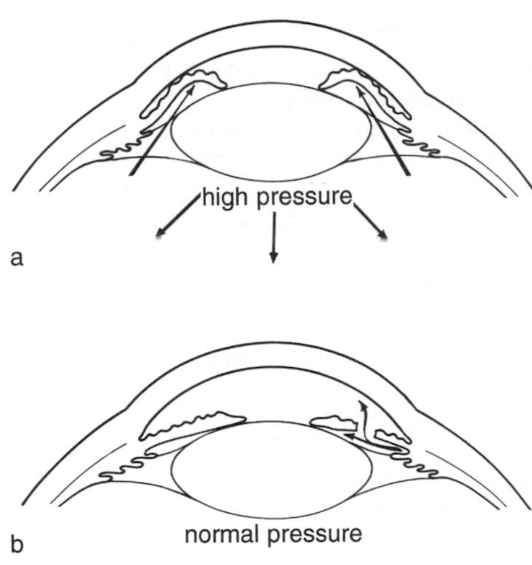

Figure 18.8 Diagrams illustrating how angle closure glaucoma arises. **(a)** The pupil margin comes into close apposition with the anterior lens capsule. Aqueous humour (arrows) is unable to pass into the anterior chamber and the peripheral iris billows forward so that it comes into contact with the cornea. This, in turn, prevents drainage of aqueous humour through the trabecular meshwork; **(b)** A peripheral iridectomy relieves the pupil block, and allows aqueous to enter the anterior chamber.

the sooner treatment is implemented the better the prognosis.

Signs and Symptoms

Patients with acute closed-angle glaucoma characteristically present with severe pain in one eye associated with redness of the eye and blurring of vision.

Clinical examination reveals a fixed, mid-dilated, oval pupil, redness of the eye, predominantly around the limbus (otherwise known as circumlimbal injection), hazy cornea and a shallow anterior chamber. The fixed pupil is principally due to ischaemia caused by a high intraocular pressure. The normal cornea maintains its clarity by the action of the endothelial cells, which pump water from the cornea into the anterior chamber. The raised intraocular pressure diminishes the function of the endothelial cells and results in waterlogging of the cornea (i.e. oedema), which gives rise to a halo effect when looking at a bright light. Occasionally, patients may also present with nausea, vomiting and abdominal pain, which is attributed to an associated vagal response.

Medical Treatment

The initial treatment of acute closed-angle glaucoma comprises measures to reduce intraocular pressure. This is achieved medically by the intravenous injection of acetazolamide (250–500 mg) and/or intravenous mannitol, the osmotic action of which is responsible for diminishing the volume of the vitreous and decreasing intraocular pressure. Glycerol flavoured with orange juice may be given orally as an alternative osmotic agent. The reduction in intraocular pressure results in the blood supply to the internal structures of the eye being restored. At 30–40 min after administration of these agents pilocarpine (2%) is instilled to constrict the pupil at such a time as the pupillary sphincter would be responsive to this drug. The result of this is to draw the iris centrally and thus break the pupil block effect which gave rise to the acute closed-angle glaucoma in the first place.

All patients with acute glaucoma are admitted to hospital for treatment. This causes obvious anxiety regarding admission, the treatment and the visual prognosis. The education of the patient needs to begin in the Accident and Emergency Department, where he will probably be given the initial intravenous injection of acetazolamide. During the initial admission period the education and support given by the nurses he comes into contact with must be consistent.

Problem	Goal	Nursing intervention
Pain due to raised intraocular pressure.	Intraocular pressure within acceptable limits – thus pain reduced.	1. Explain to the patient in simple terms what has happened to his eye. 2. Ensure administration of intravenous acetazolamide and explain its effect. 3. Give adequate oral analgesia as required if pain persists while intraocular pressure is reduced. 4. Ensure administration of prescribed drops and instruct patient in safe instillation.
Anxiety due to loss of vision and uncertainty of prognosis.	Patient understands that prompt treatment is likely to reduce the long-term effect of rise in intraocular pressure.	1. Reiterate why the vision is disturbed. 2. Explain the reasons for the treatment. 3. Ensure patient understands the necessity for prompt treatment. 4. Explain the reasoning behind the treatment to the unaffected eye.
Nausea and vomiting due to pain.	Intraocular pressure controlled, thus reducing the nausea.	1. Explain to patient the reason for the nausea and the effect of the treatment. 2. Follow above plan to control intraocular pressure. 3. Give antiemetics as prescribed. 4. Offer mouth washes as required.

The high rise in intraocular pressure is usually uniocular but often prophylactic treatment to the other eye is given in the form of pilocarpine drops, and surgery or pulsed yttrium-aluminium-garnet (YAG) laser may be performed on both eyes. Again this needs to be backed up by careful explanation to the patient.

The patient's general condition often improves dramatically following initial treatment and the consequent drop in the intraocular pressure. It is often at that stage that he starts verbalizing some of his questions and anxieties.

Surgical Treatment

In those patients in whom the episode has been short-lived and there is no evidence of visual field defect (which would be indicative of either long-standing or previous attacks of closed-angle glaucoma) the treatment of choice is peripheral iridectomy or iridotomy. The rationale of such treatment is that, even if pupillary block were to occur, a bypass route for the flow of aqueous is provided which prevents the development of angle closure (Figure 18.8(b)). Patients who have visual field loss or in whom the attack of acute closed-angle glaucoma lasted for more than 24 hours are treated by a surgical drainage procedure such as trabeculectomy with the rationale that there is likely to have been an occlusion to the outflow of aqueous at the level of the trabecular meshwork. Those patients who are refractory to medical treatment are treated by one of these two surgical procedures as a matter of urgency. If necessary, the intraocular pressure is reduced in theatre before surgery by the use of osmotic agents (e.g. mannitol) and appropriate anaesthetic measures which reduce intraocular pressure.

Anxiety in the patient will always be somewhat reduced by an understanding of what the procedure involves and what the prognosis is likely to be.

Postoperative care is again similar to that following a trabeculectomy with particular note being made by the medical staff that the intraocular pressure has been satisfactorily brought under control.

Laser treatment may be the choice of treatment rather than surgery. In this case the pulsed YAG laser is used to create a hole in the iris – an 'iridotomy'. The same explanation needs to be given here as for patients who are to undergo trabeculoplasty, as full co-operation cannot be expected without explanation and understanding.

The patient should be encouraged to instil his own drops prior to surgery or laser treatment, as he is likely to be on some form of postoperative treatment following discharge. The more supervised practice he is given the safer and more willing will be his instillation of treatment following discharge.

Chronic Closed-Angle Glaucoma

In some patients who demonstrate the typical manifestations of chronic open-angle glaucoma (namely persistently raised intraocular pressure without pain, visual field loss and cupping of the optic disc), gonioscopy reveals closure of the iridocorneal angle. This condition is uncommon and is known as chronic closed-angle glaucoma. The treatment in this situation is trabeculectomy. Such patients may also require long-term topical medication to maintain acceptable intraocular pressures.

Secondary Glaucoma

Any pathological process which gives rise to occlusion of the trabecular meshwork may result in raised intraocular pressure and consequent damage to ocular structures. These conditions include the following:

1. raised pressure due to blood in the anterior chamber (hyphaema) – the erythrocytes block the trabecular meshwork;
2. inflammation exudates or inflammatory cells in the anterior chamber resulting from iridocyclitis;

3. tumour cells in the angle of the anterior chamber;
4. lens protein (usually inside macrophages) in patients with mature cataract or traumatic lens rupture.

Thus either cells or cellular debris may block the pores of the trabecular meshwork and result in glaucoma. Most commonly the intraocular pressure tends to be high (50–70 mmHg). This leads to congestion, pain, corneal oedema and visual loss, in addition to the underlying ocular conditions. The clinical signs and symptoms are similar to acute closed-angle glaucoma.

Patients who have been subject to recurrent or persistent iridocyclitis may develop multiple posterior synechiae in which the pupillary margin becomes adherent to the anterior lens capsule. If this takes place for the full 360° of contact, the failure of flow of aqueous through the pupil results in iris bombé and secondary angle closure. The treatment for this condition is peripheral iridectomy or YAG laser iridotomy.

CONGENITAL GLAUCOMA

Congenital glaucoma is rare. It is caused by a developmental abnormality of the angle of the anterior chamber which results in inadequate drainage of aqueous. This abnormality may be inherited or it may be caused by some other intrauterine disturbance. It is usually a bilateral condition. The developing tissues of the eye of a baby are soft and the raised intraocular pressure gives rise to expansion of the globe, known as 'buphthalmos'. The deep layers of the cornea (Descemet's membrane and endothelium) are less extensible. As the globe expands, splits occur in Descemet's membrane. This gives rise to oedema and opacification of the cornea. The corneal damage is painful and gives rise to photophobia and lacrimation. A baby with this condition will characteristically lie with its head buried in the pillow because of sensitivity to light.

If the condition is not treated the persistently raised intraocular pressure results in cupping and damage of the optic nerve head, leading to optic atrophy and blindness. Enlargement of the eyeball causes short-sightedness; opacities in the cornea and amblyopia may contribute to the impairment in vision.

TREATMENT

Treatment for congenital glaucoma is surgical. In many cases goniotomy is performed. This is an operation in which a cut is made in the angle between the iris and the cornea under direct vision through a gonioscopic lens. This divides the abnormal tissue which is causing the glaucoma and the intraocular pressure is controlled. Procedures routinely carried out on adults such as tonometry and gonioscopy are impossible unless performed under general anaesthetic.

Parents of these children require support and education as to the reasons for the recurrent anaesthetics. They also need education as to how to observe for signs that a baby may demonstrate due to a rise in intraocular pressure.

Problem	Goal	Nursing intervention
Anxiety of the parents due to diagnosis and the fear of being unable to instil treatment.	Parents are educated about treatment and have established relations with hospital such that any worries can be voiced. Able to detect rises in the intraocular pressure, and therefore further visual impairment.	1. Explain condition to parents, at a level understood by them. 2. Give careful instructions as to how to put drops in baby's eyes. 3. Explain how baby will demonstrate signs of pain, by restlessness and rubbing eyes in his pillow. 4. Explain the effect and importance of treatment. 5. Ensure rapport established with nursing staff and time taken to answer any questions and allay fears as much as possible.

With early diagnosis, careful monitoring and modern surgical expertise the prognosis for this condition is reasonable. Nevertheless it is still a cause for visual morbidity. A thorough appraisal of parent education and relevant support for this condition can be found in Chapter 1.

19

The Lens

Steve Vernon and Linda Whittaker

Chapter Summary

Functional Anatomy

The healthy human adult lens (Figure 19.1) is a biconvex transparent body situated in the anterior compartment of the eye and supported through 360° by the zonule (suspensory ligament of the lens). It lies behind the iris, approximately 3 mm from the cornea. The transparency of the lens, so necessary for accurate focusing of an image, depends on the protein structure within the individual lens cells. These are continually being formed; thus the lens is the only part of the eye to grow throughout life.

The lens capsule is a transparent elastic membrane laid down by the lens epithelium. The capsule is thickest anteriorly and thinnest posteriorly, a feature important in extracapsular surgery. The lens epithelium consists of a single layer of cells of the anterior capsule which continue to divide and produce new lens fibres which are, in fact, elongated cells. At the age of 65 the lens is one-third larger than at the age of 25. The central fibres are compressed to form the nucleus, which becomes harder and yellower as the lens ages. The nucleus is surrounded by the cortex, which consists of multiple layers of lens fibres rather like layers of an onion. The zonule consists of straight, non-elastic fibres running from the ciliary epithelium of the ciliary body to the region around the equator of the lens. With the ciliary body relaxed for distance vision, the lens contributes about 17 dioptres to the refractive power of the eye. A contraction of the ciliary muscle relaxes the zonular fibres and allows the lens to take on a more spherical shape. This increases the refractive power by up to 15 dioptres and focuses the eye on a near object, a process termed accommodation. The relative inability of the older lens to change its shape leads to the condition **presbyopia**, which typically starts in middle age.

Classification of Cataract

Pathological conditions of the lens can be divided into four major categories.

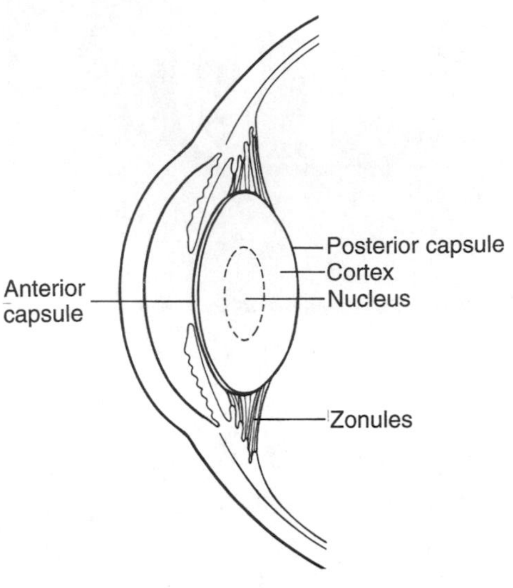

Figure 19.1 The crystalline lens.

Congenital Abnormality of Size, Shape or Position

This may cause blurred vision, because of the associated optical error, or glaucoma.

Acquired Change in Position

During a change in position, as in traumatic dislocation of the lens, the lens becomes dislocated, the iris is free to move in an anterior/posterior direction and the tremulous appearance is termed **iridodynesis**. If the dislocation is complete, the lens may fall backwards into the vitreous cavity or migrate through the pupil into the anterior chamber, where it may cause an acute rise in intraocular pressure.

With a dislocated lens, whether traumatic or secondary to a general disorder such as Marfan's syndrome, the main problem that the patient experiences is that of blurred vision and diplopia due to the altered location of the lens.

Problem	Goal	Nursing intervention
Patient complaining of blurred vision due to altered location of the lens.	Patient will report relief from visual disturbances and be able to maintain normal independence levels.	1. Explain that visual disturbances are due to the lens being located in an abnormal position. 2. Provide occlusion for the affected eye or occlude lens of spectacles. 3. Warn patient of effect of field loss on occluded side so that he can mobilize safely. 4. Ensure patient understands information given.

Congenital Abnormality in Clarity (Congenital Cataract)

This may be an isolated hereditary abnormality, associated with chromosomal abnormalities such as Down's syndrome or metabolic abnormalities such as galactosaemia, or following maternal infection in pregnancy, for example with rubella.

There are many excellent paediatric books which deal efficiently with the general care of children in hospital and promotion of bonding between mother and baby, and aspects of that will not be discussed here. This section will concentrate specifically on the effects of the cataracts themselves and promotion of visual development. The child may be referred to an ophthalmologist with suspected cataracts after the parents or health visitor have noticed white pupils or a squint. When parents realize that their child has a visual impairment, it is quite normal for them to go through a grieving phase for their 'lost' healthy child. It is important for the ophthalmic nurse to recognize this and, where possible, to assist them through this process. Blame may be placed by the parents on general practitioner, health visitors, hospital doctors, each other and even on chance and this should be recognized as part of the grieving process.

A child admitted into hospital for cataract surgery may be of any age, from a few weeks old to the teens. With congenital cataracts, the trend nowadays is to operate as soon as possible so that visual development is not delayed. The importance of admission as near as possible to operating time, providing facilities for parents to stay, involving parents in the care of their child while in hospital and ensuring the stay in hospital is as short as possible is well documented in paediatric textbooks and research articles. Support for the parents of the child with congenital cataracts should also be considered by the ophthalmic nurse.

Problem	Goal	Nursing intervention
Parents unsure of treatments and expected visual prognosis, because of lack of knowledge.	Parents will state that their knowledge is at a level acceptable to them and will feel able to ask any questions that they feel are important within 24 hours of child's admission.	1. Build up interpersonal relationships with parents. 2. Explain when surgery is scheduled and provide means for them to accompany child to anaesthetic room if desired. 3. Explain expected length of stay in hospital. 4. Detail care that parents can give, i.e. bathing, feeding, playing. 5. Explain preoperative preparation for surgery and postoperative care. 6. Provide opportunities for parents to ask questions and answer them effectively. 7. Include child in explanations if of age where language is understood.

Preoperative preparation for surgery is similar to preparation for any other type of surgery – fasting, bathing, weighing, urine testing. Specialist procedures, such as lash cutting if required, are preferably carried out when the child is anaesthetized. Principles of asepsis are utilized and adapted to the child when dressings are performed, but the procedure itself can cause anxiety, especially in toddlers.

Problem	Goal	Nursing intervention
Child apprehensive about having drops instilled because of fear of the unknown.	Child will know what to expect and why drops need to be instilled prior to the procedure.	1. Explain need for topical medication. 2. Allow parents into the treatment room if child wishes. 3. Provide demonstration on 'teddy' or doll so child can see what is going to happen. 4. Ensure drops are instilled as quickly as possible, but safely, so that the child doesn't become distressed by waiting. 5. If possible, teach the parents to instil drops.

Following surgery, refractive correction may be used fairly quickly in order for vision to be stimulated. This is usually done by either spectacle correction or the use of contact lenses. It is important that parents be given information regarding the refractive correction method chosen and its importance.

Problem	Goal	Nursing intervention
Parents unsure of the care required for ophthalmic correction with spectacles, because of lack of knowledge.	Parents will state that they feel confident in caring for the child prior to discharge from hospital.	1. Explain importance of ensuring that visual correction is worn in order to allow development of vision. 2. Explain side effects of spectacle correction, i.e. increased magnification, distortion of peripheral field and subsequent possible loss of balance until child adjusts to them. 3. Advise on cleaning glasses with soap and water to allow for maximum light to enter eye. 4. In younger children advise on using elastic to keep spectacles in place.
Parents unsure of the care required for ophthalmic correction with contact lenses, because of lack of knowledge	Parents will state that they feel competent in caring for the child's contact lenses prior to discharge home.	1. Explain importance of hygiene prior to inserting lenses. 2. Explain how often lenses must be removed and cleaned, depending on type used. 3. Show location of lens on eye surface. 4. Demonstrate removal and insertion of lenses and allow parents to practise skill until they feel competent. 5. Instruct on what to do if lens becomes lost or displaced.

In a child who has had congenital cataracts, it is usual to expect some delay in the development of vision. It is an important part of the ophthalmic nurse's role to provide information to the parents on how best to stimulate vision in their child, using the methods outlined in Chapter 1.

Finally, it is important to ensure that the parents don't become overprotective toward their visually handicapped child. Safety is important, but the child should be allowed to explore its environment and learn from it.

Problem	Goal	Nursing intervention
Potential problem of parents becoming overprotective towards their visually handicapped child through fear of injury.	Parents will be aware of safety aspects but will allow their child to explore her environment and so learn from it.	1. Explain safety measures needed to be taken, i.e. no sharp edges on toys, use of fire guards, avoidance of trailing flexes, use of cooker guards, use of safety plugs. 2. Explain importance of allowing child to explore environment. 3. Explain that some bumps will be inevitable and that they occur in all children. 4. Provide a firm 'no' for danger areas such as fires and cookers.

Depending on the age of the child, guidance should be given to the parents on helping their child achieve normal developmental milestones, but explanations should be given that some of these may be delayed due to the initial delay in the development of vision. Other problems may arise, depending on the individual child, and whether other handicaps are present, as can be the case in children with congenital cataracts. Parents should always feel able to contact the hospital if any problems arise or they are worried about any aspect of the child and its care.

Acquired Abnormalities of Clarity

This is much the largest group, most of which are termed 'senile cataracts'. However, trauma (including eye surgery), electromagnetic radiation, abnormalities in metabolism and nutrition and certain drugs may cause the formation of cataracts, as may other intraocular diseases, in particular uveitis.

Nursing care required by patients admitted for cataract surgery may have similar or widely differing aspects – each patient should be treated as an individual and his needs assessed accordingly, but other considerations may apply according to the type of cataract the patient has acquired.

If, for example, the patient has bilateral senile cataracts he may be considerably affected in daily living tasks even though one cataract is usually more advanced than the other. In contrast, the patient who has a unilateral traumatic cataract may have normal vision in the unaffected eye and may only be hindered in carrying out daily living tasks by the restrictions that are imposed on him postoperatively as a result of the surgery. The diabetic patient may have problems in controlling his diabetes because of this reduction in vision and his subsequent inability to administer his own insulin, test his urine and adhere to his dietary requirements. Similarly, systemic disorders such as rheumatoid arthritis and Parkinson's disease may affect mobilization while in hospital and lead to the patient being unable to comply with topical medication on discharge. Problems that are specific to cataract patients will be dealt with here whereas other problems relevant to all ophthalmic inpatients are covered in Chapter 7. Finally, it is essential for the nurse always to consider further problems that may be specific for her patient alone. Despite the differing causes of cataract development, the principles of care for the patient undergoing surgery are the same, whatever the cause.

Symptoms and Signs of Cataract

A cataract is any opacity in the lens and symptoms will therefore depend on the density, size and position of such opacities within the lens. Symptoms are also subjective and two patients may vary in the nature and severity of symptoms, although they have similar cataracts. Young children will not and patients of low intellect may not complain of poor vision and it is common for an elderly patient not to notice a gradual loss of acuity in one eye. They may present with any combination of the following:

1. decreased acuity: this is usually of gradual onset and is greater for distance vision than near vision in early cataracts;
2. dazzle and glare: certain early cataracts cause this symptom, which tends to be worse in bright sunlight or when driving at night;
3. a general dimming of the vision: an overall increase in density of the lens will reduce the quantity of light reaching the retina and give this symptom;
4. a change in refractive error: early cataracts often cause the patient to attend the optician more regularly as a

change in lens density alters the refractive power of the lens;

5. double vision and multiple images: cataracts are the commonest cause of monocular diplopia (double vision in one eye);
6. squint: a uniocular congenital cataract may be the cause of a squint in a child and occasionally an acquired cataract leads to a squint in an adult.

Signs of Cataract

A mature white lens may be easily seen in the usually dark pupil. Early opacities can be identified with a slit-lamp or using the ophthalmoscope, where they stand out as dark against the red background (red reflex).

Management of Cataracts

All treatment is aimed at improving the patient's quality of vision and will include careful assessment and therapy for amblyopia in children.

Prevention

Congenital Cataracts

This includes genetic counselling, rubella vaccinations in girls to prevent congenital acquisition of virus by a fetus, the screening of babies for galactosaemia (an inborn error of metabolism causing an irreversible cataract and mental retardation) and general advice against taking drugs in pregnancy.

Acquired Cataract

This includes good diabetic control in diabetes, the wearing of ocular protection at work and when playing sport, good protection of the eye during head and neck radiotherapy, the prevention of dehydration in gastrointestinal diseases, particularly in hot climates, and the prevention of overuse of cataractogenic drugs, especially steroids.

At present research into drugs which may delay or arrest the progression of cataracts is being pursued, as certain compounds have been shown to delay cataract formation in animal models.

Treatment to Alleviate Symptoms

General and Optical

Shielding the eye from extraneous light by the use of peaked caps or hats, together with darkened spectacle lenses, can reduce dazzle and glare in bright sunlight. An increase in illumination, however, may be necessary for reading in the home (Chapter 2), and accurate refractions (tests for spectacles) may delay the need for surgery in early cataracts.

Surgical

Surgical intervention should be considered when symptoms significantly interfere with the functional needs of the patient and when the potential benefits of surgery outweigh the risks. A careful evaluation of possible ocular conditions contributing to the visual impairment should be made, in particular co-existing chronic simple glaucoma and senile macular degeneration.

Most patients admitted for cataract extraction will have been on the waiting list for admission to hospital and will have received notification of their impending admission. However, the length of time of notification prior to admission may vary from a few days to a week or two and so some patients may be more prepared psychologically than others. Presurgical assessment clinics are increasingly used shortly before planned surgery for inpatients and day cases. In addition, it should never be assumed that a patient who has already had one eye operated upon will automatically experience less anxiety than someone admitted for the first time. The reverse situation quite often applies and therefore assessment should always be on an individual basis.

Although most patients are aware they are coming into hospital because they have a cataract, what they actually understand cataract to mean often differs from what it actually is. The most common description given by patients is of a skin over the front of the eye rather than a cloudiness of the lens which lies within the eye. They therefore have a further lack of knowledge in that they do not realize that the operation will result in a wound to the eye. Although this misconception is common, it should never be taken for granted that their knowledge is non-existent or incorrect and this area should be covered on patient assessment by asking the patient to explain his understanding in his own words. If a lack of knowledge is identified and the patient is not aware of his condition and treatment then steps should be taken to rectify this.

Problem	Goal	Nursing intervention
Patient doesn't understand meaning of cataract, because of misconception.	Patient will explain the meaning of cataract within 24 hours of admission.	1. Establish knowledge base. 2. Prepare and present teaching session to cover: (a) location of lens within the eye; (b) causes of cataract relevant to patient; (c) reasons for preoperative investigations; (d) reasons for surgery; (e) correction of aphakia postoperatively. 3. Evaluate teaching session. 4. Reiterate information as necessary. 5. Rectify any misunderstandings.

Visual symptoms experienced by patients who have a cataract vary greatly and therefore care given should be relevant to the visual loss experienced by the individual patient. However, a common symptom experienced by patients is dazzle or glare. This can be very uncomfortable for the patient and nursing intervention should be given to help overcome the problem.

Problem	Goal	Nursing intervention
Patient experiences 'dazzle and glare' from bright lights due to irregular refraction of light rays.	Patient will report no undue discomfort during preoperative period.	1. Establish which lighting situations cause most problems. 2. Incorporate use of blinds on windows to reduce direct sunlight. 3. Advise patient not to sit in direct sunlight. 4. Provide sunglasses for use in adverse lighting conditions. 5. Ensure ward lighting is maintained at comfortable levels. 6. Evaluate effectiveness of intervention.

Diabetic patients with an acquired cataract will need a plan of care regarding control of diabetes with insulin/tablets/diet as usual so that healing is encouraged and not delayed due to increased blood sugar levels.

Patients will usually have been scheduled for an intraocular lens implant prior to surgery. In order to calculate dioptric power of the implant for each individual patient, biometry may be carried out preoperatively. This involves measurements being taken with ultrasonic equipment and patients will need to be prepared for this procedure as they may not understand what it entails.

Problem	Goal	Nursing intervention
Patient unprepared for biometry because of lack of knowledge.	Patient will be able to state what biometry entails prior to the procedure being carried out.	1. Explain need for procedure. 2. Outline procedure: (a) patient will sit at machine resembling slit-lamp; (b) local anaesthetic drop will be instilled; (c) patient will be required to sit still and fix his vision straight ahead; (d) patient will hear the machine clicking as measurements are taken; (e) the lens strength required will be estimated. 3. It is important to explain that insertion of the lens in theatre may not always be possible at the time of the cataract operation, and that it can be done as a secondary procedure if the surgeon thinks it appropriate.

For further preoperative care for the patient undergoing cataract extraction refer to Chapter 6 for day surgery and Chapter 7 on the principles of inpatient care.

Methods of Cataract Extraction

Intracapsular

This method of cataract surgery, where the lens is removed in total, is now rarely performed in the UK. The necessary rupture of the zonule may be aided by the enzymatic action of alpha-chymotrypsin, especially in the younger patient. The lens is usually removed with a cryoprobe, which uses liquid nitrogen to provide a rapid freezing effect.

Non-traumatic lens capsule forceps are available as an alternative to the cryoprobe as a means of grasping the lens.

Extracapsular (Figure 19.2)

In this method the anterior capsule is multiply punctured (capsulotomy) or torn (capsulorhexis) and the nucleus and cortex are removed. The posterior capsule is left intact, acting as a barrier to vitreous protrusion through the pupil. Many methods of removing the lens nucleus and cortex are available, including phacoemulsification, but the desired end result is similar: a clear, intact posterior capsule supported by the zonule. Extracapsular surgery is contraindicated in dislocated lenses.

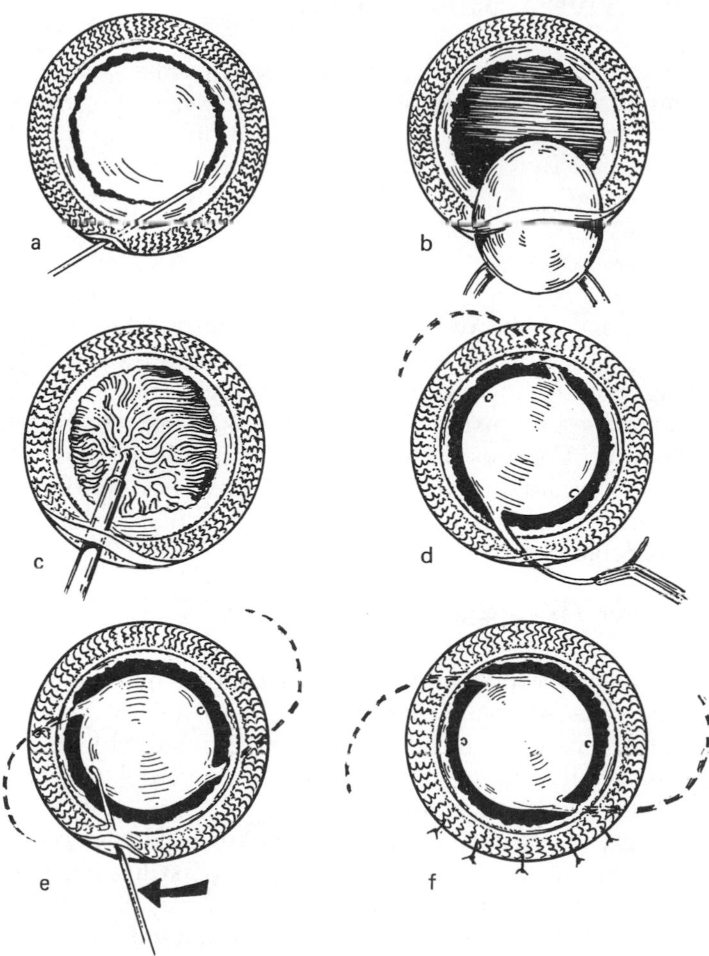

Figure 19.2 The stages of extracapsular cataract extraction. **(a)** Anterior capsulotomy. **(b)** Expression of the lens nucleus. **(c)** Aspiration of the cortex. **(d)** Insertion of the lens implant. **(e)** Dialling the lens implant. **(f)** Wound closure with interrupted sutures.

Lensectomy

The use of guillotine cutting instruments with or without ultrasonic fragmentation has become popular in certain conditions. These instruments, principally designed for cutting membranes and vitreous, can be used to break up nuclei as well as to aspirate soft lens material. They enable a lens to be removed with only a small wound in the eye and are used mainly for congenital cataracts and following trauma.

Operative Complications

In general, the more complex the procedure the greater the potential for complications. The consequences of operative complications may not become apparent until the postoperative period. Two immediate problems are worthy of particular mention.

Vitreous Loss

This can usually be avoided by a careful surgical technique, in particular, by avoiding extraneous pressure on the eye during surgery. If it occurs, an anterior vitrectomy should be performed to ensure that no vitreous is left adherent to the wound. Vitreous loss does not contraindicate insertion of a lens implant, but the visual result may be compromised by an increased risk of postoperative macular oedema or retinal detachment.

Expulsive Haemorrhage

This is a rare complication that may occur when the eye is opened. The intraocular contents are extruded through the wound because of a rapid increase in intraocular blood volume, usually following a choroidal vessel rupture. Blindness of the eye is the result.

If an expulsive haemorrhage occurs during the operation, it is important to explain to the patient what has occurred and the visual prognosis. This explanation may have to take place fairly soon after the operation, especially if the patient has had a local anaesthetic, as he may be fully aware that something has gone wrong and his anxiety levels may be

Problem	Goal	Nursing intervention
Poor visual prognosis due to expulsive haemorrhage occurring in theatre.	Patient will report that he understands reasons for sight loss and will know of services, both statutory and voluntary, that can be approached for help if required, by the date of discharge.	1. Reiterate doctor's explanation that during surgery the eye has bled badly and that is why he has a pressure pad and bandage *in situ*. 2. Explain that because of this unexpected complication the visual outcome from the operation will be very poor. 3. Allow the patient to verbalize fears and worries and also include the relatives in discussions as this will have a direct effect on the family. 4. If vision poor in other eye, once patient feels ready to take in information, advise patient and relations of services available and contact medical social worker to visit.

See also retrobulbar haemorrhage in Chapter 9.

increased if he is left uninformed. In some instances, where the patient has low or no vision in the fellow eye, registration as blind or partially sighted may have to be considered in the future and the patient will need to be referred to Social Services and informed of voluntary or statutory agencies that may be approached for assistance.

Refer to Chapter 7 on principles of inpatient care for postoperative care and management following intraocular surgery.

Postoperative Complications

Infection

Intraocular infection is a very serious but rare complication of any intraocular procedure. It usually becomes apparent between 12 and 72 hours following surgery and symptoms consist of a worsening of vision and severe pain. The lids and conjunctiva may be swollen, the cornea cloudy and a hypopyon may be present. Successful treatment requires positive identification of the causative organism by anterior chamber tap or vitrectomy and intensive antibiotics. The earlier effective treatment is instituted the better the prognosis, although visual results are usually disappointing.

Wound Breakdown

This may be associated with iris prolapse, either due to faulty surgical technique or from postoperative trauma, which includes eye rubbing. A further visit to theatre is usually necessary. A shield (cartella) may be worn at night for at least 2 weeks to help prevent this complication.

Corneal Endothelial Cell Loss

If trauma to the endothelium is severe during surgery, corneal oedema may not clear postoperatively. If the trauma is moderate the cornea may clear only to go cloudy months or years following the surgery, and a corneal graft may be necessary to restore vision. The use of viscoelastic materials such as sodium hyaluronate has proved effective in protecting the endothelium during intraocular manipulations.

Retinal Detachment

A 2% incidence of retinal detachment rate following intracapsular lens extraction is often quoted. This figure appears to be much reduced with extracapsular lens extraction.

Pupil Block Glaucoma

If the iris becomes adherent to the anterior vitreous face or the implant, such that aqueous cannot reach the anterior chamber, an acute high pressure in the eye ensues. It may be prevented by performing peripheral iridectomy(ies) during surgery.

Astigmatism

Unless carefully sutured, the wound may induce distorted vision secondary to astigmatism. High degrees may require suture removal or resuturing of the wound.

Cystoid Macular Oedema

This is a collection of fluid at the macula, reducing central vision, and is commoner with intracapsular extractions or vitreous loss and in eyes with postoperative inflammation.

Posterior Capsule Opacification

Lens fibre growth following extracapsular extraction may produce a layer of cells over the posterior capsule. If this covers the visual axis, acuity will be reduced and the posterior capsule will need to be incised. This can be performed surgically with a sharp knife via the limbus or pars plana, or with the cutting YAG laser. Both of these procedures may produce complications in themselves and the need for capsulotomy must be carefully considered.

Correction of Aphakia

When the lens or the eye is removed the eye cannot focus for near or distance (unless the eye is highly myopic). A correcting lens of suitable power must therefore be employed. There are three methods of correction of aphakia, which are also discussed in Chapter 12. All have their advantages and disadvantages and the patient should be assessed on an individual basis.

Aphakic Glasses

High-power positive lenses in spectacles may be used to focus objects on the retina. However, objects look approximately 25-30% larger than usual and peripheral vision is distorted and constricted. This form of correction is not suitable if the fellow eye is phakic and has good vision, as the difference in image size between the eyes cannot be tolerated. However, many patients who are aphakic in both eyes cope well once they adapt to the spectacles.

When correction of aphakia is to be with spectacles, temporary aphakic spectacles can be issued while the patient is on the ward.

However, because of the distortion caused by these, the patient may experience some problems which the nurse can help overcome.

Problem	Goal	Nursing intervention
Patient unable to adjust to aphakic spectacles because of distortion created.	Patient will be able to move safely around the ward at his normal level of independence before his discharge home.	1. Explain magnification, distortion and constriction of peripheral vision. 2. Allow patient to use spectacles initially while sitting down in order to get used to the visual effects. 3. Place articles, e.g. box of tissues, cold drinks, buzzer, on bedside tables and encourage patient to judge distances. 4. When patient feels ready, escort him around the ward, ensuring safety, until patient feels able to mobilize independently. 5. Emphasize that care must be taken with steps and pavement edges when outdoors.

Contact Lenses

These may be hard or soft and worn on a daily-wear or extended-wear basis. They give a full field, minimal distortion and may be used in one eye when the other has good vision. However, some patients cannot manage the manipulation involved in daily-wear lenses, while extended-wear soft lenses may induce corneal vascularization and ulceration.

Patients other than babies who are to have their aphakia corrected with contact lenses are not usually fitted with them until at least 6 weeks after surgery. In the meantime, if they have good vision in the unaffected eye, they will have to use this one eye for vision, as giving aphakic spectacles in this instance would cause an imbalance. By using one eye only, problems can occur which are similar to those occurring with a patient who has restricted visual field due to one eye being occluded (Chapter 7). In this instance, in addition to the care to be taken while the patient is on the ward, it is advisable to warn him that he must take extra care when crossing the road to make sure nothing is approaching from his 'blind' side and also when mobilizing around the home to avoid, for example, bumping into furniture and catching pan handles when they are on the cooker (Chapter 12).

Intraocular Lenses

This is the method of choice for the patient with senile cataracts. The vision will usually need to be 'fine tuned' with thin spectacle lenses for near or distance vision, or both, following surgery, although bifocal implants have recently been introduced. Lens implants bring their own short- and long-term complications, some of which may not yet be apparent, and for this reason some surgeons limit their use to patients over a certain age. Most are manufactured from polymethyl methacrylate (Perspex). The use of new flexible materials for the central lens optic is being introduced. The required power of implant lens may be calculated preoperatively when the corneal curvature has been measured by keratometry and the lens dimensions within the eye by ultrasonography. There are many different designs, but they fall into three main categories (Figure 19.3) (Chapter 12).

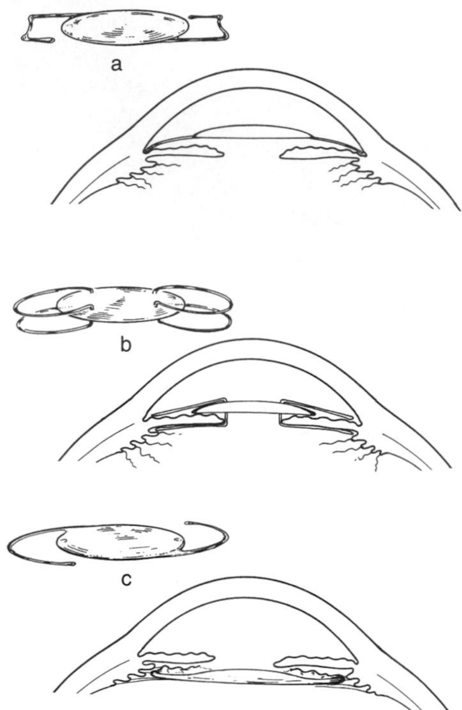

Figure 19.3 Design and position in the eye of **(a)** anterior chamber lens – now most commonly used in secondary implantation; **(b)** iris clip lens – no longer used; **(c)** posterior chamber lens.

Anterior Chamber Lenses

These are positioned anterior to the iris by placing the supporting feet in the drainage angle. They may be used after intracapsular extraction or for secondary implantation (Plate 7).

Iris-Supported Lenses

These are rarely used today because of problems of dislocation and inflammation. The lens optic is suspended from the iris by loops, either in front of or behind the iris. They were used mainly after intracapsular surgery.

Posterior Chamber Lenses

These lenses lie entirely behind the pupil. The lens may be sulcus-fixated with loops positioned between the iris and the ciliary body or 'in the bag', where all the lens is placed in the capsule of the patient's original lens. The latter relies on the integrity of the zonules for long-term stability. Posterior chamber implants are implanted following extracapsular surgery and phacoemulsification. In certain circumstances they can be sutured to the sclera behind the iris when no support exists from the capsule.

Patients receiving intraocular lens implants during surgery gain useful vision fairly quickly following surgery. Initially, there may be some corneal oedema, especially if endothelial touch occurred in theatre, but this soon settles after 2–3 days and the patient will notice improvement. As there is minimal magnification with intraocular lenses, the patient doesn't have to be taught how to cope with any visual distortion.

Prognosis for Vision Following Cataract Extraction

If corrected visual acuity alone is measured and the eye is otherwise normal, all the above procedures result in over 90% of patients attaining 6/12 or better. Modern surgical techniques have made cataract surgery much more predictable and surgery is therefore being advised with lesser degrees of cataract, particularly if an implant is planned.

Many people believe a cataract has to be ripe before it can be removed. Yet others are greatly alarmed to hear they have any degree of cataract because they fear being told they must have an operation. At the other end of the scale, some patients will be well informed and may even request a particular design of implant. Discovering the patient's preconceptions and confirming or adapting these is an important part of the specialist nurse's role.

Further Reading

Fraiberg, S. (1977) *Insights from the Blind*, Souvenir Press, London.

Kovalesky, A. (1985) *Nurses' Guide to Children's Eyes*, Grune & Stratton, London.

Weiss, T. J. (1978) *Children in Need of Special Care*, Souvenir Press, London.

20

VITREOUS AND RETINA

Grant Raymond and Karen Partington

CHAPTER SUMMARY

FUNCTIONAL ANATOMY

EMBRYOLOGY OF THE RETINA

During embryonic development the optic vesicle appears as an out-pouching of the forebrain. This subsequently invaginates to form two layers with a potential space in between (Figure 20.1).

The inner layer forms the neurosensory retina, containing photoreceptors (i.e. the rods and cones) and a complex network of nerve cells which connect the rods and cones to the ganglion cell layer (Figure 20.2). Axons from the

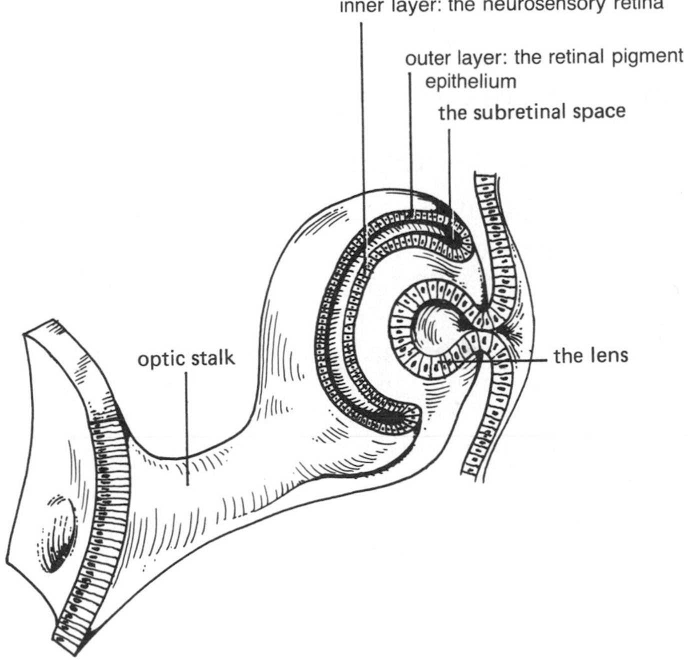

Figure 20.1 The retina in the developing eye.

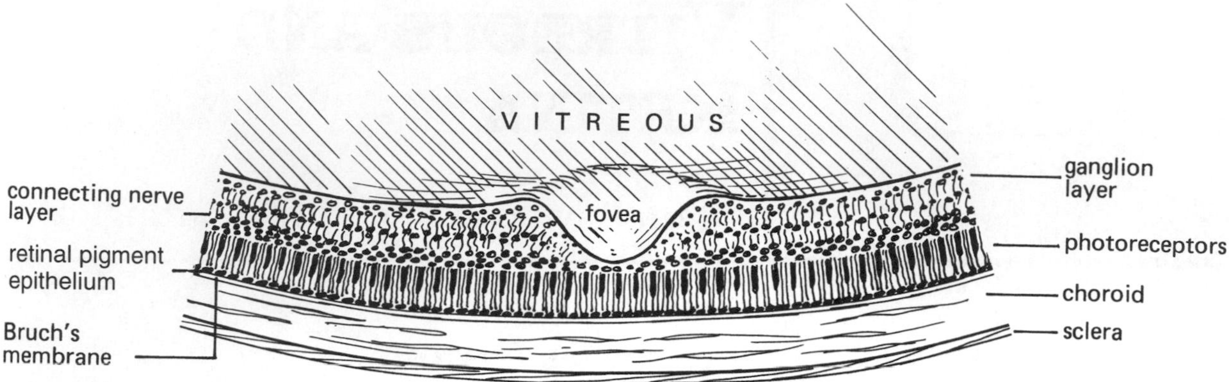

Figure 20.2 Layers of the retina.

ganglion cells travel in the plane of the retina towards the disc and form the optic nerve.

The outer layer remains as a single layer of cells known as the retinal pigment epithelium (RPE). These cells become loosely adherent to the rods and cones in the inner layer.

The potential space between these two layers (the subretinal space) is the site of fluid accumulation in retinal detachments when the neurosensory retina is displaced forwards.

Anatomy of the Retina

The retina can be divided into three regions (Figure 20.3):

1. the ora serrata, the anterior termination of the retina;
2. the midperipheral retina;
3. the central or macular region which surrounds the fovea. The fovea has only cone receptors and all the other cells in the retina are displaced so that the light falls directly on the cones. This is the area of the retina which is used for fine visual discrimination and disturbances here can cause a marked loss of visual acuity (Figure 20.2).

The optic disc is a pale pink, circular area nasal to the macula, where the optic nerve fibres leave the eye.

Blood Supply

The retina receives blood from two sources, each with its own blood/retinal barrier.

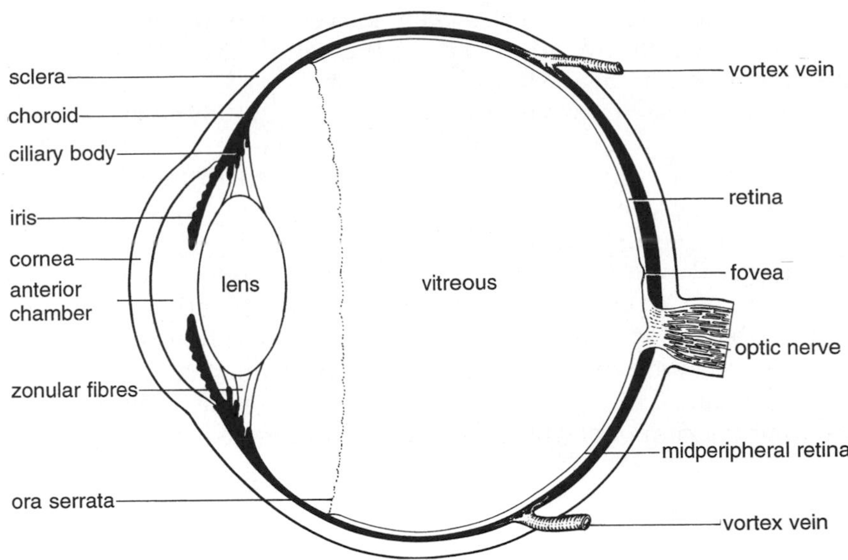

Figure 20.3 Regions of the retina.

The Choroidal Circulation

The choroid contains a mass of blood vessels, which lie between the retina and sclera, and leaks plasma through specialized capillaries (the choriocapillaris). The RPE acts as a barrier to certain substances (e.g. fluorescein) but transports some nutrients and proteins, which play an important part in the photoreceptors' response to light.

The Retinal Circulation

This circulation arises from the central retinal artery, which enters the eye with the optic nerve. Blood returns through the central retinal vein. The branches of these vessels are clearly visible on ophthalmoscopic examination and thus provide direct information about certain systemic conditions affecting small blood vessels (e.g. hypertension and diabetes). The major vessels also form landmarks which help to localize lesions within the retina. The barrier between blood and retina here is the blood vessel wall.

Physiology of the Retina

Rods and cones contain pigments (rhodopsin in rods and iodopsins in cones) which absorb light from a range of wavelengths. Light energy is then converted into nerve impulses, which are processed by the retina and make vision possible in the dark (scotopic vision).

Cones are less sensitive and function in bright illumination (photopic vision), but allow colour to be perceived. There are three groups of cones sensitive to different colours (red, green and blue). Any colour can be perceived by combined stimulation of these cells.

The macular region of the retina is primarily responsible for form and colour vision and the peripheral retina is responsible for spatial orientation. When macular function is lost the patient cannot read or sew, but retains 'navigational vision'. This means that the patient remains independent but cannot perform tasks requiring detailed vision.

The Vitreous

The vitreous is a gel-like substance filling the space between the lens and the retina. It is transparent and firmly adherent to the ciliary body and ora serrata. It is loosely adherent to the retina until the patient is approximately 60 years old, when the vitreous begins to degenerate and liquefy. This results in separation of the vitreous from the retina except at its base – the firm attachment at the ora serrata.

Investigations

The most important measure of retinal function is the visual acuity, which should be measured for distance and near vision. The retina is unique as an internal structure in how easily it can be seen. Visualization is the most useful and common way of investigating the retina. It is carried out using 1) the direct ophthalmoscope, 2) the indirect ophthalmoscope and 3) contact lenses (e.g. three-mirror lens) and non-contact lenses with slit-lamp biomicroscope examination.

Fluorescein Angiography

Fluorescein angiography is used in the evaluation of a large number of retinal disorders. It involves intravenous injection of a small quantity of fluorescent dye, which is photographed during its passage through the eye. Abnormalities may appear as an area of hyperfluorescence (e.g. due to leakage) or hypofluorescence (e.g. due to capillary occlusions). This is helpful in showing the site and nature of many retinal lesions. In many hospitals the injection is administered by the medical staff. However, with the advent of the extended role of the nurse many hospitals are now training nurses to be responsible for this procedure.

Problem	Goal	Nursing intervention
Potential medical disorder which may contraindicate immediate fluorescein injection.	To ensure the patient has no known conditions that contraindicate fluorescein injection.	1. Establish whether the patient is diabetic – if so, find out if it is controlled by tablets, diet or insulin. 2. Ask the patient if he has any heart conditions, bronchitis, asthma or hypertension. Record blood pressure. 3. Note what other medicines the patient takes. 4. Check with the patient that he is not wearing contact lenses and does not have a history of glaucoma. 5. If the patient is a young female, ensure she is not pregnant. 6. Record all relevant medical information as, in the event of a reaction to the injection, this may prove beneficial.
Patient is apprehensive through lack of knowledge regarding the procedure.	To ensure the patient understands the procedure and is willing to co-operate.	1. Explain to the patient that his blood pressure will be taken and drops instilled into his eye(s). 2. Tell him that the drops will enlarge his pupil and allow the photographer a good view of the fundus. 3. Explain that when the pupils are dilated he will be taken into the camera room, photographs will be taken and a small amount of yellow dye will be injected into his arm. As this is being done more pictures will be taken at the same time. Tell him that the flashes will be very bright but he must remain as still as possible as the dye lasts for only a short time in the eye. 4. Ensure that the patient understands that his skin will be a yellow colour for 24 hours and his urine green for 48 hours. Reassure him that this is a normal effect of the dye.

Diabetics who test their urine with Labstix should be advised to test their blood sugar instead as the dye will affect the result of the Labstix reading.

A consent form is signed in some centres by all patients. For patients under 16 years of age a consent form must be signed by the parents or guardian.

Problem	Goal	Nursing intervention
Risk of severe reaction following injection.	An uneventful procedure for the patient.	1. Observe the patient carefully throughout the procedure. 2. Ensure prompt medical attention should a reaction occur. 3. Ensure all members of the photographic unit are aware of the emergency procedure.
Potential risk of fluorescein being injected into tissues around the vein, causing severe pain to the patient.	To avoid causing pain to the patient.	1. Observe the needle site during the injection; observe for swelling under the skin or the appearance of yellow dye around the needle site.
Patient anxious about reduced vision from a dilated pupil.	To relieve anxiety and maintain safety.	1. Reassure the patient that this will last only for a few hours. 2. Advise the patient not to drive.

Electrodiagnostic Tests

Electro-Oculography (EOG)

An electro-oculogram is an electrical recording based on the standing potential of the eye. It is useful in assessing hereditary macular disease (e.g. Best's disease).

Procedure

The patient's visual acuity is recorded and electrodes are placed on the lateral and medial canthus. The patient is asked to sit in front of a large screen and, without moving his head, to follow a flashing light moving from left to right. Both eyes are tested together – initially in a dark room for 15 minutes and then in a light room for 15 minutes.

Electroretinography (ERG)

An electroretinography is an electrical recording of the response of the retina to a visual stimulus such as a flash of light. ERG is useful in the investigation of hereditary retinal diseases (e.g. retinitis pigmentosa) and in monitoring retinal toxicity associated with metallic intraocular foreign bodies.

Procedure

The patient's visual acuity is tested and recorded. Local anaesthetic and dilating drops are instilled into the patient's eye(s) and an ocular-fitted contact lens electrode is placed on or near the cornea. This enables recordings of electrical responses from various parts of the retina to be made. Reference electrodes are placed on the outer canthus and forehead.

A variety of stimulus conditions are used:

1. light-adapted: the patient sits in a light room and a high-intensity white light is used;
2. dark-adapted: the patient sits in a dark room for 10 minutes; the rods then begin to function, stimulated by a specific blue light flash;
3. flicker: a flickering light is used which selectively stimulates cones.

(It is also possible to do this test on an anaesthetized child.)

Visual Evoked Response (VER)

The VER basically measures the time taken (latency) for a light stimulus to pass along the visual pathway to the occipital cortex and also the amplitude of the response. This test may be indicated in optic atrophy, optic neuritis, unexplained low visual acuity and hysterical amblyopia.

Procedure

The patient's visual acuity is recorded and electrodes are placed over the back of the head and forehead. The patient sits in diffused light in front of a television stimulator or constantly moving chequerboard pattern. This test lasts for approximately 30 minutes.

Although ERG, EOG and VER are different tests they may all be linked to the same computer which triggers the stimuli, records the responses and provides a hard copy from which the analysis is made.

Ultrasonography

Diagnostic ultrasonography has made possible the detection of intraocular abnormalities not visualized clinically because of opacification of the cornea, lens or vitreous, and allows accurate measurement of intraocular tumours (e.g. choroidal melanoma). It uses the principle of sound waves passing through a substance and reflecting at an interface. There are two main types that use varying frequencies: A scan, which determines tissue density and composition displaying the data on a one-dimensional acoustic display, and B scan, which determines tissue morphology and produces a two-dimensional acoustic section.

Ultrasonography is most frequently performed for the following indications:

1. to assess the posterior segment of the eye for the presence of a retinal detachment or tumour when the view is obscured by cataract or vitreous haemorrhage;
2. to assess the nature of a space-occupying lesion in the eye or orbit;
3. to measure intraocular dimensions before cataract surgery in order to calculate the power of a lens implant (biometry).

Problem	Goal	Nursing intervention
The patient is anxious through lack of knowledge about the procedure.	To ensure the patient understands what is expected of him.	1. Ensure the patient is seated comfortably and is appropriately positioned. 2. Explain that a diagnostic probe covered in jelly will be gently moved over the patient's closed eyelids; meanwhile he will be instructed to look in various directions. 3. Explain that the test will take approximately 2–3 minutes from start to finish. 4. Following the scan inform the patient that results will be sent to his referring consultant and that an appointment will be made to discuss the findings.

Sometimes the scan is performed with the patient's eyelids open after an anaesthetic drop has been instilled into the eye (e.g. biometry)

Colour Vision

Defective colour vision can be hereditary or acquired. Hereditary defective colour vision occurs because one or more of the retinal photopigments are absent or abnormal; 7% of men and 1% of women have defective colour vision with poor red–green discrimination. Visual acuity is not usually affected and many such people are unaware of their poor colour perception. Defective colour vision can also be acquired. Compressive lesions of the optic nerve and optic neuritis affect colour vision, as do many macular disorders. Overdosage with dioxin and some drugs used in the treatment of tuberculosis may upset colour vision. Colour vision can quickly be assessed using pseudoisochromatic plates (Ishihara charts) or, if detailed analysis is required, the Farnsworth–Munsell 100-hue test can be used, where a patient is required to arrange subtly different coloured chips in order.

Disease of the Retina

Retinal Artery Occlusion

Occlusion of the central retinal artery causes sudden painless loss of vision. Occlusion of a branch artery causes a defect in the field of vision corresponding to the area affected.

The main causes of occlusion of the central retinal artery are emboli from an atheromatous plaque in a carotid artery in older patients and valvular heart disease in the young. Hypertension or diabetes are often associated (Table 20.1). Emboli can also originate from a blood clot accumulating in the ventricles of patients who have recently suffered from a myocardial infarct. Finally, the central retinal artery can be affected by atheroma and in cranial arteritis.

Transient loss of vision can be caused by an embolus which temporarily blocks an artery. Spontaneous dislodgement restores the circulation leaving no permanent effects. This is called amaurosis fugax, or 'fleeting blindness'.

Appearance

In arterial occlusion the retina becomes very pale and the arterioles become extremely thin. The fovea appears like a cherry-red spot in contrast to the surrounding pale retina.

Management

This condition is an ophthalmic emergency. If the occlusion is due to an embolus it can sometimes be dislodged by rapidly reducing the intraocular pressure. Treatment involves attempting to dislodge an occluding embolus into a more peripheral branch by using a variety of procedures. These include massaging the globe rapidly, administering

Table 20.1 Causes of central retinal artery occlusion

Emboli	Carotid arteries (atheroma)
	Diseased heart valves
	Myocardial infarct
	Atrial tumours
Arterial diseases	Atheroma
	Giant cell (cranial, temporal) arteritis
Associated conditions	Hypertension
	Diabetes

acetazolamide intravenously and, occasionally, anterior chamber paracentesis. However, the patient has to be seen within 6 hours of the event and treatment often proves largely ineffective even if administered promptly. Subsequent investigations are aimed at preventing further episodes, if possible, by identifying the cause and treating it.

Carotid Doppler studies and ultrasonography of the heart may be carried out to find the source of emboli. Reduction of further embolic episodes is sometimes attempted, either by surgery on the carotid arteries or with drugs that reduce platelet adhesiveness such as aspirin. Patients who have emboli from the heart may require anticoagulants.

Problem	Goal	Nursing intervention
Anxiety and fear caused by sudden loss of vision.	1. To alleviate anxiety. 2. To provide reassurance.	1. Give clear explanation of the treatment and proceedings. 2. Give the patient the opportunity to ask questions.
Anxiety due to lack of knowledge about the procedures.	1. To ensure that the patient receives adequate information. 2. To support the patient and gain his co-operation.	1. Massage of the globe – explain that his eye will be massaged by the doctor or nurse by pressing firmly through the closed eyelids with the fingertips for a few seconds and then releasing. 2. Anterior chamber paracentesis – give a brief explanation of the procedure to the patient. Ensure the patient is comfortable with his head well supported. Explain to him that local anaesthetic eye drops will be instilled to numb the area. A small needle is passed through the limbus and one or two drops of aqueous expressed. The importance of remaining still must be stressed. 3. Intravenous acetazolamide – explain to the patient that an injection will be given into a vein in the arm. Ensure that he is aware that the ensuing diuresis is an effect from the injection and a desired result.

Following a central retinal artery occlusion the patient may be admitted to a ward if an invasive procedure such as anterior chamber paracentesis has been performed.

The type of patient commonly presenting with a central retinal artery occlusion is often elderly and may therefore have other ophthalmic changes due to age, such as cataract. The sudden loss of vision in one eye coupled with diminished sight in the remaining eye may severely handicap this

Problem	Goal	Nursing intervention
Potential problem of infection following anterior chamber paracentesis.	1. To prevent infection. 2. To ensure wound heals satisfactorily.	1. Instil local antibiotics. 2. Observe and report any signs of infection.

patient, and he will require careful assessment as to his ability to cope with activities of daily living.

Retinal Vein Occlusion

Occlusion of the central retinal vein results in painless blurred or foggy vision but if severe can also cause complete loss of vision. Occlusion of a branch vein can cause considerable visual loss if the macula is involved but if a nasal branch is affected it may go unnoticed. The patient is often unaware of the condition until he rubs or shuts his good eye.

Occlusion can be due to external compression by an atheromatous plaque in the central retinal artery adjacent to the central vein. Branch veins are usually occluded where an arteriole crosses a vein. The arteriole is thickened and sclerotic in patients with hypertension. Retinal vein occlusion can also be caused by highly viscous blood. This is seen in patients with leukaemia, polycythaemia and abnormal fat metabolism (the hyperlipidaemias). Finally the condition is seen in patients with open-angle glaucoma and may be the first indication of this condition. The causes of central retinal vein occlusion can be summarized as:

1. compression by the ageing artery;
2. hypertension;
3. open-angle glaucoma;
4. hyperviscosity.

Appearance

Classically the involved retina is splashed with numerous deep and superficial haemorrhages. The veins are enlarged, engorged and tortuous. Sections of the vein may be hidden by oedematous retina. Cotton wool patches are present in severe cases.

Management

The macula may be permanently damaged, causing severe loss of vision. Recovery can, however, be complete. The main complication that can seriously threaten vision is the formation of new blood vessels. In patients with occlusion of a retinal branch vein these often stem from the retina and can cause vitreous haemorrhages. Patients with a central retinal vein occlusion are more likely to develop these vessels on the iris (rubeosis) and in the anterior chamber angle. This can progress to a severe form of glaucoma (neovascular glaucoma) which usually develops within 3 months. Argon laser treatment to the retinal periphery can prevent these problems. This treatment is only given to those patients considered to be most at risk; fluorescein angiography can be helpful to identify the retinal ischaemia present in this group of patients.

Retinopathy of Prematurity

Retinopathy of prematurity is a bilateral abnormality of retinal blood vessels. It occurs almost exclusively in premature infants who have a birth weight of less than 1500 g or who have been born at less than 32 weeks gestation. Under these circumstances the later stages of development of retinal blood vessels in the periphery can become arrested.

A ridge of tissue develops at the extent of the peripheral retinal vessels. It contains arteriovenous communications and in severe disease new vessels develop with fibrous tissue proliferation from that region. This can lead to vitreous haemorrhage and traction on the retina with dragging of the retinal vessels and macula towards the temporal periphery. In its most severe form it can present as a white pupil, from fibrous tissue proliferation behind the lens (retrolental fibroplasia).

Glaucoma, uveitis, cataract, retinal detachment or phthisis bulbi can also occur months or even years later.

Management

Treatment is based on prevention, by careful monitoring of the oxygen concentrations the premature baby is given. Peripheral cryotherapy or indirect laser treatment is now thought to improve the outcome in some of the more severe cases of this disease.

Problem	Goal	Nursing intervention
Potential problem of low birth weight infants requiring oxygen supplement.	To prevent the onset of retinopathy.	1. Careful monitoring of oxygen concentrations must be undertaken. 2. The pupils should be widely dilated to allow indirect ophthalmoscopy by the medical staff to detect any abnormality or early stages of retrolental fibroplasia.

In view of the potential for late complications from retinopathy of prematurity, regular ophthalmic examination should be undertaken and the parents of the child should be made aware of the importance of attending for eye examinations.

RETINOBLASTOMA

Retinoblastomas are malignant retinal tumours affecting young children. The majority of cases are reported in the first 3 years of life. The condition is often hereditary. It may develop from multiple foci within the eye and, in one third of patients, affects both eyes. The tumour appears as a pale pink or white mass with newly formed blood vessels on its surface. Usually the tumour is diagnosed when it is large enough to cause a white pupil ('cat's eye'). Occasionally patients can present with a squint that has resulted from reduced vision in that eye. Careful examination under anaesthesia is necessary in patients in whom the condition is suspected.

In very advanced unilateral retinoblastomas enucleation is still often required. Other treatment options include radioactive plaque treatment and proton beam therapy. Photocoagulation or cryotherapy are sometimes used to treat small tumours. Repeated examinations under anaesthesia are required until the child reaches at least 7 years of age.

The prognosis is now much improved, with a current overall survival rate of 80–90%. Genetic counselling is important to the parents of an affected child who themselves need to be examined, along with other siblings.

Problem	Goal	Nursing intervention
Parents (and child) anxious because of impending surgery.	1. To alleviate anxiety. 2. To gain family co-operation.	1. Involve the parents in the care and ensure that the child is not isolated from his family. 2. Explain simply the routine procedures. 3. If desired, the parents may carry or accompany the child to the theatre doors.

The parents will require support while the child is undergoing surgery. They should not be allowed to feel isolated and must have access to the nursing staff. The opportunity should be taken to prepare them for the return of their child to the ward, by explaining that a pad and possibly a bandage will be applied and that the child may still be drowsy or tearful.

Problem	Goal	Nursing intervention
Potential problem of haemorrhage postoperatively.	1. Prevent haemorrhage. 2. Promote healing.	1. Observe the socket and pad at each dressing to ensure that there is no excess bleeding or discharge. 2. Clots observed must not be dislodged as this may lead to further bleeding. 3. Report excess bleeding to the medical staff.
Parents may feel responsible for their child's condition and may feel they have neglected their child in some way.	To remove any feelings of guilt.	1. Explain as simply as possible the causes of the condition. 2. Encourage the parents to express any feelings of anger; offer support and advice. 3. Encourage parents to remain on the ward with their child during her stay in hospital. This will give them time and opportunity to ask questions.
Parents apprehensive due to lack of knowledge regarding the artificial eye. Concerned about loss of body image.	1. To remove anxiety. 2. To educate the parents. 3. To establish a good relationship between the parent, child and ocular prosthetist.	1. Arrange for the ocular prosthetist to see the child and parents preoperatively. 2. Ensure that a nurse is present at this visit, to facilitate later reinforcement of the information given.
Parents may be afraid of handling the shell or fitting it into the socket.	1. To reduce anxiety. 2. To enable them to become proficient at insertion and removal of the shell.	1. Explain simply the principles involved. 2. Teach the parents how to insert the shell by demonstrating first; ensure the child has his head well supported – either by lying flat or sitting up. (a) Wash hands, clean the socket and shell with saline. (b) Place the shell on the upper part of the cheek and distract the child so he is looking in an upward direction. Lift the upper lid and gently push the shell up into the socket, allowing the lower lid to flick into position over the lower edge of the prosthesis. Ensure the shell feels comfortable and wash hands. 3. To remove the shell use either a digital technique or an extractor. (a) Ask the child to look up if she is old enough, or distract her attention to gain her co-operation. (b) Use a digital technique to retract and evert the lower eyelid. (c) As the patient looks down the prosthesis may be either expelled or easily removed. (d) Ensure the parents feel confident with the procedure.

Problem	Goal	Nursing intervention
Parents are anxious that the tumour may develop in the remaining eye, affect their other children or affect future pregnancies.	To reduce anxiety and reassure them.	1. Reassure parents by explaining that repeated examinations of the unaffected eye will be carried out to permit the detection of any possible tumour in its early stage. 2. Explain that any other children they have will also be regularly screened. 3. Discuss their fears and anxieties, and future problems that may affect them. 4. Genetic counselling will be necessary, for which they may be referred.
Parents may feel isolated following the discharge of their child.	To remove feelings of isolation and to help them adjust to the situation.	1. Reassure them that they are not alone. Explain about support groups and meetings where parents and children can gather to discuss and solve problems.

Genetic Counselling

Genetic counselling is a specialized branch of medicine and its purpose is to give information to those at risk of transmitting a hereditary disorder. In some cases it is possible to reassure individuals that they have no risk of transmitting the disorder. In other cases, recent advances have offered the possibility of prenatal diagnosis at an early stage of pregnancy, but this is only possible in a few instances. With retinoblastoma some facts are clear; for example an individual with bilateral retinoblastoma has a risk of about 50% of transmission to any children. Any patient can seek genetic counselling by asking the treating ophthalmologist or general practitioner to refer him to a genetic clinic.

Retinal Detachment

Retinal detachment refers to the separation of the neural retina from the retinal pigment epithelium. This results from an imbalance between the forces of adhesion and separation. Most frequently this traction is due to age-related collapse of the vitreous. Holes can develop in areas affected by certain retinal degenerations, for instance lattice degeneration. A break where the retina disinserts from the ora serrata (i.e. its peripheral limit) is called a dialysis and is often due to blunt trauma. Two important groups of patients at risk of retinal detachment are myopes and those who have had cataract surgery, particularly where vitreous loss has occurred.

A retinal detachment occasionally results from an underlying tumour. This is most commonly a metastatic lesion or

Table 20.2 Causes of retinal detachment

1. Where there is a hole (rhegmatogenous):	Myopia	
	Cataract surgery	
	Retinal degenerations	
	Dialysis	– blunt injury
2. Where there is no hole (non-rhegmatogenous):	Traction	– diabetes
		penetrating injury
		sickle cell disease
	Serous fluid	– tumour
		inflammation

a choroidal melanoma. Detachments may also result from vitreous traction in diabetes and after penetrating injury. The causes of retinal detachment are summarized in Table 20.2.

Clinical Features

Flashing lights and a shower of 'floaters' often mark the onset of a retinal detachment. Floaters are often described as being black spots or threads which appear to move within the eye. Patients may describe seeing a shadow or curtain. Some still, however, only attend when the macula is affected, resulting in serious visual loss. Macular involvement means that, even if treatment is successful, central vision does not usually return to normal. A detached retina usually has a greyish crinkled appearance and the vessels are more tortuous as they pass over the billowing surface.

Management

If a retinal hole is detected before any detachment occurs it is sometimes possible to 'seal' the retina and choroid around the hole with argon laser therapy or cryotherapy. These procedures can be potentially performed under local anaesthesia as an outpatient or day patient procedure.

Although some retinal detachment repairs (e.g. pneumatic retinopexy) may be performed as an outpatient or day surgery procedure, the majority require at least a short hospital admission.

Patients with a retinal detachment threatening the macula require urgent surgery and posturing to prevent extension. When a retinal detachment involves the macula, surgery is relatively less urgent and posturing of reduced benefit.

Surgery is aimed principally at relieving vitreous traction and closing any retinal hole (or holes). This results in the absorption of subretinal fluid, thereby allowing the retina to return to its normal anatomical position. The scleral buckling procedure which has become established as the

Problem	Goal	Nursing intervention
Patient anxious due to sudden loss of vision.	To ensure the patient is aware of what has happened and understands the procedures to follow.	1. Give the patient a simple explanation of what has occurred. 2. Explain that admission is necessary prior to surgery. 3. Explain that bed rest may form part of the treatment to prevent further detachment. 4. Give the patient the opportunity to ask questions.
Enforced positional bed rest to prevent further detachment.	To allow the patient to become aware of his limitations and thereby gain his co-operation and maintain the appropriate position.	1. Advise the patient of his limitations regarding mobility particularly if his macula is still attached and threatened. If the patient has a superior detachment he may be nursed lying flat with one pillow, or if the detachment is inferior he will be nursed upright in a bed or chair. 2. Explain that the prescribed position will help prevent further extension. 3. Explain to the patient that he will be required to posture postoperatively if intraocular gas or silicon oil is injected during surgery.
Boredom due to immobility and reduced vision due to mydriatics.	To reduce boredom with acceptable and appropriate activities.	1. Identify the patient's recreational habits. 2. Facilitate appropriate recreational activities, e.g. talking books, personalized radio, increased visiting.

'gold standard' for simple rhegmatogenous retinal detachment repair involves indentation of the outer coats of the eye in the vicinity of the hole in order to oppose the choroid to the detached retina. This objective is achieved in several stages, under either general or local anaesthesia.

1. The conjunctiva is incised (through 360° if necessary) and the extraocular muscles are located. Once sutures are placed under the muscles it is possible to move the eye to the desired location, both to visualize the fundus and to gain access to the area of sclera overlying the hole.
2. A cryoprobe is placed on the sclera and in this way the surgeon can see, using the indirect ophthalmoscope, when the probe underlies the hole. At this point the cryoprobe is switched on to induce an inflammatory response which will result in chorioretinal adhesion.
3. One of a variety of explants is now selected and, after checking that the explant is in the correct position and of the correct size, it is permanently secured with non-absorbable sutures. In order to allow closure of the hole in this way, it may be necessary to release subretinal fluid by puncturing the sclera and choroid under the detached retina. The amount of indentation required to

achieve retinal apposition and relieve vitreous traction may be such that an encircling band is placed around the globe.

4. In complicated detachments, for instance where conventional surgery has failed, it may be necessary to relieve vitreous traction from within the eye by performing a vitrectomy. Retinal apposition may even then only be achieved by the additional measures of an indenting explant and internal tamponade using air, gas or oil.

POSTOPERATIVE CARE

Patients posturing postoperatively (generally, those with an internal tamponade) should be encouraged to sit out of bed

Problem	Goal	Nursing intervention
First dressing: patient is anxious about the postoperative results, i.e. has his vision returned?	That the patient will have realistic expectations about the visual results following surgery.	1. Following removal of the pad and bathing the eye, explain that the vision will be blurred because of the dilating drops and that the eye will be inflamed as a result of surgery. 2. Reassure the patient that chemosis of the conjunctiva and oedema of the lids will subside and are not a permanent feature.

to posture and to mobilize for 15 minutes out of every hour to avoid the complications associated with bed rest and restricted mobility. Patients who have had retinal detachment or vitreous surgery frequently experience pain for 3–4 days postoperatively. The patient should be prepared for this preoperatively and appropriate analgesics should be administered as prescribed.

Problem	Goal	Nursing intervention
Patient is concerned about the potential problem of redetachment following discharge.	To reassure the patient. To outline the ways he can assist towards reducing the possibility of further detachment.	1. Explain to him that he will have regular medical supervision. 2. Remind him that he must not lift heavy items, must avoid strenuous exercise and should instil correct drops at regular intervals as advised by the consultant. 3. Explain the importance of attending regularly for outpatient appointments and returning to the hospital should he encounter any problems.

Diabetic Retinopathy

Diabetes mellitus is a complex and widespread disorder of metabolism in which insulin is either absent (juvenile-onset) or decreased (maturity-onset). Diabetes occurs in 1–2% of the population.

1. The incidence of blindness is approximately 20 times greater in diabetics than in non-diabetics.
2. The incidence of diabetic retinopathy is more closely related to the duration of the disease than to any other factor.
3. Approximately 2% of all diabetics become blind.
4. Diabetic retinopathy is the commonest cause of blind registration in people between the ages of 20 and 65 years.

The severity of the retinopathy is related to the duration and control of the patient's diabetes. Other known risk factors include hypertension, smoking and pregnancy. The retinopathy involves the small retinal vessels and capillaries, especially in and around the macula. Diabetic maculopathy is the commonest cause of visual loss associated with diabetic eye disease. Retinopathy is somewhat artificially divided into background (non-proliferative), pre-proliferative and proliferative retinopathy.

Background (Non-Proliferative) Diabetic Retinopathy

This occurs when small vessels and capillaries develop areas of weakness in their walls, resulting in the development of microaneurysms which can be seen clinically as tiny red dots. These vessels tend to leak, causing localized oedema. Eventually exudates develop, which are yellow–creamy-white lesions in the retina, representing lipid deposits. Haemorrhages are also common. If they are superficial they are described as flame-shaped, and when deep they tend to pool into dot or blot haemorrhages.

Preproliferative Diabetic Retinopathy

This represents the most severe stage of non-proliferative diabetic retinopathy. The risk of progression to proliferative disease is very high. It is characterized by the presence of venous beading and/or significant areas of large retinal blot haemorrhages, multiple cotton wool spots and/or multiple intraretinal microvascular abnormalities.

Proliferative Diabetic Retinopathy

This occurs when the capillaries eventually become occluded and is more common in insulin-dependent diabetics. The reduced blood supply to the retina leads to the formation of new blood vessels, which develop particularly at the optic disc. Retinal or disc new vessels can bleed into the vitreous. Fibrous tissue will also proliferate alongside these new vessels and adhere to points along the surface of the retina. This tissue matures and subsequently contracts, pulling on the points of attachment to cause tractional retinal detachments. The end stage of diabetic eye disease is neovascular glaucoma, when the trabecular meshwork is irreversibly blocked by new vessels in the drainage angle.

Management

Good control of blood sugar levels has a beneficial influence on the development of most complications of diabetes, including retinopathy. Background retinopathy can cause marked loss of visual acuity if oedema and exudates spread into the fovea. Despite this loss of macular function, patients will preserve their navigational vision.

Patients with proliferative retinopathy, however, can lose navigational vision if a vitreous haemorrhage or tractional detachment develops. Vitrectomy may be required to clear haemorrhages, facilitating intraoperative laser treatment and surgical correction of tractional sequelae.

Problem	Goal	Nursing intervention
Patient is anxious regarding the possibility of losing his sight.	To increase the patient's knowledge of the disease process and thereby gain compliance with treatment.	1. Try to explain simply what diabetic retinopathy means. 2. Stress the importance of regular ophthalmic examinations. 3. Patient needs to be taught that short-term elevation in blood glucose levels can cause temporary visual disturbances.
Patient is unaware of how he can help to slow down the progression of diabetic retinopathy.	To teach the patient how he can help preserve his sight and prevent complications.	1. Explain that at present there is no medical cure for diabetic retinopathy but that certain measures may be helpful. 2. Patient should be told that good initial metabolic control will not prevent retinopathy but may help to slow down the progression.
Potential problem of systemic disorders which may contribute to diabetic retinopathy.	To prevent further complications where possible.	1. Encourage patient to attend regular diabetic clinics. 2. Advise the patient to have his blood pressure checked regularly – strict control of hypertension is important to avoid further adverse effects to the retinal circulation.

Ocular complications of diabetes can generally be treated effectively if the condition is diagnosed early enough. Although diabetic retinopathy is most often a bilateral disease the severity may differ greatly from one eye to the other. Patients with diabetic retinopathy often face systemic complications simultaneously and will require understanding, sympathy and advice from the nurse concerning all aspects of care.

LASER TREATMENT

Laser stands for **l**ight **a**mplification by **s**timulated **e**mission of **r**adiation. It is a highly concentrated beam of light that is used to cause a small retinal burn. Panretinal photocoagulation or ablation may stabilize proliferative diabetic retinopathy and entails the application of a few thousand laser burns outside the vascular arcades. The exact mechanism by which laser treatment modulates the growth factor imbalance associated with neovascularization is unknown. Laser treatment may cause some loss of peripheral and night vision but aims to preserve central and colour vision. In addition, focal or grid-pattern laser burns may be applied to regions of retinal thickening associated with diabetic maculopathy.

NURSING CARE OF A PATIENT UNDERGOING LASER TREATMENT

The term 'laser' conjures up different images for individual patients. Showing them the laser room prior to treatment

Problem	Goal	Nursing intervention
Patient is anxious because of lack of knowledge.	1. To reduce anxiety by giving clear explanations. 2. To gain the patient's confidence and co-operation.	1. Explain to the patient that the treatment involves directing a specialized light beam towards the affected area of the eye. 2. Explain that the pupil(s) will need to be dilated to allow a clear, full view of the fundus. Remind the patient that his vision will be slightly impaired by the drops, and bright laser light. His vision may take a few days to return to normal. 3. Ask the patient if he has any questions.
If the patient is a diabetic there is a potential problem of hypoglycaemia caused by stress and anxiety.	1. To prevent hypoglycaemia.	1. Ascertain the patient's medical condition and find out if he is insulin- or tablet-dependent. 2. Ensure that the patient has eaten and taken normal medication prior to the treatment. 3. Check to see if the patient feels comfortable and has no hypoglycaemic symptoms, e.g. cold, clammy skin or tremor.

can help to dispel any preconceived ideas they may have. Many patients having laser treatment will have been examined on a slit-lamp previously and will be familiar with the equipment. If the patient understands that the laser machine is a modified slit-lamp with special attachments he will have a better idea of what is expected of him.

Problem	Goal	Nursing intervention
Patient is concerned that treatment may be painful.	To reassure the patient that treatment is not usually painful, but may be uncomfortable.	1. Explain that anaesthetic drops will be instilled to numb the front of the eye. Tell the patient that the drops will sting initially, but for only a few seconds. 2. Explain the procedure briefly; tell the patient that a special contact lens will be positioned on the front of the eye. This allows the doctor to view the fundus in greater detail and also helps to keep the eyelids open. 3. Flashes of a very bright light will be experienced during the treatment, which may be uncomfortable.
Patient apprehensive, unaware of what is required of him.	To ensure that the patient understands how he can assist with the treatment.	1. Explain that it is very important to remain as still as possible at the slit-lamp. 2. Ensure that the patient understands that he must inform the doctor if he needs to cough or move position. 3. Explain what the doctor is doing at each stage; if the patient understands why a procedure is being carried out he will be more co-operative. 4. Ensure that the patient knows what to expect, i.e. that he will see rapid flashes of light and hear a clicking sound while the machine is being operated.

Following laser treatment patients may notice a short-term darkening of colour, occasionally a red tint over their vision and a dull ache for several hours. Reassure the patient that the colour abnormalities are temporary and advise him to take a mild analgesic if the ache does not subside.

Age-Related Macular Degeneration

The retinal pigment epithelium (RPE) cells are never replaced. When they age, they deposit material in the underlying membrane which accumulates to form **drusen**. These are small yellowy-white spots in the retina which may eventually enlarge to become confluent with their neighbours. In themselves they do not affect vision, but they are signs of disturbed metabolic function by the RPE cells with age. Eventually areas of the RPE layer become atrophic and may disperse pigment into the macula. This is called macular degeneration and affects fine central vision, causing difficulty, for example, with reading and sewing.

The Disciform Response

Some patients may go on to develop an abnormal blood vessel membrane which arises from the choroid (i.e. subretinal neovascular membrane). This can leak fluid which lifts the central retina, causing the patient to complain of distorted and blurred vision. If these membranes bleed, a disciform macular scar subsequently forms.

Management

A fluorescein angiogram may be required to define the presence and extent of a subretinal neovascular membrane. This membrane can sometimes be destroyed by the argon, krypton or diode laser if seen in its early stages. There is a high incidence of the other eye being similarly affected at a later date. Patients must be warned regarding early symptoms and the need to self-monitor with an Amsler grid and return immediately if any central blurring or distortion occurs.

Problem	Goal	Nursing intervention
Anxiety due to loss of vision.	To relieve anxiety. To gain co-operation with tests and investigations.	1. Explain to the patient that investigations will be performed to establish the cause of his loss of vision. 2. Explain to the patient that it will be necessary to check central vision, measure the intraocular pressure, dilate the eye and use lenses to examine the retina. 3. Reassure the patient by ensuring he receives adequate information and has the opportunity to ask questions.

Those affected severely by age-related macular degeneration will need assistance with low-vision aids and blind registration. It is important to encourage these patients to use suitable magnifying devices to maximize their residual visual function.

Hereditary Retinopathies

Retinitis Pigmentosa

This condition primarily affects rods but eventually results in impairment of all visual cells. Patients first notice that they have difficulty in seeing in the dark, usually in their teens. The peripheral field of vision slowly erodes away, leaving tunnel vision.

Ophthalmoscopic examination reveals the characteristic 'bone-corpuscle' pigment proliferation in the retinal periphery and attenuated arterioles. Eventually the optic disc develops a yellowish, atrophic appearance. The course of the illness varies considerably and is related to the hereditary pattern. Rarely, this is associated with systemic diseases, which need to be excluded.

Electrodiagnostic tests are sometimes performed to confirm a diagnosis and may be of use in assessing other members of the family. This is important in working out the hereditary pattern in order that genetic counselling can be undertaken. Apart from supportive measures there is no widely accepted treatment for this condition.

Best's Disease

This is a macular dystrophy which is dominantly inherited, in other words there is a one in two chance of a child of the affected person developing the disease. The macula is occupied by a light orange deposit that looks like the yolk of a fried egg. This material eventually disperses to look 'scrambled', causing severe disruption of fine central vision.

Stargardt's Disease

There is also a macular dystrophy which is recessively inherited, in other words the parents are not affected but both carry a defective gene. It results in progressive atrophy of the macular pigment epithelium, with associated visual loss. Vision deteriorates insidiously in adolescence. There are often associated multiple, fishtail-like, pale lesions in the retinal periphery.

Acquired Immune Deficiency Syndrome (AIDS)

This is an apparently new disease caused by the human immunodeficiency virus (HIV), which infects lymphocytes in the blood. It is estimated that by the year 2000 over 100 million people in the world will be infected. It is only transmitted by sexual contact, by drug addicts sharing their needles or by needlestick injury. Some haemophiliacs became infected because of contaminated blood products. There is a high incidence in promiscuous homosexual men. Patients affected have antibodies to the virus and can therefore be detected. The majority of individuals infected eventually develop a deficiency in their immune defences and thus develop AIDS. Of those that do, many will die of opportunistic infections or Kaposi's sarcomas. The virus has been demonstrated in tears and all corneal donors are now screened for antibodies. Care must be taken with contact lens work in the infected individual.

Retinitis

Patients with AIDS may develop cotton wool spots, which are asymptomatic, or they may have blurred vision from a retinitis which presents with intraretinal haemorrhage and retinal necrosis. This retinitis is most commonly due to cytomegalovirus (CMV). Patients with CMV retinitis respond to the antiviral agents ganciclovir and foscarnet given intravenously. Nevertheless, the condition is a serious threat to the vision of AIDS patients.

Nursing Care

It is important that nurses be aware of their own prejudices before attempting to help a patient suffering from AIDS to cope with the situation in which they find themselves. The patient will need psychological support throughout his stay in hospital and also when discharged into the community. It is therefore essential to establish a good relationship with the patient to gain his confidence and trust.

Patients, families and partners will need help and support throughout this time and practical advice with regards to problems which may arise. It is advisable to refer to AIDS counsellors in situations where the nurse feels unable to undertake the role due to lack of knowledge or psychological and emotional inadequacies.

Conditions of the Vitreous

Vitreous Detachment

With age the vitreous liquefies and collapses. Separation of the vitreous from the retina occurs, except at the ora serrata. Disruption of the vitreous is usually noticed by the patient, who sees black moving particles, called floaters, in his field of view.

The vitreous may, however, remain attached at certain points to the peripheral retina. The traction of the detaching vitreous on these residual points of adhesion stimulates the retina so that the patient sees flashing lights. This traction may cause retinal tears, which can lead to a retinal detachment. A common site for persistent attachment of the vitreous is to retina overlying a superficial vessel. Tears at these sites can damage an underlying vessel and cause a vitreous haemorrhage.

Floaters and flashing lights are considered as warning signs. A thorough examination of the retina should therefore be performed.

Asteroid Hyalosis

Hundreds of stellate opacities are suspended throughout the vitreous. They appear creamy-white, sparkle and arise from degeneration of the vitreous. They are of no significance, rarely cause symptoms and require no treatment.

Synchysis Scintillans

Cholesterol crystals are seen in this condition as glittering white crystals in eyes that have degenerated after long-standing inflammation or vitreous haemorrhage.

Vitreous Haemorrhage

This most commonly arises from a retinal break or new blood vessel growth. The haemorrhage often arises when the vitreous detaches from the retina. Bleeding into the vitreous can also result from the rupture of the fragile new blood vessels that can develop as a response to retinal ischaemia in conditions such as diabetic retinopathy, central retinal vein occlusion, sickle cell retinopathy and retinal vasculitis.

Vitreous haemorrhage can also result from trauma and spontaneously from tumours. Occasionally, a haemorrhage is related to hypertension or a bleeding diathesis alone.

The nursing care given to patients with vitreous haemorrhage must differ depending upon the cause, but a generalized outline of the care required can be given. The patient presenting with a recent vitreous haemorrhage may be admitted and postured sitting bolt upright overnight with both eyes padded. This allows the haemorrhage to settle inferiorly, often allowing visualization with the indirect ophthalmoscope of any underlying retinal tears or pathology. These lesions may be treated with indirect laser or cryopexy to prevent development of a retinal detachment or further haemorrhage, depending on the underlying cause.

In many cases the haemorrhage will resolve or settle, allowing vision to improve. When the haemorrhage persists ultrasound allows monitoring for the presence of underlying retinal detachment, development of a posterior vitreous detachment or localization of an intraocular foreign body. Definitive vitrectomy surgery can then be planned, depending upon the circumstances of the case concerned. The prognosis following vitrectomy is often limited by the underlying condition and is frequently difficult to predict preoperatively.

VITRECTOMY

Vitrectomy is the surgical removal of the vitreous. The procedure usually involves endoscopic access to the vitreous chamber via the pars plana using three separate entry ports (Figure 20.4):

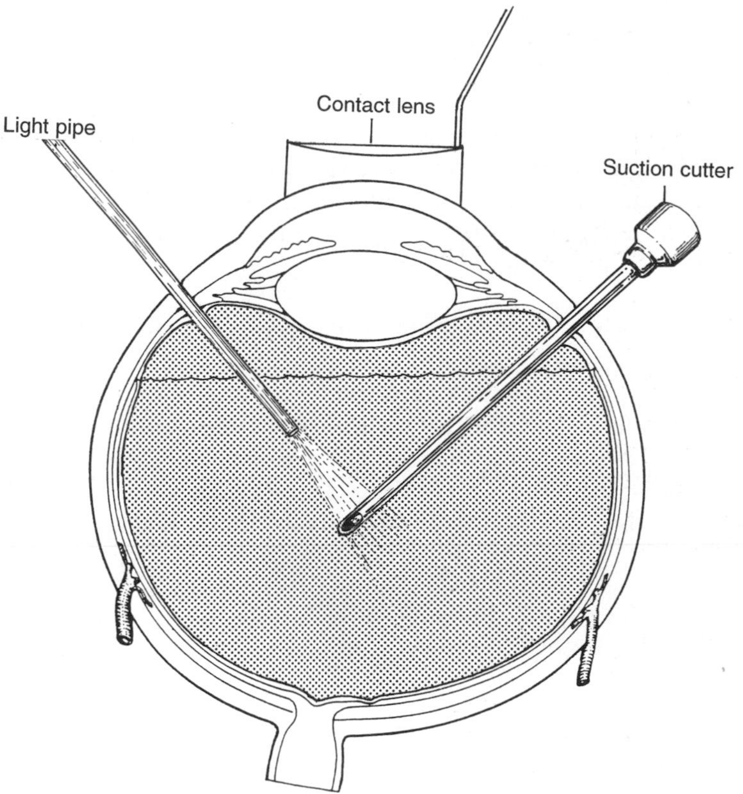

Figure 20.4 Surgical approach in vitrectomy. The infusion line to maintain intraocular pressure is not shown.

1. an infusion line to maintain intraocular pressure;
2. for entry of a suction cutter;
3. for a fibreoptic probe for illumination.

The surgery is carried out under the operating microscope. The anterior vitreous is usually visible using the normal light source from the microscope. When the central and peripheral parts of the vitreous are being removed a contact lens is placed on the surface of the eye and illumination is provided by the fibreoptic light source. Indications for a vitrectomy are:

1. removal of vitreous opacities, e.g. vitreous haemorrhage following branch vein occlusion;
2. as part of the repair of a complicated retinal detachment, e.g. removing the scar tissue associated with proliferative vitreoretinopathy;
3. in the management of severe diabetic disease, e.g. to remove vitreous haemorrhage, relieve tractional retinal detachment and gain access to the retina for further laser treatment (which may be performed intraoperatively with an endolaser probe);
4. removal of intraocular foreign bodies. Fine scissors and forceps may be utilized to cut and manipulate tissue and foreign bodies under direct visualization. In some cases the patient's lens may also need to be removed if a cataract prevents sufficient visualization of the posterior ocular structures.

In 'simple' vitrectomy (e.g. for vitreous opacities) the vitreous is replaced with infusion fluid. In more complicated situations the vitreous cavity may be filled with either gas or silicone oil to produce an internal tamponade to facilitate reattachment of the retina. Postoperatively the patient will be required to posture so that the buoyancy of the intraocular gas or oil closes any retinal breaks, aiding chorioretinal adhesion from intraoperative cryotherapy or laser. Posturing face down or cheek to pillow also minimizes contact between any intraocular gas and the patient's crystalline lens, which may lead to cataract formation.

Preoperative Care

Problem	Goal	Nursing intervention
Patient is anxious through lack of knowledge about impending surgery and investigations.	To relieve anxiety by discussing the aims of surgery and ensure the patient understands why preliminary investigations are necessary.	1. Reassure the patient by simply describing tests such as ultrasound scanning of the eye which will assess the degree of haemorrhage or presence of an unseen retinal detachment. 2. A preoperative visit from a theatre nurse may help to alleviate anxieties. 3. Discuss with the patient his fears and anxieties; offer advice and support.
Patient is unaware of how he can contribute to his care.	To educate the patient and gain his co-operation.	1. If gas or silicone oil exchange is to be used, it may be beneficial to show the patient the postoperative position he will have to maintain for a number of days. If possible, ask the patient to practise either lying face down (a pillow under his abdomen will provide support and lessen the problem of backache) or sitting in a chair leaning forward over a bed table. (The latter position will help alleviate problems such as chest infection.) 2. Explain to the patient that the position is necessary to facilitate the success of the retinal surgery and prevent problems such as cataract formation. If the patient understands the rationale for his treatment he will be more co-operative.

Very often the vitrectomy patient is a diabetic and therefore may have many of the problems associated with diabetes. The routine pre- and postoperative care of a diabetic patient undergoing vitrectomy is the same as that for other forms of surgery, involving general anaesthesia with monitoring of intravenous infusion and measuring of blood sugar levels.

Postoperative Care

Problem	Goal	Nursing intervention
Patient distressed because of pain in the eye.	To relieve the patient's pain and to ensure that there are no complications.	1. Give regular prompt analgesia. 2. Explain that, because of the nature and length of surgery, some pain or discomfort is expected but should be relieved by analgesia. 3. If severe pain persists, contact the medical staff – it may be due to raised intraocular pressure.
Patient is concerned about the outcome of surgery and whether it has been successful.	To give support and to ensure the patient understands that he may not regain good vision.	1. It is very important to ensure that the patient is prepared psychologically prior to removing the eye patch for the first time. Ensure that the patient's expectations are realistic. 2. Inflammation of the eyelid and chemosis of the conjunctiva may be present; explain that this will subside and become less tender. 3. When the surgeon examines the eye, remain with the patient. The nurse should be present when he is told of the possible prognosis and can offer comfort and support if the prognosis is poor.
Patient finds it difficult to maintain face-down position and encounters problems eating and drinking.	To make the patient as comfortable as possible.	1. Encourage him to alter his position from lying face down to sitting upright with head forward on a pillow over an overway, and *vice versa*. 2. Allow him to mobilize to the toilet and for exercise for 15 minutes in every hour (discuss this with medical staff first). 3. Allow the patient to sit up for meals. Patients often find eating while lying down causes indigestion and discomfort. The use of a high chair to sit in and a low table for food will enable the patient to keep his head inclined forward.
Patient is unaware of his limitations on discharge.	To ensure that the patient understands the reason for the limitations imposed, to gain his co-operation and compliance.	1. Explain that he will be unable to travel by aeroplane until the bubble has absorbed (if he has had intraocular gas exchange, e.g. SF6). 2. Tell him he must not lift heavy weights. 3. He must not return to work until given permission from his eye surgeon. 4. Advise him to wear dark glasses if he is photophobic. 5. Remind him to instil drops and ointments as prescribed. 6. Remind him to keep all Outpatient Department appointments. 7. Advise him to contact the hospital immediately should any problem arise.

Outpatient follow-up can take weeks, months or even years. Some patients regain good vision, while others have a residual degree of visual handicap. For those patients who lose vision in one eye there will always be some fear of similar problems occurring in their remaining eye. They must therefore be advised to seek prompt medical attention should they experience any ocular symptoms.

21

Orbit, Optic Nerve and Visual Pathways

Robert Doran and Deirdre Donnelly

Chapter Summary

Functional anatomy

Congenital orbital disease

Acquired orbital disease

Visual pathways

Functional Anatomy

The orbits are the two cavities in the front of the skull that hold and protect the eyes and their associated nerves, muscles and blood supply. Each orbit is roughly the shape of a four-sided pyramid lying on its side with its apex pointing backwards and its base open to the front.

Seven bones contribute to the walls of the orbit (Figure 21.1). At the anterior opening the bones forming the margin are thickened. Elsewhere, the orbital walls are very thin bony plates, which separate the orbit from other cavities in the skull and face. The orbit is related above to the frontal sinus and the anterior cranial fossa. On the medial side are the nose and ethmoid sinus; laterally is the temporal fossa and below lies the maxillary sinus. Disease arising in the paranasal sinuses may easily involve the orbit via the thin intervening walls. The bony walls are continuous anteriorly

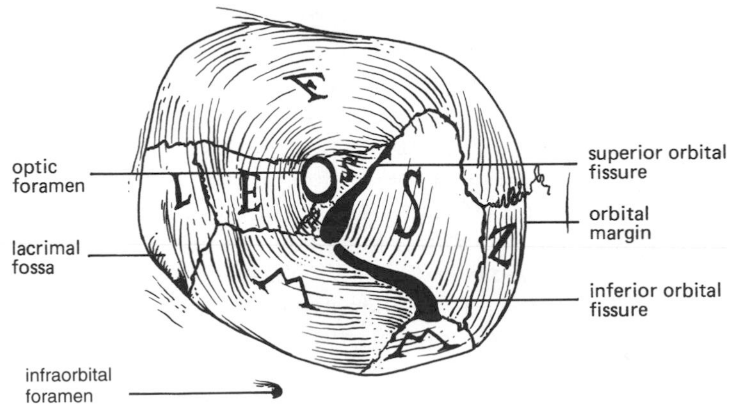

Figure 21.1 Frontal view of the bones of the left orbit. The bones, in order of decreasing area, are: (F) frontal; (M) maxilla; (Z) zygomatic; (S) sphenoid; (E) ethmoid; (L) lacrimal; (P) palatine (mnemonic – Forty Mad Zebras Sat Eating Lolly Pops).

with the periosteum on the face and at the orbital apex with the dura mater lining the cranial cavity.

The contents of the orbit are as follows:

1. eyeball (globe);
2. six extraocular muscles (four recti; two obliques);
3. optic nerve and meninges;
4. ophthalmic artery and branches;
5. ophthalmic veins (draining to cavernous sinus);
6. cranial nerves III–VI;
7. ciliary ganglion and ciliary nerves;
8. lacrimal gland;
9. lacrimal sac;
10. orbital fascia and fat.

There are three openings at the orbital apex which transmit structures vital to the eye. They are:

1. the optic foramen;
2. the superior orbital fissure;
3. the inferior orbital fissure.

The optic foramen is the anterior opening of the optic canal which carries the optic nerve and the ophthalmic artery.

The superior orbital fissure transmits the motor nerves to the extraocular muscles – the oculomotor nerve (III), the trochlear nerve (IV) and the abducent nerve (VI) – and also three sensory nerves to the eye, eyelids and facial skin. These are the lacrimal, frontal and nasociliary branches of the ophthalmic division of the trigeminal nerve (V). Sympathetic nerve fibres also gain access to the orbit through the optic foramen and the superior orbital fissure.

The inferior orbital fissure gives passage to two sensory branches of the maxillary division of the trigeminal nerve (V). Ophthalmic veins drain through both orbital fissures and may act as a route of spread of infection from the face to the cavernous sinus or to the pterygoid venous plexus.

The eyeball is held in the middle of the orbital opening by the tone of the six extraocular muscles, and by orbital fascia and fat. The orbital fascia surrounds the globe to form Tenon's capsule and also envelops the anterior bellies and tendons of the extraocular muscles. Between the muscles, the fascia is condensed into bands called check ligaments which act as shock absorbers to allow smooth rapid eye movements. Inferiorly, the condensed fascia is in the form of a sling beneath the eye known as Lockwood's ligament.

Fatty tissue fills available space in the orbit. It is confined in front by the orbital septum on the deep surface of the eyelids. Inside the cone-shaped space between the recti muscles it is soft and mobile to accommodate the optic nerve and central retinal artery during eye movements.,

Congenital Orbital Disease

Congenital conditions of the orbit, such as microphthalmos (small eye) and anophthalmos (absence of the eye), meningocele and encephalocele (herniation of part of the contents of the cranial cavity into the orbit) are thankfully rare.

Parents of children with congenital conditions are likely to be distressed and worried about their child as well as anxious to know about his condition and about what the future holds for him. Many parents in this situation also feel that they are in some way responsible for their child's condition.

The nurse who is caring for the child and his parents at the time can help to alleviate some of their worries by giving them the information they desire.

Problem	Goal	Nursing intervention
Parents of a baby with a congenital orbital condition are naturally worried what the future holds for their child. Anxiety is increased because they feel they may be responsible for their child's condition.	To relieve parental anxiety and guilt by giving relevant information.	1. Ensure that both parents have had the opportunity to talk to medical staff about their child's condition, its possible cause and its prognosis. 2. Ensure that the parents have understood what the doctors have told them by asking them to repeat what the doctor said. 3. Encourage them to ask any further questions they may have. 4. Allow and help them to express their feelings openly. Attempt to answer any particular problems or queries that may arise. 5. Ensure that the parents fully understand what the future holds for their child in terms of eyesight, cosmetic appearance and general health. Tell them what help is available to deal with these issues. 6. Give parents information on any self-help groups for parents of children with this condition and encourage them to contact these organizations. 7. Give them the name of someone at the hospital to contact if in need of further help and advice. 8. Attempt to relieve feelings of guilt by emphasizing to parents that this is not their fault. However, if the problem is genetically inherited, ensure that they are referred for genetic counselling.

Acquired Orbital Disease

Space in the orbit is limited. Any tumour or increase in the size of the tissues will tend to push the eye forward, causing proptosis. In severe proptosis the cornea may not be fully protected by the lids and urgent treatment may be necessary to protect the cornea by suturing the lids (tarsorrhaphy) or decompressing the orbit.

The diagnosis of proptosis and its underlying cause should follow a method such as that outlined in Table 21.1. A careful history is obtained of the onset and duration of the proptosis with details of any variation or other associated symptom such as pain or diplopia. Evidence provided by previous facial photographs may be very useful.

Examination begins with assessment of the position and symmetry of the eyes and lids. This may reveal lid lag or lid retraction, which are common findings in dysthyroid orbital disease. The eyes are examined for any sign of episcleral vessel enlargement, which may be associated with raised orbital venous pressure, and for corneal ulceration due to exposure. Sight may be at risk in proptosis because of optic nerve damage so assessment of vision by acuity tests and visual fields is particularly important.

Proptosis may be unilateral or bilateral and is measured with a ruler by reference to the lateral bony orbital margin. Normally the apex of the cornea does not protrude more than 20 mm beyond this point. A difference of 3 mm or more between measurements for the two eyes may signify unilateral proptosis. A special rule (exophthalmometer) is used to achieve the most reliable measurement (see Figure 10.4). The interpupillary distance and vertical position of the eyes is also measured. Horizontal or vertical eye displacement may indicate the position of an orbital mass; for example, a lacrimal gland tumour tends to push the globe down and medially.

Palpation of the orbit may reveal localized swelling and will show how tense the orbital tissues are. A pulsatile swelling suggests an arteriovenous anastomosis in the cavernous sinus and an associated orbital bruit may be audible

Table 21.1 Diagnosis of proptosis

History and photographs
Observation of eyes and lids
Measurement in three dimensions
Visual acuity and visual fields
Eye movements and tonometry
Palpation and auscultation
Pupil and fundus signs
Cranial nerves in the orbit
Special investigations

with the stethoscope over the eye or forehead. A tense but soft reducible swelling may be due to orbital venous varices, which increase in size on straining or stooping.

Eye movements may be limited in proptosis either by mechanical restriction or by nerve or muscle weakness, and alignment of the eyes should be tested in the nine cardinal

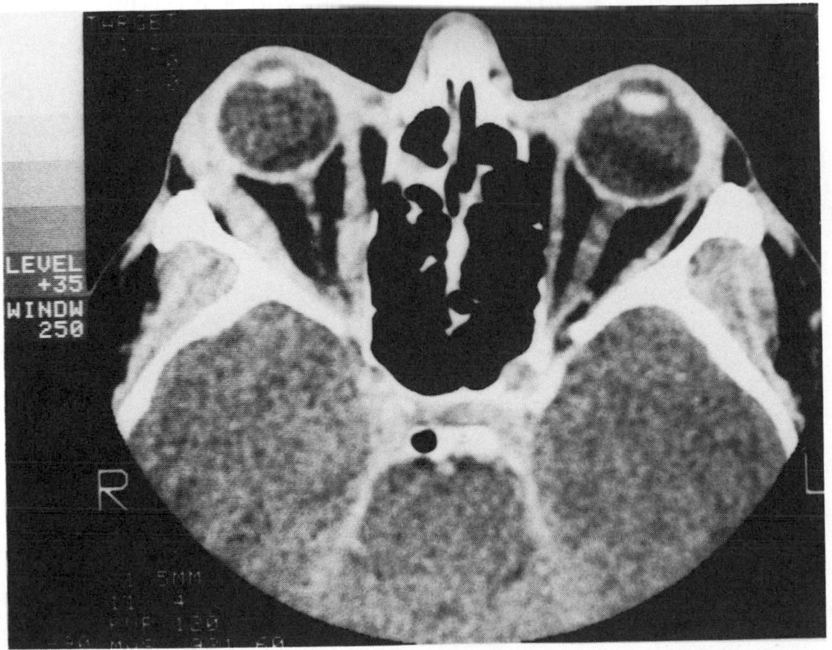

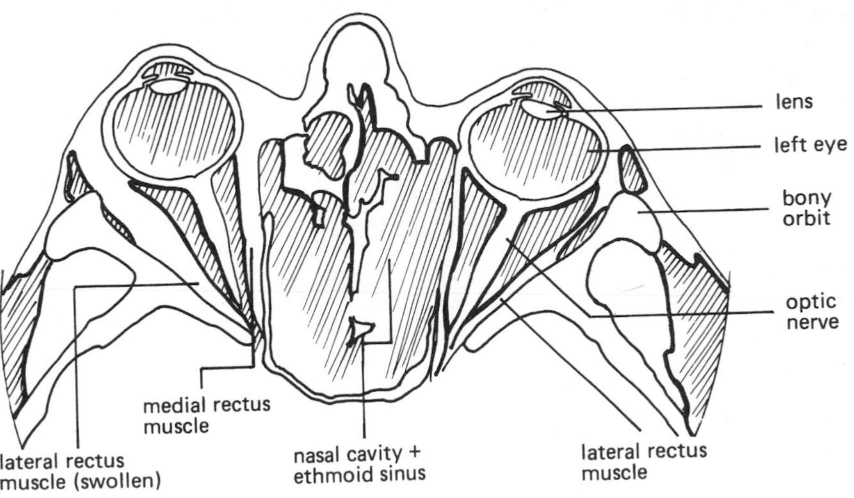

b

Figure 21.2 **(a)** Horizontal CT scan of skull and orbits in a patient with dysthyroid eye disease. **(b)** Note proptosis and swelling of lateral and medial rectus muscles of right eye (on left of diagram).

directions of gaze (Chapter 22). If diplopia is noted, a Hess test is performed, together with a field of binocular vision (Chapter 22). The trigeminal nerve is assessed by testing corneal sensation. Raised intraocular pressure measured when the eye is deviated compared to when looking straight ahead is due to failure of a muscle to relax and is another common feature of dysthyroid eye disease. After testing the pupillary responses, the fundi are examined for signs of pressure on the optic nerve (optic disc pallor or oedema) or on the posterior globe (choroidal folds).

Special investigations include plain X-rays, venography and ultrasound. The most useful special investigations are orbital computerized tomography (CT) scan (Figure 21.2) and magnetic resonance imaging (MRI). This will often demonstrate the position and full extent of orbital tumours and the size and position of the extraocular muscles and optic nerve. It is also useful in showing whether there is bony involvement in any disease process.

Dysthyroid Eye Disease

Much the commonest cause of both bilateral and unilateral proptosis is thyroid disease. It is due to a lymphocytic infiltration of the extraocular muscles and associated oedema of orbital tissues. It is usually associated with a currently or previously overactive thyroid gland. Signs may be mild to severe and include proptosis, squint, lid retraction and lid lag on downward gaze. It is more common in females but may be particularly severe in males.

Problem	Goal	Nursing intervention
A patient with bilateral exophthalmos is complaining of sore, uncomfortable eyes. Potential risk of corneal ulceration.	To relieve patient's discomfort and prevent complications arising from corneal exposure.	1. Explain to the patient why he is experiencing eye discomfort by telling him about his condition and how it affects him. Ensure he understands explanation given. 2. Monitor control of thyroid disease. Give medication to control condition as prescribed. 3. Instil eyedrops as prescribed to relieve lid retraction and also to maintain an adequate tear film over the cornea. 4. Teach the patient how to instil the drops and ensure he is able to do this safely. Ensure he is aware of the purpose and frequency of the drops. 5. Monitor the condition of the cornea and the effectiveness of the drops in improving patient comfort and preventing corneal damage.

Guanethidine eye drops, for lid retraction, and hypromellose may help eye comfort. The course of the eye disease is chronic and variable. The important complications are optic nerve compression in the apex and corneal exposure. The medical treatment in advanced cases includes high doses of oral corticosteroids and radiotherapy. Surgery for exposure includes lateral tarsorrhaphy and advancement of the upper and lower eyelids.

Proptosis and a lateral tarsorrhaphy can be unsightly and the patient may be very concerned about this and afraid that people will stare at him. It can be a great help to the patient to discuss this aspect of his condition with a nurse, who can also suggest ways of dealing with this problem.

Problem	Goal	Nursing intervention
Patient is worried about the appearance of his eyes because of proptosis or a tarsorrhaphy. Anxious and embarrassed that people will stare at him.	To help patient to come to terms with his appearance by suggesting ways in which he can improve his appearance.	1. Encourage the patient to voice any concerns he has about his appearance. Reassure him that it is not unusual to be concerned about this and that it is a perfectly normal worry. 2. Suggest ways in which the exophthalmos can be disguised – by not accentuating the eyes with make-up or, if the patient wears glasses, by getting lenses with a slight tint. 3. Suggest ways in which a tarsorrhaphy can be disguised, e.g. by wearing dark glasses or sunglasses. Point out to the patient with a tarsorrhaphy that once the sutures have been removed and the swelling has subsided, his eyes will look better. 4. Encourage the patient to act normally and to carry on with his normal lifestyle. Point out that his appearance will be far more noticeable if he does not act normally but tries to hide. 5. Reassure him by reacting towards him as you would to any other person, without staring at his eyes. Encourage relatives and friends to act similarly.

Orbital Decompression

If systemic steroids cannot be given or have failed, surgical decompression of the orbit may be needed to prevent visual loss. Occasionally, this is done for cosmetic reasons alone. Removal of orbital bone allows more room for the soft tissues. The operation is performed through an orbitotomy (see later). There are a variety of other anatomical approaches, which usually require collaboration with facciomaxillary, plastic or neurosurgeons. It is always a major procedure, for which the patient must be adequately prepared.

Problem	Goal	Nursing intervention
Lack of knowledge of what surgery involves and of the effect it will have means that the patient is unable to make an informed decision.	To inform patient of what surgery and aftercare involve, so that it is possible for him to give an informed consent.	1. Explain to the patient that the purpose of the operation is to prevent permanent damage to his eye and loss of vision. 2. Outline what the operation involves, namely removing a part of the orbital bone from both eyes to relieve the proptosis. 3. Point out that the operation will take 2 hours or more under general anaesthetic. 4. Explain that his eyes will be bruised and sore after the operation and that both his eyes will be padded. 5. Make clear to him that if he experiences any pain postoperatively, the nursing staff will take immediate action to relieve this and make him comfortable as soon as he reports it. 6. Encourage the patient to ask questions about the operation and the care he will receive, and attempt to answer these queries as far as possible. 7. Ensure that the patient has understood what he has been told and that he is able to give an informed consent before the operation is carried out.

Orbital decompression surgery often involves operating on both eyes at the same time. This creates a problem for the patient in the short-term as both his eyes will be padded on his return from theatre.

Problem	Goal	Nursing intervention
Patient is unable to see following orbital decompression surgery as both his eyes are padded. Unable to carry out activities of daily living independently.	To help patient to carry out the activities of daily living he would perform himself if he could see.	1. Point out to the patient prior to the operation that both eyes will be padded after the operation, at least until the first postoperative dressing is carried out on the day after surgery. Give him the opportunity to experience this 'double-buffing' before the operation so that he knows what it is like. 2. After the operation, assist the patient with activities of daily living such as washing, eating and drinking for as long as he is unable to see. 3. Always introduce yourself by name when

Problem	Goal	Nursing intervention
		approaching the patient and when talking to him. Reassure him that he will receive all the help he needs while his eyes are padded. Emphasize that he need not be afraid to ask for help by always responding at once to any request. 4. Prevent the patient from coming to any harm while his eyes are padded by removing any potentially hazardous items or obstacles from his immediate environment.

Orbital Tumours

Orbital tumours may be benign or malignant. Benign tumours include dermoid and epidermoid cysts and a mucocele which arises in an adjacent sinus. Cysts grow very slowly from embryonic islands of dermal tissue that are congenitally misplaced in the orbit. They tend to be smooth, firm and solitary and anchored to the bone near a suture line. They contain fluid and debris derived from skin structures (e.g. hair and sebaceous secretions) and may communicate with the cranium. Inflammatory masses, such as sarcoid and pseudotumour, may imitate benign neoplasms.

True neoplasms may arise from any of the tissues present in the orbit. Of importance are those of the nerves, muscle and lacrimal gland. The commonest are the benign haemangioma of vascular tissue and the malignant rhabdomyosarcoma of childhood. Those with large vascular (cavernous) spaces may become calcified. Those composed of smaller vessels may be associated with an angioma on the face or lids (strawberry naevus).

Tumours of lymphoid tissue are also common, and are difficult to classify; some, like lymphoid pseudotumour, are benign and contain mature lymphocytes, while lymphoid tumours, including lymphosarcoma, Hodgkin's disease and leukaemic infiltrates, may show variation in cell type. The exact diagnosis will depend on the results of haematological examination of peripheral blood and bone marrow as well as biopsy of the orbital mass and lymph nodes if any are involved.

Optic nerve glioma is a slow-growing tumour in children which may also involve the chiasma. It usually causes visual loss and proptosis and may lead to further intracranial damage. Meningioma may arise from the covering of the optic nerve and spread to involve the optic disc. More commonly, this tumour originates from the area of the sphenoid bone and then may grow to press on the optic nerve. Neurofibromas are also found and, in the case of neurofibromatosis, are associated with multiple nerve tumours elsewhere in the body.

Secondary tumours of the orbit may spread from the globe (e.g. retinoblastoma, choroidal melanoma) or from the nose or sinuses (e.g. nasopharyngeal carcinoma). Other tumours spread by blood-borne metastasis. The commonest are from the lung in men and from the breast in women.

The correct diagnosis of the type of orbital tumour is sometimes only achieved by performing an orbital biopsy.

Treatment

Sarcoid and inflammatory pseudotumour may improve greatly on systemic steroid therapy and this treatment may be used as a diagnostic trial. Tumours such as lymphoma are sensitive to radiotherapy, whereas rhabdomyosarcoma may respond to radiotherapy or antimetabolite chemotherapy. Surgery may be aimed at biopsy, removal of discrete masses or reducing the bulk of tumour, as may be necessary with meningioma.

Problem	Goal	Nursing intervention
Patient has a small growth in his orbit which has been diagnosed as a benign orbital tumour. He is worried in case this is life-threatening and is not sure what should be done about it.	To relieve unnecessary patient anxiety by giving information.	1. Explain to the patient that the orbital tumour is benign and therefore not life-threatening. Point out that as it is not increasing in size or causing him any problems, it therefore does not require any treatment. 2. Talk to him about his feelings and any worries he has had about this tumour and reassure him again that it is harmless. 3. Point out that, although the tumour is not causing any harm at present, if he should notice any increase in size, any visual disturbance or any change in pigmentation of the eyelids or surrounding skin, he should report these changes immediately to his doctor. Emphasize that this does not necessarily mean that the tumour has become malignant, but that its increased size can cause damage by compressing the eye itself or by cutting off its blood supply.

The nursing care required by patients with malignant tumours also varies, depending on whether the lesion is a primary or a secondary tumour. For all patients, and those who are close to them, the diagnosis of 'cancer' gives rise to a whole host of reactions, including anger, fear, depression, shock and denial.

Problem	Goal	Nursing intervention
The patient and his family and friends are extremely shocked, upset and frightened because the patient has been diagnosed as having a malignant orbital tumour.	To give the patient and his family the chance to express their feelings. To provide comfort, advice and support at this time.	1. Talk to the patient and his family about their feelings. Allow them to express these and work through them, e.g. by crying, etc. 2. Try to comfort and support the patient and his family and to help them begin to come to terms with the problem. 3. Help the patient to cope with any feelings of disbelief he may have, particularly if he has experienced no visual symptoms or pain. 4. Explain what treatment is required and ensure that the patient understands. 5. Give the patient the opportunity to be alone with his thoughts if he desires this. However, for the patient who does not wish to be alone, ensure that someone is with him at all times to give him the emotional support he needs. 6. Give advice and support to the patient's family and friends where needed.

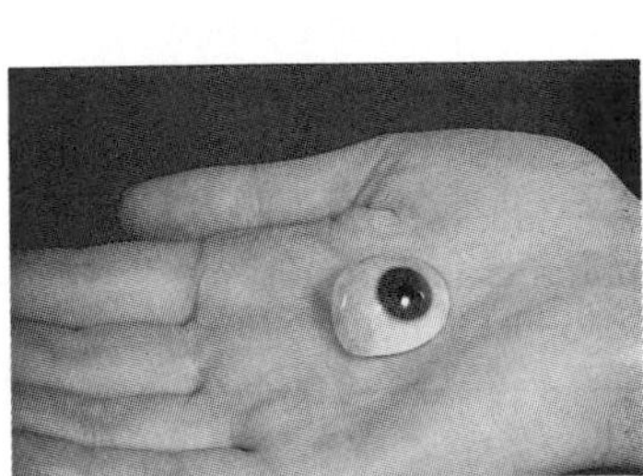

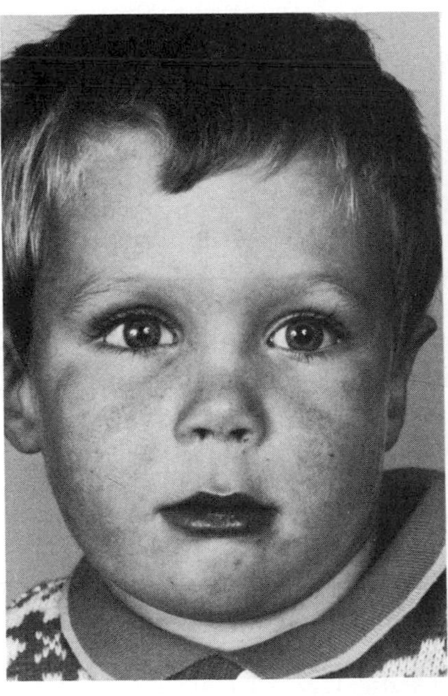

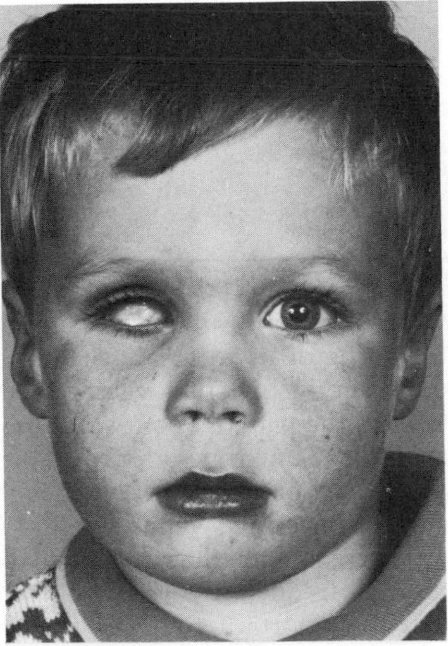

Figure 21.3 **(a)** An ocular prosthesis removed from the socket. **(b)** Child with and without an ocular prosthesis. (Courtesy of Mr Robin Brammer.)

If the tumour is confined to the globe it is possible to eradicate the tumour by removing the eye (enucleation). In fact, the commonest indication for enucleation is malignant melanoma of the choroid (Chapter 17).

The cosmetic appearance of the person who has had an enucleation can be greatly improved by the fitting of an artificial eye (Figure 21.3). This is a specialized task and one

Problem	Goal	Nursing intervention
Patient is about to have an enucleation and is distressed and depressed about his appearance once his eye has been removed.	To help patient to adjust to his altered body image.	1. Spend time preoperatively with the patient and give him the chance to express his feelings and voice his fears about his appearance following the operation. Adopt a sympathetic attitude towards him and take the time to listen to what he wants to say. 2. Provide emotional support to help him to cope with his grief. 3. Emphasize the more positive aspects of the situation and the necessity of the operation; that he will be alive and healthy afterwards. However, at the same time continue to acknowledge that it is perfectly normal for him to grieve over his loss. 4. Outline the aftercare that he will receive. Describe what this involves. 5. Ask someone who has been through this operation in the past to talk to the patient. 6. Tell him that his eye will look like a black eye after the operation and that the wound is not immediately obvious. 7. Encourage the patient to look at his eye postoperatively, but allow him to do this in his own time. Suggest that he wears dark glasses initially if he is worried about how it will look to other people. Encourage him to socialize again gradually after the operation. 8. Assess his reaction after the operation and plan his further care accordingly. 9. Involve ocular prosthetics if available.

which is carried out by an ocular prosthetist. Preparation for the fitting of an artificial eye begins in the preoperative period when the patient is visited by the ocular prosthetist, who talks to the patient about what the fitting and wearing of an artificial eye involves and what the finished result looks like.

The first prosthesis, or shell, is fitted within 2–3 days after surgery once any swelling around the socket has subsided, in order to maintain the size and shape of the socket. This initial fitting is frequently carried out by the ophthalmic nurse.

It is important that the patient knows how to insert, remove and clean this shell prior to discharge from the ward if infection and discomfort are to be avoided and if he is eventually to become accustomed to handling and wearing an artificial eye. Once the patient can successfully handle the prosthetic shell he will be able to cope with an artificial eye, as the principles of handling and caring for this are the same as for the shell.

At first, however, the idea of handling and wearing the prosthetic shell can be distasteful and difficult for the patient:

Problem	Goal	Nursing intervention
A patient who has had an enucleation does not know what fitting and wearing an artificial eye/shell involves. Needs to learn how to care for the shell prior to discharge home. Patient also finds the idea of a shell initially distasteful.	To teach the patient how to wear and care for his artificial eye/ shell and to help him to adjust mentally to doing this.	1. Explain what inserting the shell or artificial eye involves and illustrate this by use of diagrams and pictures. 2. Explain what caring for the shell or artificial eye involves and how often it will need to be removed for cleaning, etc. 3. Allow the patient to insert and remove the shell or artificial eye for himself under supervision, giving him adequate time and privacy to do this. Explain that although he may find it difficult and distasteful at first, he will soon get used to it. 4. Practise insertion, removal and cleaning of the shell several times, until the patient is confident of his ability to do this unsupervised. 5. Advise him to contact the ward again after he has been discharged, if he has any problems at home. Provide him with written instructions on how to manage the shell prior to discharge.

A patient undergoing an enucleation requires the same physical preoperative nursing care as a patient undergoing any other extraocular surgery. The main fear of a large number of patients who are about to undergo an enucleation is that the wrong eye will be removed. It is part of the nurse's role to reassure the patient that this will not happen and also to ensure that there is no possibility of it occurring.

Problem	Goal	Nursing intervention
Patient is very worried in case the wrong eye is enucleated.	To ensure correct eye is removed and reassure patient of this.	1. The eye to be removed is identified by both nurse and patient prior to the operation and this is checked carefully with the information in the notes and on the consent form. If any discrepancies are discovered, these are always sorted out before the operation is allowed to commence. 2. The nurse ensures that the doctor clearly marks the eye to be removed with an arrow prior to the patient going to theatre, and ensures that this arrow is still prominent at the time of going to theatre. 3. The patient is reassured by the nurse by informing him of the number of checks that are made prior to the patient going to theatre, and in theatre as well, in order to prevent any mishap occurring.

Following the operation, during the postoperative recovery period, the biggest risk to the patient's well-being is haemorrhage occurring from the severed blood vessels in the socket. It is important that the nurse on the ward observes closely for this potential complication and acts promptly should any bleeding occur.

Problem	Goal	Nursing intervention
Potential risk of shock following severe blood loss if a haemorrhage occurs in the socket following an enucleation.	To minimize the risk of haemorrhage and to take appropriate action to prevent blood loss if a haemorrhage does occur.	1. Observe dressing every half-hour at least following surgery, for the first 4–6 hours, looking for any signs of fresh bleeding. 2. Nurse patient lying on his operated side to maximize the pressure on the dressing. 3. If fresh bleeding occurs, do not disturb original dressing but apply extra firm padding and bandaging on top of this. Inform medical staff immediately.

Infection is another potential problem following an enucleation.

Problem	Goal	Nursing intervention
Potential risk of infection developing in socket following enucleation.	To prevent infection postoperatively.	1. Carry out all postoperative surgical dressings using an aseptic technique. 2. Observe socket each day for signs of infection or discharge. Keep socket clean by washing/irrigating with a sterile normal saline solution. 3. Instil antibiotic ointment or drops as prescribed. 4. Advise patient against touching, rubbing or wiping his lids, particularly with dirty hands or tissues. 5. Teach the patient always to wash his hands before and after instilling medication and inserting or removing the prosthetic shell.

Some of the patients who require an enucleation will be children. This is naturally a very traumatic time for both the parents and the child. The impact on the child will very much depend on his age and also on his sight in the other eye. The parents may need counselling and will need advice about practical topics, such as the child's education, if he is severely visually handicapped by the loss of his eye. The nursing care needs of the family in this situation must be assessed on an individual basis. Self-help groups for parents of children with a similar problem may be able to help the parents to accept the situation and cope with this distress.

Evisceration

In some rare cases when the eye is severely infected (e.g. if the patient has panophthalmitis) it is necessary to perform an operation called an evisceration in order to prevent the infection back-tracking along the optic nerve to the brain. It is only carried out if all medical and antibiotic treatment has failed to control the infection.

A surgical incision is made around the limbus, the cornea is removed and the contents of the eye are scooped out with an evisceration scoop. The sclera and conjunctiva remain and the optic nerve is not cut.

This operation will have the same psychological impact on the patient as an enucleation as it means essentially that he has lost his eye. The patient undergoing an evisceration will therefore require similar nursing care to the patient undergoing an enucleation and the problems created by loss, altered body image, altered vision and the cosmetic appearance of the eye afterwards all need to be discussed by the nurse with the patient.

There is, however, the additional problem of the potential risk of cross-infection and, for this reason, the patient will need to be isolated and barrier-nursed in a similar manner to the patient with orbital cellulitis. The care plan covering the potential risk of the infection causing orbital cellulitis to spread further would also apply for the patient undergoing an evisceration.

Exenteration

Malignant tumours which have spread from the globe to the orbit and some primary orbital tumours necessitate exenteration. This is the complete removal of the orbital contents. The orbital walls, if intact, require skin grafts either from the lids with the margins excised or from elsewhere.

This is an extremely devastating and extensive operation to carry out and would be valueless and damaging to the patient if it were carried out without first checking that the tumour has not already spread beyond the orbit and that the orbital tumour is not itself a secondary spread from a tumour in some other part of the body.

However, 70% of orbital tumours are of a primary nature. It is nevertheless important to carry out a comprehensive series of tests, mainly X-rays and blood tests, before going ahead with the operation.

Problem	Goal	Nursing intervention
Patient is unaware of why he is to undergo a series of investigative tests, what these tests are and what they are for.	To reduce anxiety caused by lack of knowledge and uncertainty. To help the patient to prepare for tests.	1. Explain to the patient and/or his family what tests are required and why they have been requested. 2. Make clear what the tests may find and also what is likely to happen should the tests prove negative. 3. Prior to each test, explain to the patient what it involves, how long it will take, what he will feel and what he will be expected to do during each test. Ensure he understands the explanation given. 4. Ensure that the patient is comfortable during and after each test. 5. Ensure that the findings of the tests and the implications of these findings are made clear to the patient and/or his relatives.

If, following the findings of this extensive testing, it is decided by doctor and patient to go ahead with the exenteration, the preparation and nursing care required preoperatively are similar to that required by the patient undergoing an enucleation. The extent of the psychological problems experienced may be much greater, however, as the disfigurement resulting from an exenteration is much greater. The same principles of providing sympathetic emotional support, and the opportunity for the patient to express how he feels, apply.

The prosthesis required following an exenteration is much more extensive than the artificial eye and includes the eyelids and even orbital bone. These prostheses are frequently attached to spectacles. Improved cosmesis can be achieved with 'osseointegrative' techniques.

The considerable loss of tissue resulting from an exenteration means that in many cases a skin graft is required. The donor site is normally on the inner thigh or the upper arm and must be an area where there is minimal growth of hair, in order to be cosmetically acceptable.

The nurse must make sure that the patient understands that he may need a skin graft and prepare the donor site for grafting.

The postoperative problems of a patient in the early stages of recovery following an exenteration are similar to those of a patient recovering from an enucleation – haemorrhage and infection. Most patients who have undergone either type of operation are usually given a course of systemic and topical antibiotics postoperatively.

Problem	Goal	Nursing intervention
Patient is unsure whether a skin graft is needed, where the skin is taken from and why it may be needed.	To ensure that patient understands why the skin graft may be carried out and what it involves.	1. Explain to the patient that a skin graft may be necessary to replace some of the skin lost during the operation. Ensure he understands. 2. Tell him where the skin graft will be taken from and how big it will be. 3. Give him an estimate of how long the donor site will take to heal.
Loss of skin during exenteration means that the patient needs a skin graft in order to minimize disfigurement and promote healing. Potential problem of infection and rejection if donor site is not properly prepared.	To minimize disfigurement by skin grafting. To prevent infection or rejection of graft by preparing donor site properly.	1. Ensure donor site is clearly identified and marked. 2. Explain to the patient how the donor site is to be prepared and why this is being done. 3. Prepare donor site as requested by surgeon, shaving and cleansing if it is ordered.

The surgical dressing of a patient who has undergone an exenteration is generally left *in situ* for up to 7 days after the operation. The first postoperative dressing is then carried out by a member of the medical staff and may warrant another visit to theatre.

Fitting a prosthesis following an exenteration is very specialized work and is normally carried out solely by an ocular prosthetist. Mishandling of this delicate situation could cause a delay in the patient's ability to accept and adjust to the prosthesis.

Chemotherapy and/or radiotherapy may also be required by these patients and the care and support needed during this treatment should be planned and given accordingly.

Patients who have had either an enucleation or an exenteration are often discharged home fairly quickly following surgery (within 2–4 days after an enucleation and 10–14 days after an exenteration), in an effort to get them to resume their normal lives as quickly and with as little disruption as possible. The patient's problems – particularly those of a psychological nature – are by no means resolved by the time of discharge. Further help may be required with learning to handle and care for the prosthesis, and further psychological support may be needed to help the patient to cope with his loss, altered appearance and altered vision. He may also need advice concerning employment, driving, etc. if the loss of an eye affects the work that he does. Such advice and support is obviously important on a long- as well as a short-term basis.

Problem	Goal	Nursing intervention
Patient is about to be discharged home following exenteration. Risk of further emotional, psychological and practical problems developing or being realized after discharge. Rejection if donor site is not properly prepared.	To provide emotional support for the patient and practical help after discharge.	1. Inform district nurse of patient's impending discharge home, pointing out any potential problems the patient may have. Inform the patient's general practitioner of his treatment and discharge. 2. Talk to the patient and talk about the type of problems he may experience when he gets home. Reassure him that he can always seek advice from hospital staff if he needs it, give him the ward's phone number so he can contact ward if necessary. 3. Explain that the district nurse will call initially to see how he is getting on. 4. Arrange follow-up medical and ocular prosthetic department appointments and ensure that the patient has written information about these to take home. Invite him to visit the ward again after he has been discharged. 5. Assess the patient's psychological condition and reaction to his operation, and refer to a social worker for further counselling if appropriate. 6. Ask the patient if he feels the operation will affect his job in any way. If he is worried about this, ensure that the social worker is also aware of this. 7. Give him advice on driving, etc. – point out that although it is not advisable for him to drive until he has had time to recover from the operation and adjust to unilateral vision, there is no reason why he should not be able to drive again in the future.

Orbital Trauma

Blows to the orbit may lead to haemorrhage or fracture. Blow-out fractures of the orbital floor or medial wall often result from blunt injuries to the eye. The signs are soft tissue swelling, enophthalmos (eye sunken in or down) and limitation of eye movement in upward gaze. There will be paraesthesia of the cheek if the infraorbital nerve is involved. Plain X-rays may confirm that orbital tissues around the fracture site are prolapsed into the adjacent sinus. CT scans are proving to be particularly helpful in evaluating the need for surgery and its planning.

Treatment is usually conservative unless there is obvious enophthalmos or there is diplopia in primary gaze. If this is marked or persists for more than a few days surgical exploration of the fracture and repair with a silicone prosthesis is required.

Problem	Goal	Nursing intervention
Patient has sustained a blow-out fracture of the orbit within the last 24 hours.Potential risk of neurological Injury also having been sustained.	To monitor patient's condition for first 24 hours after sustaining a head injury to ensure that no further damage has occurred.	1. Explain to the patient that the blow he sustained to his eye has fractured the orbital floor and that there is always a possibility of further symptoms developing within the first 24 hours which could indicate a more serious injury. 2. Admit the patient to the ward until the initial 24 hours are past and put him on strict bed rest. 3. Carry out neurological observations at regular intervals to assess his neurological state and report any abnormalities to medical staff. 4. Reassure patient that he is all right if no further problems arise and allow him to go home once he has been medically reviewed. 5. Should any neurological problems occur, treat appropriately and obtain a medical referral to a neurologist.

It can be a very frightening thing for the patient with a blow-out fracture to realize that he has double vision. The patient needs to be reassured that this is only a temporary problem and will resolve.

Problem	Goal	Nursing intervention
A patient with a blow-out fracture complains of double vision, especially on looking up. He is anxious and worried about this as he does not know how long it will last.	To relieve anxiety.	1. Explain to the patient the reason why he is experiencing double vision. 2. Reassure him that this is likely to pass of its own accord, within 2 weeks in most cases. 3. Explain that if it does not resolve in this time, a small operation may be required and the double vision will be corrected in any case. 4. Advise him to contact the hospital again if he is at all worried. Arrange for him to have the progress of the recovery from his injury monitored as an outpatient.

If the fracture, muscle entrapment and diplopia do not resolve of their own accord within about 10 days and surgical repair is considered necessary, it is the responsibility of the nurse to ensure that the patient understands why surgery is necessary and what it involves.

Occasionally the medial wall of the orbit is fractured. The patient is normally symptomless until he blows his nose,

Problem	Goal	Nursing intervention
Patient has been told that he needs an operation to correct a blow-out fracture. Lack of knowledge about what this involves has caused unnecessary anxiety and uncertainty.	To relieve anxiety and prepare mentally and physically for theatre.	1. Tell the patient that the purpose of the operation is to correct his double vision by repairing the fracture. 2. Explain that this involves freeing the trapped muscles from the fracture and placing an implant on the floor of the orbit to prevent the muscles from becoming trapped again. 3. Ensure that the patient has understood the explanation. Ask him if he has any queries and try to answer these if possible.

causing air to escape via the fracture from the sinuses into the orbit and the eye to puff up dramatically (surgical emphysema). When this happens the patient usually presents himself hurriedly at the ophthalmic Accident and Emergency Department.

A carefully taken history is valuable in helping to confirm the diagnosis.

Problem	Goal	Nursing intervention
Patient has presented in A & E with marked puffiness around one eye which has developed suddenly. He is very worried about what has caused this and how serious it is.	To ascertain cause of symptoms and reassure patient by telling him what has caused his symptoms and how they can be treated.	1. Examine the eye, eyelids and skin covering the orbital area. Crinkling of trapped air on palpation indicates probable medial wall fracture. 2. Take a detailed history from the patient, asking when he first noticed the symptoms, what he was doing at the time and whether he has had any blow to the eye or surrounding area recently. 3. Once the patient has been examined by the doctor, outline the probable diagnosis to him. Reassure him that this will resolve of its own accord in time and that there will be no after-effects from the injury. 4. Explain that an X-ray will be needed to confirm the diagnosis, tell the patient what this will involve and organize X-ray. 5. Tell the patient not to blow his nose for several weeks. 6. Reassure patient and advise him to contact the hospital again if he should have any further worries.

Penetration of the orbit may result from almost any object which is either sharp or which has been projected at high speed. Perforating injuries are commonly caused by scissors, knives, air-gun pellets and glass (e.g. following a road traffic accident). History-taking is vital in order to alert staff to the possibility of orbital penetration. The injury may require surgical exploration to remove a foreign body or haematoma. Preoperative assessment of vision and optic nerve function is essential.

Problem	Goal	Nursing intervention
Patient has suffered a perforating orbital injury. Potential risk of complications occurring or treatment being inappropriate if cause of injury is not firmly established at the outset.	To determine cause of injury and thus plan appropriate treatment and care for the patient. To promote a speedy and uncomplicated recovery.	1. Tell the patient that, in order to treat the injury in the best way, it is important to know what has caused the injury, when it happened and what the patient was doing at the time. 2. Record the history in the nursing Kardex and inform medical staff. 3. Reassure the patient that the most appropriate course of treatment can now be initiated.
Patient is agitated and frightened by the apparent delay in commencing treatment of his orbital injury that is due to his being asked to undergo X-rays, vision and other tests.	To relieve patient's agitation and fear by telling him why the tests are necessary before treatment is commenced.	1. Tell the patient what tests he is being asked to undergo. 2. Explain that the purpose of these tests is to determine the extent of the injury and how best to treat it. Point out that if these tests were not carried out at this stage it would be difficult to plan the care and treatment he needs. 3. Explain what each test involves, how long it will take and what he will be expected to do during it. 4. Reassure the patient that the delay in commencing treatment will not cause any further harm. 5. Ensure that the patient is informed of the results of the tests and what these mean. 6. Help to relieve the patient's agitation and anxiety by talking to him, reassuring him and giving him the emotional support he needs.

Treatment also depends on the nature of the material responsible for the injury and whether any of this has been retained in the orbit. If an inert or blunt-edged substance remains in the orbit, it may be decided to leave this *in situ*. If the substance is made of woody or vegetable matter, or if the injury has been caused by an animal bite, a course of antitetanus injections should be given and antibiotic treatment instituted.

An X-ray may be requested if it is suspected that a radio-opaque substance such as a metal fragment has been retained in the orbit. The treatment to be given must be explained to the patient by the nurse.

Problem	Goal	Nursing intervention
Patient is unaware of what the treatment for his orbital injury will consist of. This lack of knowledge is causing anxiety and may potentially result in poorer compliance with treatment and aftercare.	To ensure treatment is carried out safely and well. To relieve patient anxiety by giving information and also to improve patient's ability to comply with treatment.	1. Explain to the patient what treatment he is being given, why this is being done and how long the course of treatment will take. 2. Point out what his role is in carrying out the treatment, e.g. taking antibiotics or completing a course of injections. 3. Tell him why this course of treatment has been taken for him and explain what follow-up he will need. 4. Ensure patient is able as well as willing to carry out his part in the course of treatment required.

An attempt may be made to remove a retained fragment of magnetic material from the orbit by using a large electromagnet in theatre to draw a fragment back out along its original portal of entry. If this is successful then the extent of the damage caused by the injury is minimized as no additional surgical wound has been made to remove the fragment.

If this is unsuccessful, or if the retained fragment is not magnetic, the foreign body may be removed in an operation called an orbitotomy. The nurse should always ensure that the patient knows what this involves.

Problem	Goal	Nursing intervention
Patient is to have an orbitotomy to remove a foreign body from the orbit. He is frightened and anxious about this. His anxiety is compounded by his lack of knowledge of what this operation involves.	To relieve patient's anxiety and fear and to prepare him mentally and physically for theatre.	1. Explain to the patient that a foreign body has been retained in the orbit following injury and that he needs an operation to remove this in order to prevent it from doing any further damage. 2. Explain what the operation involves, how he will be prepared for it, when the operation will be carried out and what postoperative care he will need. 3. Talk to him about any worries he has and help him to deal with these. Reassure him.

Orbitotomy

There are three anterior routes employed in orbital surgery.

1. A conjunctival and Tenon's capsule incision is most familiar to the ophthalmic surgeon and allows access to the globe and interior optic nerve within the muscle cone.

2. An incision through the eyelid and orbital septum may be made in any quadrant but the view is limited and great care is needed to maintain haemostasis.
3. A periosteal incision at the orbital margin, approached via the lid, gives access to any part of the orbit by reflecting the periorbital tissue.

The patient is prepared for surgery in the same way as a patient undergoing any other extraocular operation under general anaesthetic. It is particularly important in this case, however, to ensure that the wound and the surrounding area are thoroughly cleansed before surgery begins, as one of the main complications following a penetrating orbital injury is infection.

Problem	Goal	Nursing intervention
Risk of delayed healing and the development of further complications postoperatively.	To prevent infection and so minimize the risk of other complications arising.	1. Commence patient on a course of antibiotics preoperatively if prescribed. 2. Clean the wound and the surrounding area as well as possible prior to surgery. 3. Use an aseptic technique pre- and postoperatively when carrying out any ophthalmic dressing or care. 4. Advise the patient against touching the wound with his hand or a tissue, etc. and also not to touch or rub the surrounding area, and explain that this is to minimize the chances of any infection developing. 5. Give topical antibiotics as prescribed. 6. Monitor the condition of the wound and patient, observing for redness, inflammation, pain, discharge or raised body temperature. Inform medical staff should any of these signs occur. 7. Monitor optic nerve integrity by checking visual acuity and pupil responses to light, as directed.

Further blood loss and haemorrhage occurring behind the newly repaired surgical wound is another possible complication of surgery carried out to remove a foreign body.

The development of a haemorrhage behind the wound needs to be avoided as the swelling could cause proptosis and could also cause permanent damage to the patient's vision by exerting pressure on the optic nerve and on the globe itself. In some cases an orbital drain will be placed *in situ* to try and prevent this complication and its consequences.

Problem	Goal	Nursing intervention
Potential risk of damage to or loss of vision occurring after an orbital wound has been repaired if a haemorrhage or blood clot develops behind the wound and is unable to escape, or if the orbital wound drain inserted to help prevent this fails to drain.	To prevent damage of the eye or loss of vision after orbital surgery.	1. Monitor and empty orbital wound drain as ordered and observe the colour and amount of drained fluid. 2. Ensure that the drain is securely anchored and prevent pulling on the drain by attaching the drainage tubing firmly to the patient's temple or cheek with tape. Anchor the drainage bottle firmly to prevent it from falling off the patient's bed and pulling on the drain. 3. Maintain bed rest while the drain is *in situ* and help the patient to carry out the activities of daily living that he would normally carry out for himself were he not confined to bed and handicapped by the presence of the orbital drain. 4. Explain the purpose of the drain to the patient and advise him only to move his head slowly and gently in order to avoid pulling on the drain or causing it to dislodge. 5. Observe for any signs of haemorrhage, e.g. swelling of the orbital tissues. Report this, or any increased volume of drained fluid or fresh blood in the drain, to medical staff. 6. Use an aseptic technique when handling the drain and drainage bottle. 7. Remove drain using aseptic technique when risk of further haemorrhage has passed.

The length of stay in hospital of a patient who has had an orbital wound repaired will vary, depending on the nature and extent of the injury and its repair.

When the patient is ready for discharge it is important to ensure that he knows how to prevent further complications and promote healing by carrying out the prescribed after-care. The preparation for discharge is similar to that required by any other postsurgical ophthalmic patient – ensuring that the patient will receive the drops he has been prescribed and knows what follow-up is needed, etc. He should also be made aware of what signs of potential complications he should look for, such as redness, pain and discharge indicating infection, and what he should do if any of these occur.

Orbital Infection

A bacterial infection of the eyelids (periorbital cellulitis) is a serious condition requiring urgent attention, especially if it

Problem	Goal	Nursing intervention
Patient suffering from orbital cellulitis. Risk of potential complications if infection either goes untreated or spreads because inadequately treated.	To prevent further spread of infection. To promote resolution of orbital cellulitis.	1. Give systemic and topical antibiotics as prescribed. Explain to patient that these are necessary to resolve his condition and also to prevent the infection from spreading further. 2. Monitor patient's condition for improvements or deterioration. Report any worsening in symptoms, e.g. increased pain, rigor or delirium, to medical staff immediately. 3. Check pupils hourly, or as instructed.
Patient is feverish and feels unwell because of orbital cellulitis.	To reduce fever and increase patient comfort and recovery.	1. Put patient on bed rest and encourage him to get plenty of rest while he is feeling unwell. 2. Monitor his temperature and pulse 2-hourly. 3. Keep patient cool by tepid sponging and by covering him with the minimum of bedclothes. Use a fan to cool him down further if needed but ensure the fan does not blow directly on to the patient. 4. Change the patient's bed and nightclothes as often as needed if he is hot and sweating. 5. Encourage the patient to drink at least 2 litres of fluid daily. Maintain a fluid balance chart. 6. Ensure that his immediate environment is peaceful and conducive to rest. Ask him if there are any ways in which he could be made more comfortable. 7. Report any significant changes in temperature to the medical staff. 8. Restrict the number and length of visits so that the patient is not overtired by this.
Patient complaining of severe pain around his eye which is worse when he moves his eyes.	To relieve pain and make the patient more comfortable.	1. Observe for signs and/or complaints of pain and give analgesia as prescribed. 2. Monitor effect of analgesia half an hour after administration and again before next dose is due. Encourage the patient to say if the pain returns and ask him about the effect of the analgesia. 3. Explain to the patient that one of the symptoms of orbital cellulitis is pain on moving the eyes. Suggest that he attempts to move his eyes as little as possible until the inflammation has subsided. Advise him to move his head rather than just his eyes when he wants to look at something. 4. Ensure that the patient is able to get enough sleep and rest to cope with the pain. Make him comfortable so that the pain is minimized.

occurs in young children. Even more serious is orbital cellulitis, when the infection finds its way behind the orbital septum.

The features of both conditions are similar: a sudden onset of eyelid swelling, redness and chemosis. If the infection is within the orbit the eye may be proptosed and mobility reduced. The patient will be febrile and in pain. There may be a history of trauma, though this may be as trivial as eyebrow plucking.

Admission, full examination, skull X-ray and a full blood count and blood culture are necessary. The origin of the infection, especially in the child and teenager, is often the sinuses. An ENT opinion is, therefore, required as drainage of sepsis may be required.

An important but rare differential diagnosis is cavernous sinus thrombosis which may follow facial sepsis. Systemic antibiotics are required as is urgent neurosurgical consultation.

Medical treatment for orbital cellulitis consists primarily of intensive systemic and topical antibiotic therapy. The nurse ensures that the patient receives this treatment and monitors its effect on decreasing the patient's temperature and the swelling. It is important that the nurse monitors the control of the infection and is aware of potential complications.

Proptosis may develop if the swelling of the orbital tissues is marked. If this occurs then the nursing care planned must also include measures to prevent the complications of proptosis. The swelling of the tissues in orbital cellulitis can be reduced to some extent and the inflammatory reaction localized by the application of heat.

Problem	Goal	Nursing intervention
The patient's lids and the surrounding orbital tissues are very swollen because of orbital cellulitis. Risk of damage occurring to the eye if the proptosis becomes any more severe.	To prevent damage to the eye by relieving the swelling.	1. Explain to the patient that some of his symptoms are caused by swelling and that therefore it is advisable to reduce it. Tell him that this can be done by applying heat to the eye. 2. Point out that during this treatment the patient will simply be asked to lie down and that although he will feel heat around his eye, it will not hurt or scald him. Tell him that if he does feel that it is too hot he should say so and the heat source will immediately be withdrawn. 3. Apply heat locally to the swollen area (e.g. by hot spoon bathing or using a Maddox heater) without allowing the heat source to come into contact with the skin. Carry out this treatment 4-hourly or as ordered. 4. Monitor the effectiveness in reducing swelling and relieving symptoms.

Severe orbital cellulitis may damage vital structures at the apex, resulting in paralysis of the extraocular muscles, caused by involvement of the III, IV and VI cranial nerves, and decreased vision – the orbital apex syndrome.

Nursing care is the same as for orbital cellulitis. Particularly if the patient is a child, it is important to inform the parents or relatives of the potentially serious and life-threatening nature of this development.

Abscess formation is another complication of orbital cellulitis. The treatment of this is by surgical incision and drainage.

The types of infection causing orbital cellulitis and cavernous sinus thrombosis are contagious and it is important to prevent the spread of infection to any other person. This is particularly important if the patient is in hospital on an ophthalmic ward where postsurgical patients are also present. To prevent cross-infection the patient with orbital cellulitis or cavernous sinus thrombosis should be isolated.

Problem	Goal	Nursing intervention
Risk of cross-infection on ward if patient with orbital cellulitis comes into contact with other patients.	To prevent cross-infection.	1. Isolate the patient with orbital cellulitis in a single room or side ward. 2. Explain to the patient that it is necessary for him to stay in this room in order to prevent the spread of infection to any other patient. 3. Employ the principles of barrier nursing when carrying out his care, wearing aprons when giving care and washing the hands thoroughly before and after giving care. 4. Ensure that the equipment used to nurse the patient with orbital cellulitis is reserved for his use only and is not used for other patients unless it is first sterilized. 5. Use an aseptic technique when carrying out ophthalmic dressings and care. 6. Advise the patient not to touch or rub his infected eye. 7. Instil topical antibiotics as prescribed. 8. Help the patient to find diversion activities to occupy his time, talk to him and keep him company. 9. Restrict the number of visitors allowed in his room.

Vascular Disorders

Orbital Venous Varices

These may result from a congenital venous malformation and so they often present in childhood. They manifest themselves as a soft, reducible swelling and can cause proptosis. The proptosis may be more marked, or only present, on straining, or crying in the case of a child. There is the risk of corneal exposure if the proptosis is marked, in which case it warrants the same treatment as proptosis resulting from any other condition.

Particularly when the patient is a child, the parents can be very worried about what is causing the swelling.

Problem	Goal	Nursing intervention
Parents are very anxious about what is causing swelling of their child's eye and what is causing the eye to protrude.	To relieve anxiety by informing the parents what is causing their child's symptoms.	1. Ascertain what symptoms are present to establish and confirm diagnosis. 2. Once diagnosis has been confirmed, tell the parents that the swelling is due to varicose veins in the orbit and that the swelling will increase occasionally on stooping or straining. Explain that these veins are generally harmless although cosmetically not very attractive. 3. Reassure the parents about the harmless nature of this condition. However, advise them to inform the hospital and seek further advice if any permanent increase in the amount of swelling occurs, as this may indicate a haemorrhage.

Caroticocavernous Fistula

The internal carotid artery lies within the cavernous sinus, which is a venous chamber. A caroticocavernous fistula can result either from the rupture of a carotid artery aneurysm in the cavernous sinus or from a severe head injury that ruptures this vessel.

The patient presents with a pulsating proptosis (generally unilateral), swelling of the lids, dilated conjunctival and retinal blood vessels and impaired vision. A bruit may be heard over the eye.

The diagnosis is confirmed by CT scan, carotid arteriography and Doppler ultrasound studies.

Problem	Goal	Nursing intervention
Patient is suspected of having a carotico-cavernous fistula. Need to carry out CT san and carotid arteriography to confirm diagnosis. Patient is wary about these tests, not knowing what they are for or what they involve.	To prepare patient for investigative tests.	1. Explain to patient that the carotid arteriography and CT scan are necessary to confirm the diagnosis and therefore to plan appropriate action. 2. Explain what the tests will involve, how long they will take, what they will feel like and what patient will be expected to do during the tests. 3. Ask patient if he has any worries or queries regarding the tests. 4. Reassure patient and ensure that he is comfortable and safe during and after the tests.

The condition can be quite painful and so nursing care must be geared towards relieving this pain. The patient will also be worried about the prognosis for his condition and its effect on his vision.

Problem	Goal	Nursing intervention
Lack of knowledge about progress of condition and its long-term effect on vision is causing patient a great deal of anxiety.	To relieve anxiety by giving information.	1. Explain to patient that his condition may resolve itself spontaneously over several years. Point out that his vision will be impaired during this period and that little can be done to relieve this. 2. Ensure that patient is followed up regularly as an outpatient so that his condition continues to be monitored. 3. Answer any queries patient may have as well as possible. Advise him about effective pain relief if he experiences any pain.

In some cases, if vision is threatened by the fistula or if the proptosis is very severe, surgery may be warranted. An embolus is deliberately placed in the carotid artery so as to occlude the fistula.

Visual Pathways

Functional Anatomy

The visual pathways consist of the afferent nerves and nuclei subserving vision. They connect the retina of both eyes to the occipital visual cortex. They are conveniently divided as follows (Figure 21.4):

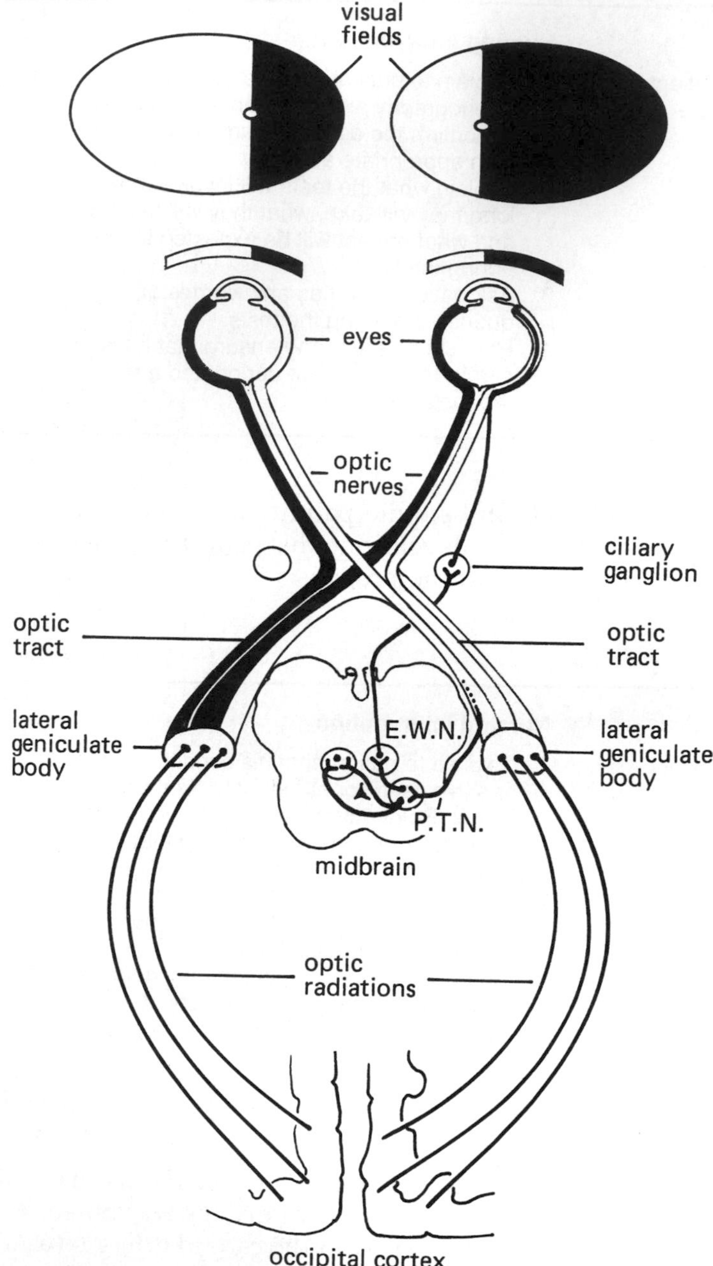

Figure 21.4 Arrangement of the afferent visual pathways from the retina to the cortex. PTN = pretectal nucleus; EWN = Edinger–Westphal nucleus.

1. optic nerves;
2. optic chiasm;
3. optic tracts;
4. lateral geniculate nuclei;
5. optic radiations;
6. visual cortex.

Each optic nerve is composed of approximately 1 million fibres which are the axons of retinal ganglion cells projecting to areas of the brain. Most fibres synapse in the lateral geniculate nucleus with neurones connecting to the visual (or striate) cortex in the occipital cortex of the brain.

Some optic nerve fibres conduct the pupillary light reflex. These fibres synapse in the midbrain (pretectal nuclei) with neurones connecting to the Edinger–Westphal nuclei on both sides.

Another small group of afferent fibres passes from the optic tract to the superior colliculus on each side, where relays connect to the ocular motor nuclei and spinal nerves to mediate subcortical visual reflexes. The route which an optic nerve fibre takes in the afferent pathways depends on the position of its ganglion cell body in the retina. Ganglion cells on the temporal side of the eye project to the brain on the same side. Those on the nasal side of a vertical line drawn through the fovea of each eye pass to the other side via the optic chiasm. Behind the chiasm, fibres come together in the optic tracts from the corresponding half retinae and are related to corresponding fields of vision in each eye (Figure 21.4).

Disease affecting the visual pathways may be localized according to the pattern of field defects present in both eyes. Pressure on the chiasm, caused, for example, by an enlarging pituitary tumour, will damage the mixed fibres from ganglion cells in the nasal halves of each retina and will lead to bitemporal field loss. The extent of field loss will mirror the chiasmal damage but even when this is total, the nasal fields will still be preserved because uncrossed fibres are not affected. Partial damage, for instance, to the lower chiasm will show field loss in the upper parts of the temporal fields (superotemporal quadrantanopia). Unilateral damage to the optic tract, lateral geniculate, radiation or cortex will cause a homonymous hemianopia. This is a one-sided loss of field in the corresponding halves of each eye. For example, thrombosis of a branch of the middle cerebral artery on the right side may infarct the optic tract and lead to left-sided homonymous hemianopia with loss of the nasal field of the right eye and temporal field of the left eye. This kind of field deficit commonly accompanies the other more obvious features of a stroke.

The Optic Disc

The optic disc or papilla is the part of the optic nerve visible within the eye. It is about 1.5 mm in diameter, round or slightly oval and pink with a distinct outline. A central depression, the optic cup, occupies about a quarter of its surface and may appear paler than the remaining rim. The central retinal artery and vein emerge from the nasal part of the cup and branch into tributaries to each retinal quadrant.

The main blood supply to the optic nerve behind the eye is from the central retinal artery and its branches. This artery, a branch of the ophthalmic artery, enters the nerve by piercing the meninges about 1 cm before reaching the globe. The optic disc tissue has a separate blood supply with its main contribution from the short ciliary arteries. These are about 10 in number and enter the back of the globe to anastomose, providing a rich source of blood to the choroid.

Congenital Conditions

Coloboma (a hole occurring in the optic disc) and opaque nerve fibres are included here. These conditions may not be noticed until the child has his eyes tested at school age (or possibly earlier if any visual difficulty is noted), as they are not immediately evident unless fundal examination has been carried out.

The parents of a child with such a congenital anomaly are likely to be shocked and upset on hearing this news, especially when they realize that it is not possible to correct their child's visual problems with, for example, glasses. A full explanation and a sympathetic approach are needed.

Problem	Goal	Nursing intervention
Parents of a child with a sight defect have been told that this is due to a congenital abnormality of the visual pathway, for which there is no treatment. Parents are shocked and upset by this news.	To help parents to cope with their feelings on hearing of their child's condition.	1. Allow the parents sufficient time and privacy to absorb the news they have been given by medical staff. 2. Talk with the parents about their problems and worries, both in the immediate future and in the long term, and listen to them sympathetically. Allow them to express their feelings. 3. Answer queries as far as possible, and refer them to books, self-help groups, etc. from which they may be able to obtain further support and information. 4. Emphasize the more positive aspects of the situation: that now the condition has been diagnosed it is possible to ensure that necessary services to help their child are contacted, e.g. partially-sighted schools, mobility officers, etc., to help the child to make the most of his residual vision. 5. Provide comfort and support for the parents and ensure that they know they can contact you or someone else at the hospital for further help if they need it.

Retrobulbar (Optic) Neuritis

Inflammation of the optic nerve behind the globe is called retrobulbar neuritis. It may rarely be caused by specific infections such as measles or syphilis. More commonly the condition is due to demyelination, which may be isolated or occur as part of a disseminated sclerosis in the nervous system.

The patient is usually a young adult female (sex ratio F:M 3:1) who notices sudden onset of reduced vision in one eye. This may be moderate, with 'clouding' and loss of colour brightness, or profound, with only perception of light remaining. There is usually an ache in or behind the eye which is worse on lateral gaze, and the visual symptoms may be worse when the body temperature is raised by exercise or a hot bath.

If the condition is unilateral, there will be a relative afferent pupillary defect and a paracentral field defect of variable pattern. The globe is often tender to palpation but the optic disc is usually normal in appearance.

Spontaneous recovery is usual within 2–4 weeks, especially after a first attack, although the pupil and field signs may still be detected. In severe cases systemic corticosteroids may be given. After initial recovery the clinical course is very variable; some patients have no further disease whereas others may suffer involvement of the fellow eye or progress to multiple sclerosis.

Optic Disc Oedema

Optic disc oedema is a term for a swelling of the optic nerve head. When this is due to raised intracranial pressure it is called papilloedema (Plate 8). The distinct outline is blurred or lost and the surface capillaries are dilated. Small haemorrhages are seen on the disc and in the retina nearby. The veins may also be swollen and oedema may spread into the macula, affecting central vision. The important causes are raised intracranial pressure, tumour involving the optic nerve, malignant hypertension and local inflammation of the eye (posterior uveitis) or nerve (papillitis).

Intracranial pressure may be raised by tumours, including aneurysms, and by encephalitis or meningitis blocking cerebrospinal fluid outflow.

Optic Atrophy

Atrophy of the optic nerve is the death or loss of nerve cells (ganglion cells), which may result from their direct damage or interference with their blood supply. The optic disc appears pale or, if the atrophic process is advanced, almost white.

Optic atrophy may be due to a rare inherited abnormality, when both discs will look pale. Most acquired optic nerve disease is unilateral and so comparison of the two discs is important. The common causes of optic atrophy are ischaemia (e.g. from ciliary vascular occlusion in cranial ('giant cell') arteritis), following retrobulbar neuritis and in advanced glaucoma.

Pupillary Syndromes

The pupil is activated by two opposing iris muscles. The size of the pupil at any moment is determined by a balance of the innervation to the two iris muscles. The constrictor pupillae muscle is parasympathetic and by contracting makes the pupil small (miosis). The nerve pathway to the constrictor is from the Edinger–Westphal nucleus in the midbrain via the oculomotor nerve and ciliary ganglion (Figure 21.4). The parasympathetic system carries impulses to cause miosis in response to an increase in light level or as part of the accommodation response to a near target.

The dilatator pupillae is sympathetic and when it contracts the pupil dilates. The nerve path to the dilatator is from the hypothalamus via the spinal cord and the superior cervical ganglion and thence in sympathetic fibres accompanying the carotid artery and its branches to the eye.

Efferent Pupil Defects

A bright light or near target presented to one eye normally leads to equal constriction of both pupils, because the nerve pathways cross over in the chiasm and in the midbrain. A parasympathetic 'efferent' pupillary lesion occurs when either the oculomotor nerve or the ciliary ganglion or the constrictor muscle (or all three!) fails to function. The pupil is larger than in the opposite eye, and a search is made for other signs of oculomotor paralysis. The same effect is caused by mydriatic eye drops like homatropine.

Horner's Syndrome

In this syndrome there is a relative miosis (smaller pupil) due to paralysis of the dilatator muscle. There is also a partial ptosis from paralysis of Müller's muscle in the eyelid. There may also be reduced sweating on the forehead and temple on the same side. The diagnosis may be confirmed by a drop of 4% cocaine in each eye. The normal pupil will dilate while the Horner's pupil remains unchanged. It is then necessary to find the level of the lesion in the long sympathetic path by further pharmacological tests.

Radiography may be required to exclude an apical lung tumour or cervical rib as the cause.

Adie's Myotonic Pupil

Adie's pupil is a benign form of unilateral efferent parasympathetic pupil defect, commonly found in females in the third and fourth decade. The affected pupil is larger than its fellow and does not react to light. On near stimulation there is a very slow and sustained pupil contraction with slow recovery. The pupil is supersensitive to 0.5% pilocarpine eyedrops, which cause constriction.

Argyll Robertson Pupil

The Argyll Robertson pupil is generally small and irregular with an absent light reflex. There may be a slow near response which is hard to demonstrate. The condition is bilateral and is typical of syphilis of the CNS. This disease is now uncommon where antibiotics are available and the pupil abnormality may rarely be caused by other lesions of the pupillary pathways in the tectum of the midbrain.

Afferent Pupil Defects

A lesion of the anterior visual pathway on one side (retina, optic nerve), besides reducing vision in one eye, will cause an afferent pupillary defect. In this case, in ordinary lighting, both pupils will be the same size. However, if a bright light is shone into the eye with an afferent defect due, say, to optic neuritis, the response of pupil constriction will be reduced on both sides compared to when the same light is moved in front of the other, healthy eye. If the light is moved briskly back to the defective side, the pupils will dilate. Partial defects can occur and comparison of the two sides is the essence of the test (swinging flashlight test).

Thus: efferent lesion = unequal pupils;
afferent lesion = unequal response of both pupils to the same light according to the side of stimulation.

Investigation and Management of the Patient with an Optic Nerve Disorder or Disorder of the Visual Pathway

It is possible to determine which part of the visual pathway has been affected by looking at the pattern of visual field loss. If the loss is in one eye only, then the problem must be affecting the optic nerve before it reaches the optic chiasma (e.g. optic neuritis, retrobulbar neuritis, optic disc oedema).

If the problem or condition affects the visual pathway in the region of the optic chiasma, bitemporal field loss (bitemporal hemianopia) is displayed. Chiasmal disease may be asymmetrical and careful examination of the temporal field in an apparently uninvolved eye may be needed to confirm the diagnosis. Any condition affecting the part of the visual pathway between the optic chiasma and the visual cortex manifests itself as a homonymous hemianopia. Interestingly, however, when this part of the visual pathway is involved the patient usually only notices a slight loss in one eye and is usually unaware that the problem is affecting both eyes.

Obtaining a history of the visual problem and determining which part of the visual pathway is involved are important first steps in identifying what has caused the visual loss.

Problem	Goal	Nursing intervention
Patient is complaining of a reduced visual field and is anxious to know what has caused this. Impossible to give him this information, however, as the nature and extent of the field loss, and the part of the visual pathway involved, are unknown.	To determine nature and extent of visual loss and which part of the visual pathway has been affected, so that patient can be given accurate information and possible treatment.	1. Talk to patient about his visual loss and obtain information about its speed of onset, when he first noticed it, whether it is constant or intermittent and whether or not there are any associated symptoms, e.g. pain. 2. Explain to patient that you need to do visual tests to measure his visual acuity and visual field so that the extent of his visual loss can be determined. Outline what these tests involve, how long they will take and what he will be expected to do during the tests. 3. Carry out the tests and report the findings to medical staff. Record the finding in medical and nursing notes. Identify the area of the visual pathway involved. 4. Reassure patient that now the problem has been identified and is being looked into, he will receive any advice and information he needs, and also treatment if this is possible.

In order to determine the underlying cause a variety of investigative tests are necessary. For example, one of the causes of optic disc oedema is raised intracranial pressure. Possible reasons for this include an aneurysm or a tumour, and a CT scan would enable the actual cause to be identified. Carotid arteriography is sometimes requested if a vascular problem is suspected of being the cause of the visual loss. A series of blood pressure readings would establish whether malignant hypertension was a likely cause of optic disc oedema.

Accompanying symptoms can also provide clues to the underlying cause and can narrow down the number of tests needed to identify the cause. Temporal pain, when associated with sudden visual loss, may indicate that the cause is ischaemia due to cranial arteritis. This suspected cause could then be confirmed by measuring the blood erythrocyte sedimentation rate (ESR). Paraesthesia or previous diplopia associated with retrobulbar neuritis suggest disseminated sclerosis as a possible reason for this inflammation. Evidence of addiction to, for example, alcohol or tobacco may provide a clue to the possible cause of an optic atrophy. Signs of nutritional deficiency may also suggest a possible reason for this condition, which may be confirmed by evidence of vitamin B_{12} deficiency.

At this stage the patient is probably bewildered. He may wonder whether all these tests are really necessary and what relevance they have to his eyes. Uncertainty about what they involve, whether they will hurt and whether something more serious may be wrong than he has been told can cause considerable anxiety.

It is important that the nurse explains to the patient what tests are required and why they are necessary, in order to alleviate this anxiety.

Problem	Goal	Nursing intervention
Patient has a condition affecting the visual pathway, resulting in visual field loss. He is anxious and uncertain about having a series of tests carried out, as he does not know what these involve or why they are necessary.	To relieve patient anxiety by giving him information about the tests. To prepare patient mentally and physically for the tests.	1. Explain to patient that it is important to determine the underlying causes of his sight loss if appropriate treatment is to be commenced. Explain that the cause can be determined by a series of investigative tests. 2. Point out what tests are required and what each of these involves. Tell him when they will be carried out, what he will be expected to do during each test, how long each test will take and what each one will feel like. 3. Ensure that patient understands the information you have given him and make sure he is clear about the part he has to play in each test. 4. Answer any queries he has concerning the tests and reassure him if he is anxious. 5. Give a step-by-step explanation to patient of what is happening as the test is being carried out. Maintain patient's dignity during each test and ensure each test is carried out safely and that the comfort of the patient is always considered. 6. Ensure patient is told of the results of the tests and what these findings mean in terms of future treatment and care.

Once the underlying cause has been identified it is of course important, wherever possible, to treat this and so prevent further sight loss as well as any other complications of the condition from occurring. The treatment given must be specific to the underlying condition. If a tumour compressing some part of the visual pathway (e.g. the optic chiasm) has been responsible for the sight loss, it may be possible surgically to remove the tumour and thus prevent further damage.

Problems caused by hypertension may respond to systematic antihypertensive drugs. The progression of optic atrophy caused by vitamin B_{12} deficiency can be halted by giving the patient a course of monthly injections of hydroxocobalamin, to replenish the body's stores of vitamin B_{12}. Halting the progression of optic atrophy caused by a toxin (alcohol, tobacco, lead, etc.) necessitates complete removal or withdrawal from the toxic agent. Cranial arteritis (a condition which produces ischaemia, leading to optic atrophy) can be successfully treated by giving the patient a course of high-dose systemic steroids.

Treatment in many cases must be carried out on a long-term basis. It is therefore going to be largely the responsibility of the patient to ensure that it is carried out. In order to promote compliance it is important that the patient understands why treatment is needed, what the prescribed treatment regime involves, why it is important and what will happen if the treatment regime is not adhered to. The nurse must also check that, as well as being willing to comply with the treatment, the patient is also physically able to comply.

It may not always be possible to provide effective treatment for every patient. Direct damage to the optic nerve through injury, such as severance of the optic nerve itself or damage to its blood supply (resulting in optic atrophy), cannot be repaired or treated in any way and the ensuing sight loss is permanent.

In conditions such as retinitis pigmentosa (Chapter 20), however, which can also cause optic atrophy, the patient must be prepared not only to accept that his current sight loss cannot be restored but also that his vision is likely to deteriorate progressively in the future.

Sometimes a visual field loss can be an early sign of a general problem. Optic neuritis, for example, is sometimes the first indication that a patient has disseminated sclerosis.

Problem	Goal	Nursing intervention
Patient needs long-term treatment for the cause of his visual loss, in order to prevent further visual loss and also to prevent any further complications arising from the underlying cause/condition. However patient is unable to carry out treatment as he does not know what is involved or why it is important.	To promote compliance with treatment regime by explaining what it involves. To prevent further complications from arising. To prevent further visual loss by treating underlying cause. To prepare patient for carrying out treatment.	1. Explain to patient that his visual loss is due to an underlying medical condition and that if further loss is to be prevented, it is important to treat this underlying cause. 2. Outline what the treatment of the underlying condition involves as well as what will/might happen if the treatment is not adhered to. Explain the frequency of the treatment regime, how long it needs to be carried out for and whether there will be any side effects from the treatment. Emphasize the role which the patient will be expected to play in the regime. 3. Ensure that patient has understood what he has been told. Give him written information about the treatment regime to back up verbal information given. 4. Explain the treatment and its importance to the patient's relatives and friends so that they can encourage patient compliance. 5. Ensure patient is physically as well as mentally capable of carrying out the treatment. If he is unable to do this himself, ensure that someone else – relative, friend, district nurse, etc. – is aware of the need for treatment and is able and willing to carry it out. 6. Monitor the effectiveness of the treatment on a long-term basis. Reinforce the importance of compliance each time patient is seen. Adjust regime as necessary and ensure patient understands changes. Discuss any problems with him.

However, it must be borne in mind that not all people with optic or retrobulbar neuritis will later go on to develop disseminated sclerosis. It may be felt necessary to prepare the patient or his relatives at this early stage for the problems he may encounter in the future. Alternatively it may be decided simply to explain that the visual symptoms will disappear and may return only transiently, while arranging medical follow-up for the patient to check whether any general symptoms occur in time.

22

ORTHOPTICS

Rowena McNamara

CHAPTER SUMMARY

In this chapter the management of patients with disorders of ocular motility will be outlined. This subject makes up a large part of the workload in any eye unit as up to 8% of the child population have developmental eye problems. Orthoptists have a unique function in this area and an understanding of their role should ensure good co-operation and communication.

Orthoptic terminology has been limited to that which the nurse is likely to meet in everyday practice.

FUNCTIONAL ANATOMY OF THE EXTRAOCULAR MUSCLES

There are six muscles attached to the globe. They are called extraocular muscles to differentiate them from the ciliary and iris muscles, which are within the eye. They act as muscle pairs, so that when one muscle contracts and shortens the other muscle of the pair relaxes and lengthens. For example, when the VIth nerve causes the lateral rectus muscle (LR) to contract, the IIIrd nerve causes the medial rectus muscle (MR) in the same eye to relax and the eye rotates outwards (Figure 22.1).

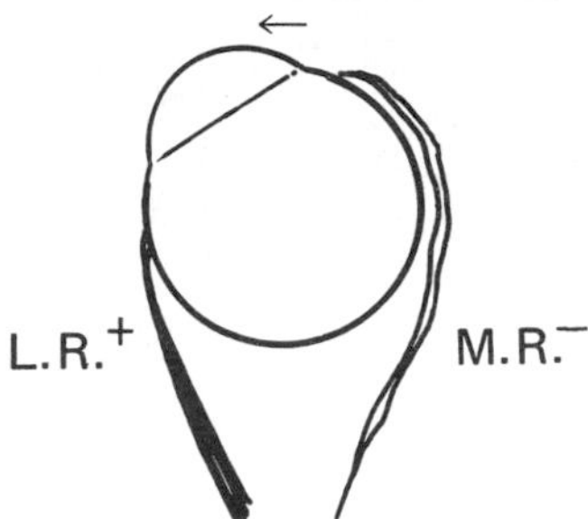

Figure 22.1 Actions of the lateral and medial rectus muscles.

Five of the extraocular muscles originate from the apex of the orbit and are attached at the annulus of Zinn (Figure 22.2). The inferior oblique muscle originates from the anterior portion of the maxillary bone of the orbit.

The direction in which each muscle pulls the eye is determined by its position in the orbit and its angle of insertion on to the globe (Figures 22.2–22.4).

The two eyes normally both point in the same direction so that an image falls on each macula (fovea). If an object moves, both eyes are rotated symmetrically to keep it in view. This involves paired eye movement co-ordinated in the midbrain.

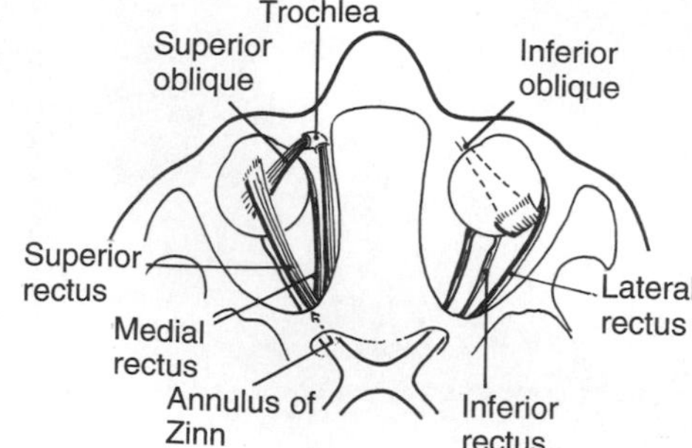

Figure 22.2 Origins of the extraocular muscles.

Action of Muscles

Horizontal Recti

These are the medial rectus and lateral rectus, which move the eye from side to side. Movement towards the nose is termed **adduction** and movement away from the nose is termed **abduction**.

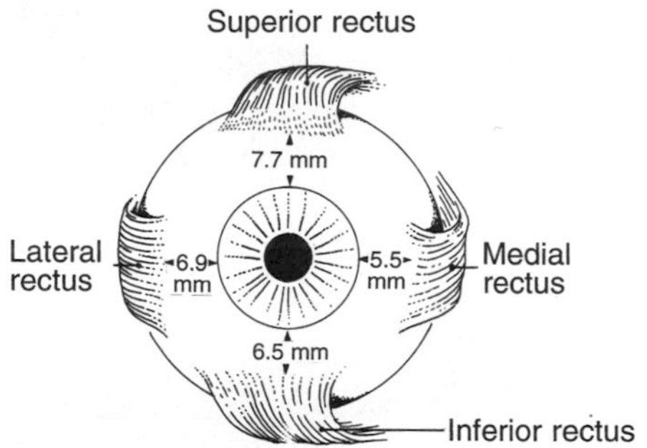

Figure 22.3 Insertions of the rectus muscles (right eye).

Vertical Recti

The superior rectus and inferior rectus muscles mainly move the eyes up and down – **elevation** and **depression** respectively.

Oblique Muscles

These comprise the superior oblique and inferior oblique muscles. When the head is tilted the oblique muscles rotate the eyes in order to keep them horizontal (Figure 22.5).

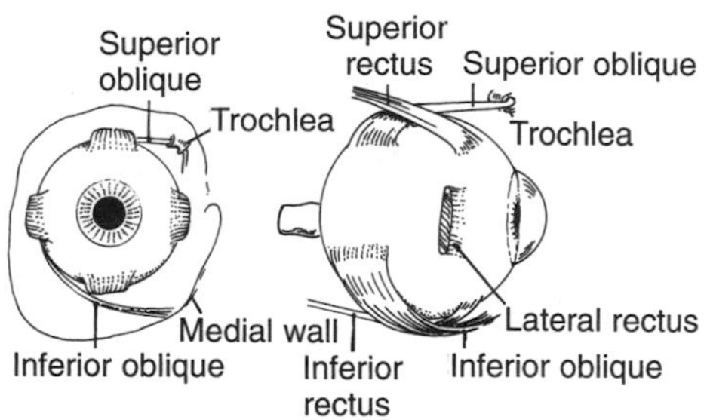

Figure 22.4 Insertions of the oblique muscles (right eye).

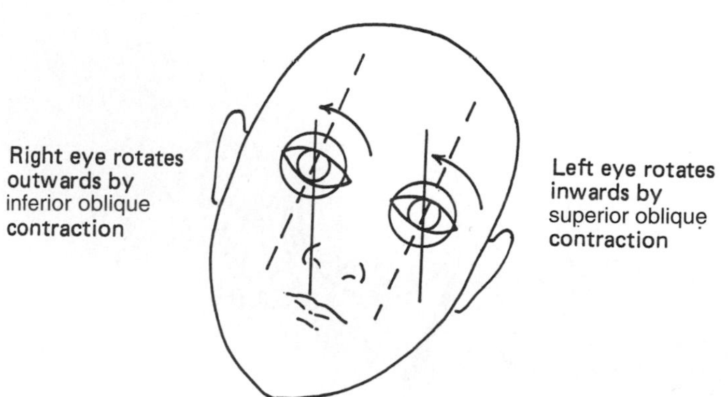

Figure 22.5 Action of the oblique muscles during head tilting.

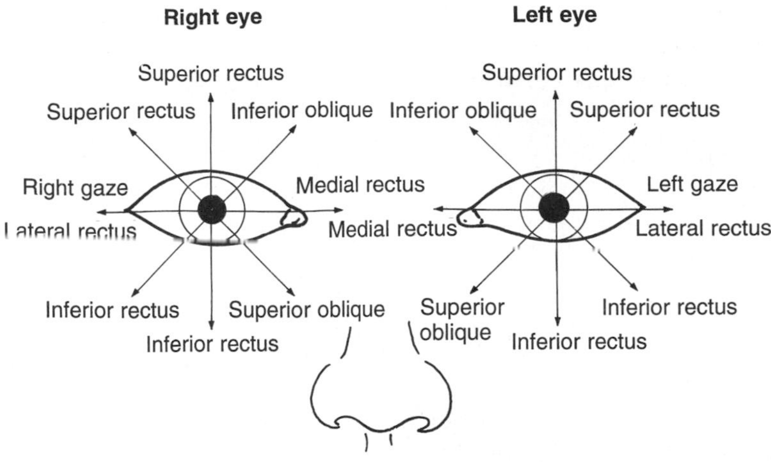

Figure 22.6 Actions of the extraocular muscles.

By asking the subject to look in eight directions, the actions of all six muscles are examined. Figure 22.6 illustrates the actions of the muscles tested in each direction of gaze. For example, looking to the right examines the right lateral rectus and the left medial rectus. Looking up and to the right examines the elevation of the right superior rectus and the left interior oblique, since the vertical action of the inferior oblique is maximum when the eye is adducted.

Squint (Strabismus)

A squint, also known as cast, turn, lazy eye or crossed eye, is the term to describe any condition where the eyes are not parallel. The two types of squint are **concomitant** and **paralytic** (incomitant).

Concomitant Squint

This is a developmental problem and is common. Since the eye muscles move the eyes as a pair, the squint will be present in all directions of gaze. A simple analogy is to think of car headlights that are not aligned straight ahead (Figure 22.7). No matter how the steering wheel is turned the lights can never become parallel.

The different types of squint are as follows.

1. One eye may turn inwards – this is **convergence** or esotropia.
2. One eye may turn outwards – this is **divergence** or exotropia.

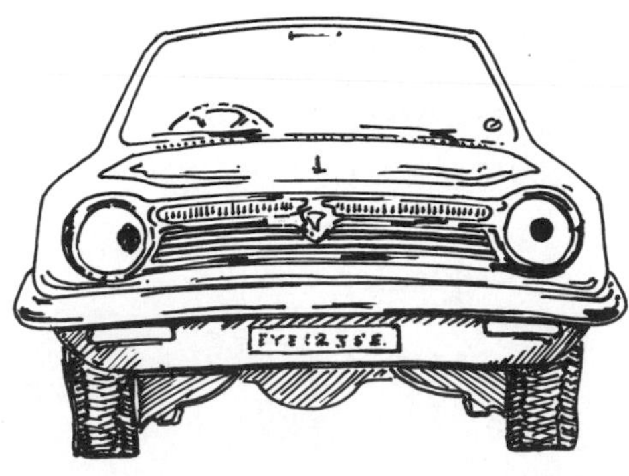

Figure 22.7 Non-aligned car headlights are like a concomitant squint.

3. One eye may turn upwards – this is **elevation** or hypertropia.
4. One eye may turn downwards – this is **depression** or hypotropia.

The squint (strabismus) can be present all the time, or it may only appear when the child is tired or ill, or concentrating on near objects. It may be obvious from birth or develop in early childhood.

When a squint is present all the time (manifest) it is referred to as a 'tropia', e.g. a convergent squint is an esotropia. In addition to the manifest squints, some people's eyes squint only when the eyes are prevented from seeing together and they are described as having a latent squint or 'phoria', e.g. a latent convergent squint is an esophoria.

Eyes in newborn babies lack co-ordination and seem to wander in different directions with very little control. By 6 months of age, however, the eyes should be parallel when viewing objects far away and rotate symmetrically towards the nose (converge) when focusing at near. Many young children have flat noses, which produce skin folds on the inner canthus known as epicanthic folds. This can give the appearance of a squint called pseudosquint (Figure 22.8).

If an actual squint is diagnosed it must be treated immediately – a child will not grow out of a true squint.

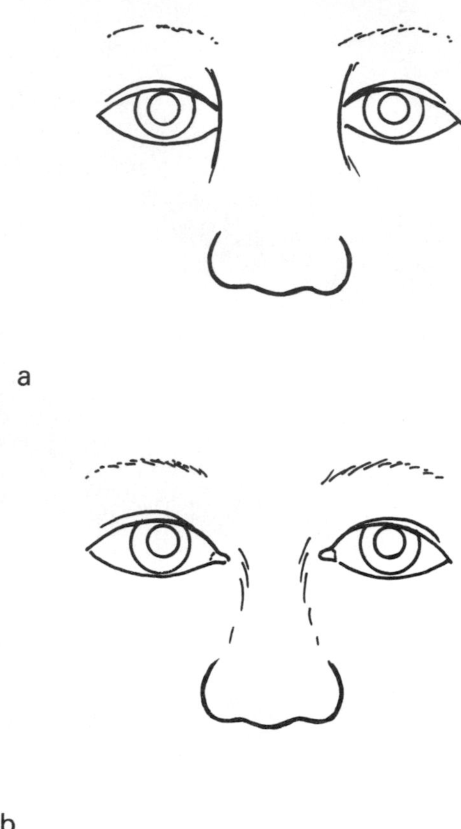

Figure 22.8 **(a)** Epicanthus. **(b)** Normal appearance as bridge of nose develops.

Mechanisms Involved in Squint

In normal vision, called binocular single vision (BSV), both eyes rotate to look at the same object (Figure 22.9(a)). As the eyes are separated in the skull, they send slightly different views of the object to the visual cortex. The two pictures of the triangle are blended in the visual cortex and associated areas by a process called fusion and the slight difference in views produces three-dimensional vision or stereopsis.

If the squint is present the straight eye still sends a clear picture of the triangle from the fovea to the visual cortex. The squinting eye, however, is pointed elsewhere and whatever falls in the path of this fovea is also sent to the visual cortex, e.g. the rectangle in Figure 22.9(b).

The rectangle is not at the same distance as the triangle and is therefore out of focus. The triangle is still in the visual field of the squinting eye but is relayed to the visual cortex from the peripheral retina. The area of the retina has far fewer cones and is incapable of sending a clear picture; furthermore, it has the property of making the triangle appear to be somewhere else. The appreciation in the cortex of the triangle in two different places is called double vision or diplopia. In order to prevent the confusion caused by see-

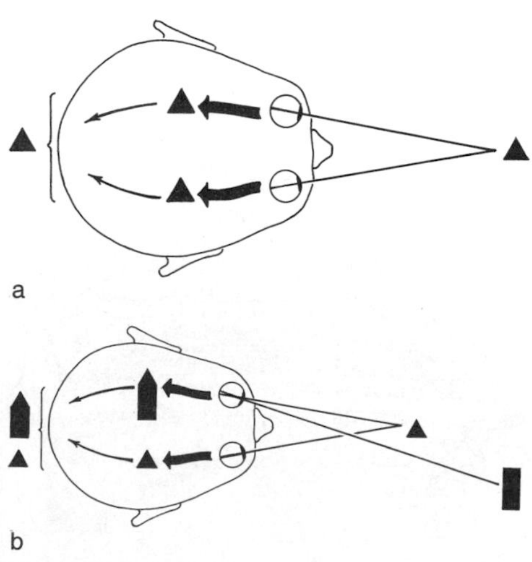

Figure 22.9 **(a)** Binocular single vision. **(b)** Squint.

ing the rectangle and the second image of the triangle, the brain ignores the pictures from the squinting eye by a mechanism called suppression. Without treatment, this suppression, together with the fact that the fovea of the squinting eye never receives a clear image, leads to **amblyopia**.

This is the critical period of visual development. Any interruption to the visual development during this time will have a permanent effect unless it is treated. The best results of treatment are obtained while the child is still in the visual development period. It is obviously vital, therefore, that children with squints are referred early, before 3 years of age, in order to reverse amblyopia.

Amblyopia

Amblyopia can be classified as follows.

1. Due to squint – termed strabismic amblyopia as described above.
2. Due to refractive error:
   (a) a difference in refractive error between eyes;
   (b) astigmatism;
   (c) a marked bilateral refractive error.
   Correction of the refractive error by wearing glasses can improve the vision in this type of amblyopia. It may be accompanied by a squint which is often barely noticeable, called a **microtropia**.
3. Due to opacities – termed **stimulus deprivation amblyopia**. A child with a congenital cataract will not receive clear images from the fovea. Thus when the cataract is removed, long periods of occlusion of the good eye are essential if vision is to develop in the other.

Orthoptic Management of Concomitant Squint

Patients can be referred by any of the personnel in Table 22.1.

Table 22.1 Reason for referral of patients with concomitant squint

Personnel	Reason
General practitioner	Squint noticed by parent, health visitor, optician, teacher
Optician	Defective vision or squint
Medical staff in casualty	Sudden onset of squint or diplopia
Community orthoptist	Failing 18-month or 3-year vision screening test
Community practitioner/ school nurse	Failing 5- or 7-year school vision test
Paediatrician	Squint or vision defect suspected in premature/handicapped children

When a patient first comes to the clinic, the orthoptist will do several tests to investigate the following:

1. **Squint**: manifest squint is diagnosed with the cover test; preventing the eyes from being used together by the cover test can also reveal a latent squint or **heterophoria**;
2. **Amblyopia**: defective vision in one eye is diagnosed using a variety of vision tests suitable for the age of the patient;
3. **Binocular vision**: this may be normal with good convergence, fusion and stereopsis, abnormal where the eyes have adapted to the squint, or completely absent.

The assessment procedure is described in the order in which the tests are generally carried out.

HISTORY

The orthoptist will ask the patient and/or parents:

1. the reason for attendance;
2. to describe the symptoms;
3. when it occurred and how often it now occurs;
4. details of any previous treatment with glasses, occlusion or surgery carried out elsewhere.

The cause of a squint in infants is often unknown, but it may be associated with the factors outlined in Table 22.2.

Table 22.2 Factors associated with squint in infants

Factor		Effect on eyes
1.	Heredity	Parents who squint are more likely to have children who squint.
2.	Refractive error	Hypermetropia (long sight) and anisometropia (different refractive error in each eye) may underlie the squint.
3.	Prematurity	Premature and low birth weight babies are more prone to reduced vision and squint.
4.	Birth trauma	Long labour and forceps are associated with lateral rectus weakness and esotropia.
5.	Illness	High temperature and infection cause eye muscle weakness, which may reveal a squint.
6.	Syndromes	Squint occurs more frequently in children with Down's syndrome, hydrocephalus, cerebral palsy, etc.
7.	Injuries	Head injury may damage the nerve supply to the extraocular muscles and produce squint.

VISION

The method used to test vision is selected by considering the child's chronological and mental age, as shown in Table 22.3. Each test gives an indication of vision but it is not until the child can manage a row of letters that the orthoptist is assured of an accurate assessment.

Vision is always tested uniocularly, using a plaster patch to occlude each eye, and with glasses if they have already been prescribed. Co-operative children with reduced vision are reassessed using a pinhole. Children with a reading age of 4 and above can read the Maclure near vision test; otherwise a reduced Sheridan Gardiner single test and key card is used to assess near vision.

Patients with nystagmus are tested with both eyes open as a patch may increase the nystagmus. This is particularly important if special education is being considered due to partial sight.

Table 22.3 Tests of vision related to a child's chronological and mental age

Age	Development	Tests
2–4 weeks	Watches mother when speaking; turns head and eyes towards light	Preferential looking; follows pen torch; corneal reflections
4–6 weeks	Smiles at mother; fixes steadily; moves eyes together over wide range	Optokinetic drum; objection to occlusion
2 months	Follows moving objects and patterns	STYCAR mounted and rolling balls
6 months	Binocular convergence; accommodation; refixation; reaches for objects	Catford drum; ability to overcome effect of a prism
10 months	Index finger approach to objects	Cake decoration; Smarties, etc.
1 year	Casting objects; pick up feeding utensils	STYCAR toys
1.5 years	Interested in book, identifies on request, names pictures	Kay and Beale Collins pictures
2 years	Post shapes; matches objects	Ffooks symbols; Sjøgren hand
3 years	Imitates cross and circle	Sheridan Gardiner singles
4 years	Matches shapes and letters	Snellen chart with key card
6 years	Reads letters and numbers	Snellen; Maclure reading book

The Cover Test

This is the main diagnostic test for detecting squint. There are two parts to the test:

The Cover–Uncover Test

Method: Shine a pen torch into the eyes and observe the reflections of the light from the cornea. If the reflections are not in the centre of the pupil in each eye, cover the eye which looks straight with an occluder and watch the other eye. For example:

1. Shine a pen torch towards the eyes. In Figure 22.10(a) the reflection from the torch is off-centre in the right eye; therefore the straight eye (left eye) is covered and the right eye watched carefully.
2. In Figure 22.10(b) the right eye has moved outwards to look at the light; the corneal reflection is now in the centre of the right eye. The left eye is turned inwards behind the occluder; this diagnoses a right convergent squint.
3. Remove the cover and observe the right eye (Figure 22.11).
   (a) Right eye turns in again, indicating reduced vision.
   (b) Right eye remains straight, indicating good vision; this is recorded as right/alternating convergent squint.

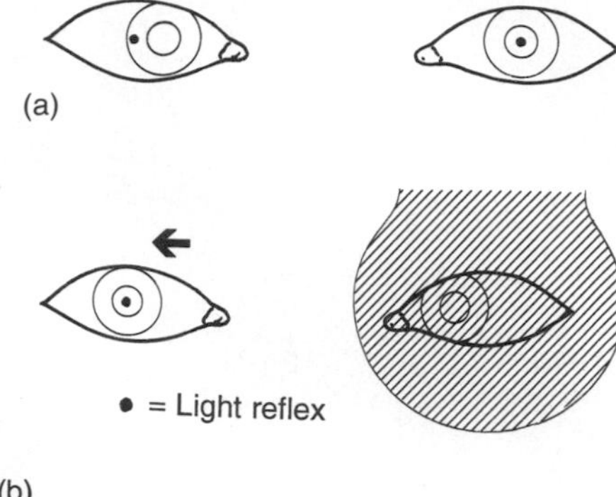

Figure 22.10 **(a)** & **(b)** Light reflex as seen in the cover test.

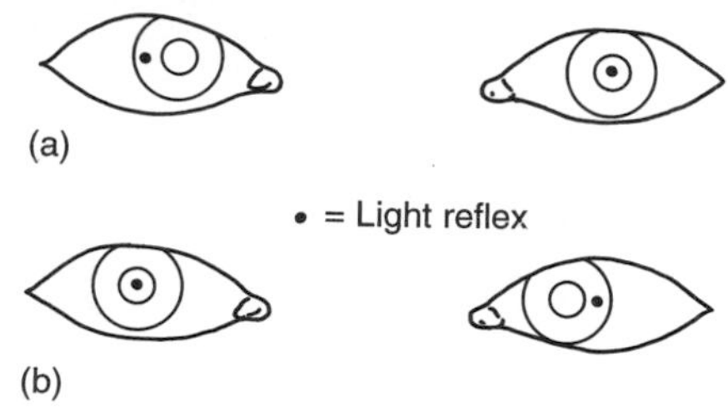

Figure 22.11 Light reflex as seen in the cover test (continued).

The orthoptist will carry out the cover–uncover test:

1. using a detailed/accommodative target after the light;
2. asking the patient to look at 0.33 m, 6 m and far distant targets;
3. with and without glasses, if worn.

The alternative Cover Test

This is used to diagnose latent squint (heterophoria). Method: As for the cover–uncover test but then occluder is moved from one eye to the other, preventing the eyes from being used simultaneously.

Ocular Movements

Weakness of any of the six extraocular muscles can cause ocular motility disorders, including squint. It is important to diagnose which muscles are weak in order to manage the disorders correctly. The orthoptist again uses a pen torch and occluder and asks the patient to follow the light while keeping his head still. The patient follows the light from the straight ahead (primary) position in eight directions. Movements of both eyes are termed 'versions' and the test is used to diagnose underaction or overaction in each position. Uniocular movements can also be tested to diagnose mechanical limitations (i.e. inability to move the eye due to tethering of the muscle). In this way the orthoptist assesses the action of all six ocular muscles in each eye.

A and V Phenomena

A fixation stick is used as a target to examine the size of the squint when the patient looks up and down. A convergent squint which increases on looking down and decreases on looking up has a V eso pattern (Figure 22.12).

Binocular Vision

Patients with perfectly straight eyes (orthophoria) have normal binocular single vision (BSV) and the two eyes correspond normally with one another (normal retinal correspondence). BSV is characterized by;

1. **convergence**: symmetrical adduction of both eyes while looking at an approaching target; this is recorded as the nearest point at which the eyes remain fixing the target, e.g. binocular convergence to 6 cm, well maintained;
2. **fusion range**: converging and diverging the eyes to maintain fixation of an object, measured using:
   (a) prisms;
   (b) synoptophore;

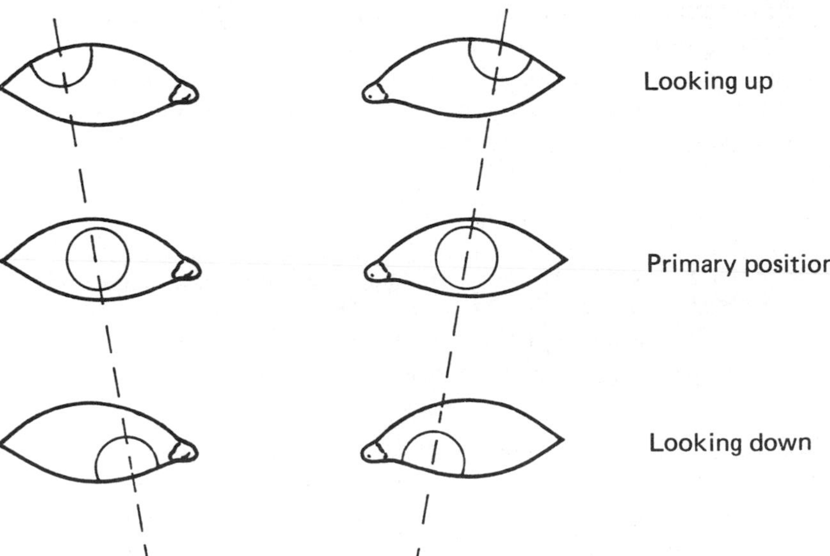

Figure 22.12 The V eso pattern.

fusion should be bifoveal, since both fovea are being used to look at the object;
3. **stereopsis**: appreciation of depth using stereotests, e.g. the TNO using red and green goggles.

It is important to establish in the child with squint whether or not potential binocular vision is present. If it is then the case requires intensive orthoptic treatment, glasses and/or surgery to achieve full binocular potential. A cosmetic case is one in which no potential binocular vision is present and glasses and/or surgery are indicated simply for cosmesis.

Abnormal Binocular Vision

Manifest squints that have been present for several years may develop an abnormal type of binocular vision. The retina of the straight eye learns to correspond with the squinting position of the deviating eye. This is termed abnormal retinal correspondence (ARC). Patients with ARC have abnormal binocular convergences and fusion, and some degree of stereopsis.

Measurement of Squint

The squint can be measured in:

1. **Hirschberg's approximation**: useful in children and when there is very poor vision in the squinting eye;
2. **prism dioptres** (Δ), using the prism cover test: the strength of prism is increased until the squinting eye no longer moves to look at the target (Figure 22.13); 1° = 2 Δ; the principle of the prism cover test in right convergent squint is shown in Figure 22.14;
3. **degrees**, using the synoptophore: the tube is rotated in front of the squinting eye until there is no movement to look at the picture in the tube.

Fixation

This is used to describe the point on the retina used to look at objects. It is normally the fovea, since it has the better visual acuity. Some squinting eyes are unable to use the fovea and are diagnosed as having eccentric fixation.

Orthoptic Treatment of Convergent Squint

Orthoptic treatment aims to:

1. restore and maintain equal visual acuity;
2. straighten the eyes;
3. make the eyes work together if possible.

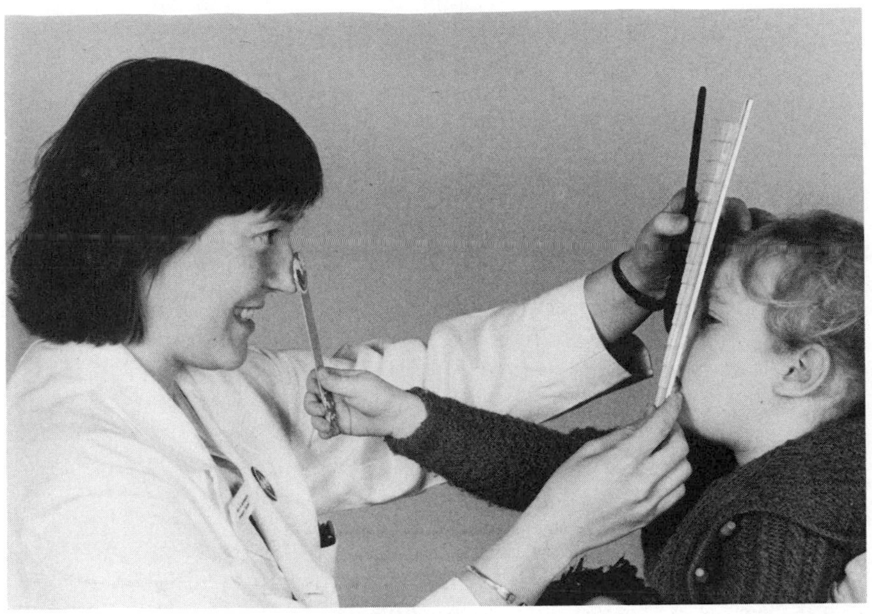

Figure 22.13 Measuring a squint with a prism bar.

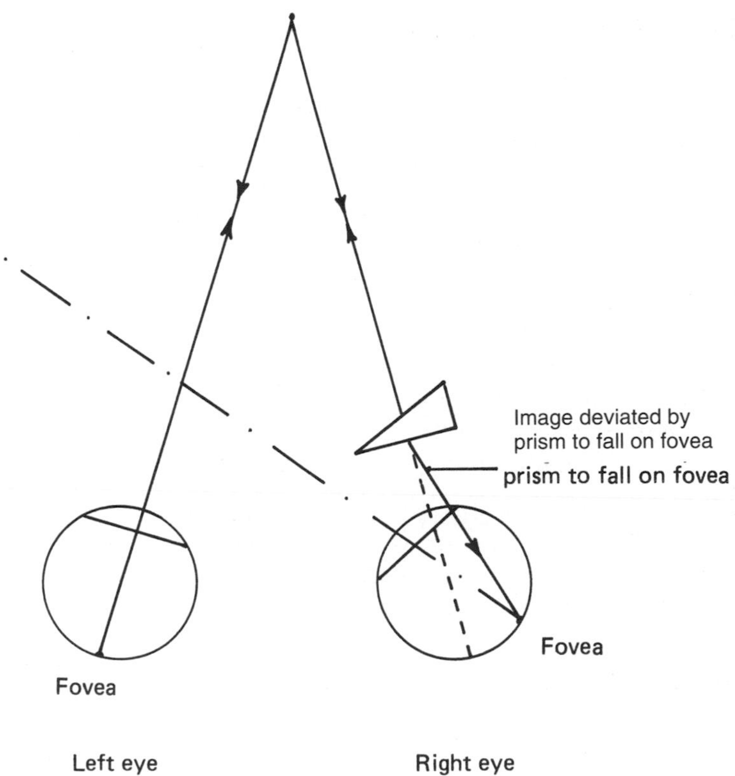

Figure 22.14 Ray diagram showing measurement of squint.

In order to fulfil these aims a number of methods are used.

Glasses

Children attending the orthoptic clinic will have a refraction performed using a cycloplegic drop (cyclopentolate or atropine). The action of these agents is first to paralyse accommodation, which would otherwise interfere with the assessment of the true refractive error, and second to dilate the pupil and allow visualization of the fundus. It must be remembered that rare conditions of childhood such as developmental anomalies and retinoblastoma may be the cause of a squint.

If there is a refractive error, glasses are prescribed to correct:

1. **vision**: amblyopia caused by refractive error can improve when glasses are worn constantly; any residual amblyopia is treated with occlusion;
2. **squint**: corrective lenses can reduce the size of a convergent squint, which in certain cases may become an esophoria.

Occlusion

Occlusion (usually involving wearing a patch) is the most effective treatment for amblyopia. The aim is to produce equal vision in each eye by occluding the better to encourage development in the poorer.

Best results of occlusion are achieved when:

1. the treatment is started soon after the onset of the squint;
2. the patient is still in the critical period of visual development;
3. the patch is worn correctly;
4. the glasses, if prescribed, are worn with the occlusion;
5. the patient attends regularly for review.

Methods: Total occlusion is achieved with Coverlet, Opticlude, Elastoplast or Micropore patches on the face or Blenderm and extension patches on glasses.

Prescribed time will depend on:

1. **level of vision in the eye**: the denser the amblyopia the longer the occlusion will be needed to improve vision;
2. **age of patient**: babies with a squint are occluded very carefully initially for 10 minutes only per day and reviewed weekly. Wearing a patch for too long at this age can damage the vision in the better eye. The exception is the treatment of congenital cataract. These babies

are occluded for many hours daily in order to treat very defective visual development. Children over 1 year can be occluded up to 8 hours daily if necessary. Occasionally, children who refuse to wear patches are admitted for supervised occlusion. Parents will need enormous support and encouragement while the child is on the ward, particularly if arm splints have been used. This can establish a patching routine that the parents are able to continue at home.

There are other less effective methods that can be used with children who will not co-operate with patching; these include CAM vision stimulator and drug therapy.

Treatment is continued until the squint alternates or the orthoptist judges that optimum vision has been reached.

Orthoptic Exercises

There are a number of types of squint for which exercises are prescribed. There are situations where a child is encouraged to appreciate the diplopia that occurs with intermittent squint, and then to avoid it by controlling the squint.

Exercises can only be successful with co-operative children who attend clinic regularly. The exercises are taught and supervised in the clinic by the orthoptist and practised at home between visits. If a nurse in the community is involved in the care of a child undergoing this treatment, she should learn from the orthoptist the purpose and method of the exercises in order to supervise and support the child and his family.

Exercises are used most frequently to help a patient control a latent squint (phoria), where the effort involved is producing blurred vision and headache.

The following is a case report to illustrate the orthoptic investigation and treatment of a patient with a symptom-producing heterophoria. It is also included to illustrate how orthoptic terminology is used in practice.

Case Report

Investigation

1. **History**: a student aged 20 attends the orthoptic clinic complaining of headaches after reading for several hours. The headaches go away after resting the eyes and began 6 months ago. When questioned about possible causes, the patient explained that he was studying hard for exams.
2. **Visual acuity**:

	R	L	
R	6/5 L	6/5	Snellen;
	6/5	6/5	Reduced Snellen (reading vision).

3. **Cover test**:
(a) near: slight exophoria with delayed recovery to BSV;
(b) distance: minimal exophoria with good recovery.
4. **Ocular movements**: appear full.
5. **Binocular vision**:
   (a) convergence: binocular to 20 cm then the right eye diverges, with diplopia;
   (b) fusion range: Eso 10 Δ; Exo 12 Δ
   (c) stereotests: TNO 120″ of arc.
6. **Measurement**:
Prism cover test: Near: 12 Δ Exo; Distance: 4 Δ Exo.

Diagnosis: Convergence weakness exophoria with convergence insufficiency, i.e. the symptoms are caused by the effort to control the exophoria and converge the eyes while reading.

Treatment

1. **Refraction**: the patient had a routine refraction (correction of small refractive errors, especially astigmatism, can often eliminate asthenopic symptoms (headache, eye strain)). Any glasses ordered should be worn prior to orthoptic treatment.
2. **Orthoptic exercises**: the patient did not have a refractive error and orthoptic exercises were commenced.
   Aim: to improve the near point of convergence; to enable the patient to read comfortably.
   The methods are:
   (a) to improve convergence by repeatedly looking at an advancing object such as a pen held in the hand, or a dot on a card;
   (b) to put up prisms of increasing strength in front of one eye to improve the convergent fusional range;
   (c) to encourage the patient to learn to converge the eyes while relaxing accommodation.

Observation

Squints can vary enormously when the child is ill, tired or upset. It is important, therefore, once the vision is equalized, to measure and assess the squint several times until an overall impression is obtained. Obvious squints will receive squint surgery before the child is teased by peers (i.e. under 3 years). In less obvious squints the parents, child, orthoptist and ophthalmologist will meet to discuss the best course of action.

Children with squints that are cosmetically acceptable who have no binocular vision are advised that their eyes are better left without surgery. It is explained that the eyes will gradually diverge in one or two decades so that an esotropia may become less noticeable. The child will generally be discharged aged 7 years and invited to return should there be any problem later. Visual acuity is monitored until discharge.

SURGERY

Surgery is performed for the following reasons:

1. cosmetically poor appearance;
2. to restore BSV in intermittent squints, particularly when they are too large to respond to orthoptic exercises.

The bulk of squint surgery is carried out on the horizontally acting muscles in children.

METHODS

1. **Strengthening**: the muscle is made to pull more effectively by cutting a piece out of it (resection), thereby shortening its length. It is reattached to the globe in the original position.
2. **Weakening**: the muscle is made less effective by detaching it from its insertion and reattaching it further back (recession). This slackens the muscle and reduces its effectiveness at pulling the eye.

Thus for a right esotropia, the right eye is swung into the primary position by recessing the medial rectus to weaken adduction, and resecting the lateral rectus to enhance abduction.

CHOICE OF SURGERY

The surgeon will vary the amount of recession and resection in relation to the size of the squint based on his own previous surgical results. In general, however, an esotropia of 20° (40 Δ) will be treated with a medial rectus recession of 5 mm and lateral rectus resection of 8 mm.

Recessing and resecting more of the muscle than the maximum above will cause limitation of eye movements. So for squints > 40 Δ the same surgery may then be performed on the non-squinting eye. It will not produce a squint in the straight eye.

Squints which are greater at one distance or position need surgery which will affect the squint more where it is greatest; for instance, for convergence excess esotropia, both medial recti are recessed.

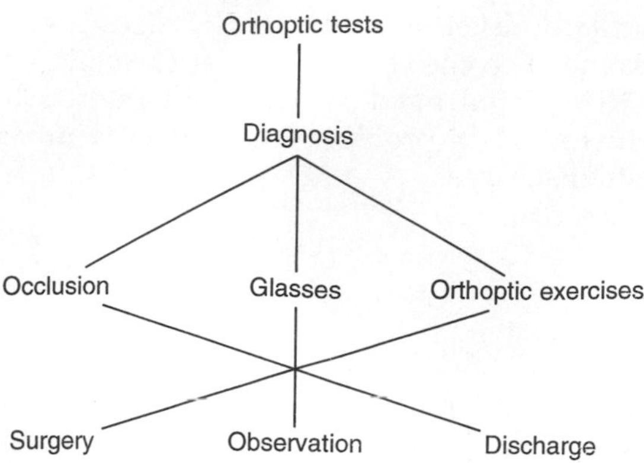

Figure 22.15 Orthoptic management of concomitant squint.

Adults Receiving Squint Surgery

The same principles apply to adults who have requested surgery for a squint they have had since childhood, with the following considerations.

1. More surgery is required as adult muscles respond less well to weakening and strengthening.
2. Where surgery was performed in childhood, reoperations are less effective and scarring becomes a problem, often limiting ocular movements.
3. The patient may experience diplopia postoperatively. This may be temporary, but in a few cases persists. The orthoptist will carry out a preoperative diplopia test to assess the likelihood of the patient appreciating diplopia. Where it is found to be a possibility it should be discussed with the patient before surgery.

A summary of orthoptic management of concomitant squint is given in Figure 22.15.

Paralytic Squint

A lesion affecting an extraocular muscle or its nerve supply will interfere with normal ocular motility.

Because any given muscle works maximally in one direction, a paralytic squint is incomitant, in other words it varies according to the position of gaze. For example, a left VIth nerve paresis impairs the ability of the left eye to abduct. The squint is greatest on looking to the left and absent on looking to the right. The diplopia produced by such a problem can be offset by turning the head to the left (i.e. in the direction of action of the weak muscle).

TYPES OF PARALYTIC SQUINT

1. **Neurogenic**: IIIrd, IVth and VIth nerve palsy may all be due to vascular lesions, injury, multiple sclerosis, etc.
2. **Mechanical**:
   (a) blow-out fracture;
   (b) Duane's retraction syndrome;
   (c) Brown's syndrome.
3. **Myogenic**
   (a) dysthyroid eye disease;
   (b) myasthenia gravis.

Thus a large number of conditions may cause a patient to complain of sudden onset of double vision. A systematic approach is required to establish which muscle(s) is malfunctioning and what the underlying cause is, and this can involve full examination, blood test and CT scan.

The following case illustrates the orthoptic investigation and management of an adult with a VIth nerve palsy.

Case Report

Investigation

1. **History**: a patient aged 45 years attends the Accident and Emergency Department complaining of double vision, worse in the distance and to the left. Image separated horizontally. The onset was sudden, on waking that morning. Past medical history:
   (a) general: patient hypertensive;
   (b) ophthalmic: no childhood squint, no glasses worn.
2. **Visual acuity**: right 6/6, left 6/6 Snellen's. This suggests no childhood amblyopia.
3. **Abnormal head posture** (AHP) (Figure 22.16): face turned to the left. The eyes are thus directed to the right, where there is single vision.
4. **Cover test**:
   (a) with AHP: near and distant slight esotropia with good recovery to BSV;
   (b) without AHP: near slight (L) esotropia with diplopia. Distant moderate (L) esotropia with diplopia.
5. **Ocular movements**: moderate limitation of left eye in abducted positions (LLR) with overactions of the yoke muscle in the other eye (RMR).
6. **Binocular vision**: with AHP convergence binocular to 6 cm; fusion range: 30 Δ Eso; 19 Δ Exo.
   Stereopsis: TNO 120″ of arc.
7. **Measurement**: prism cover tests without AHP:
   Near 15 Δ Eso
   Distant 40 Δ Eso } fixing right eye

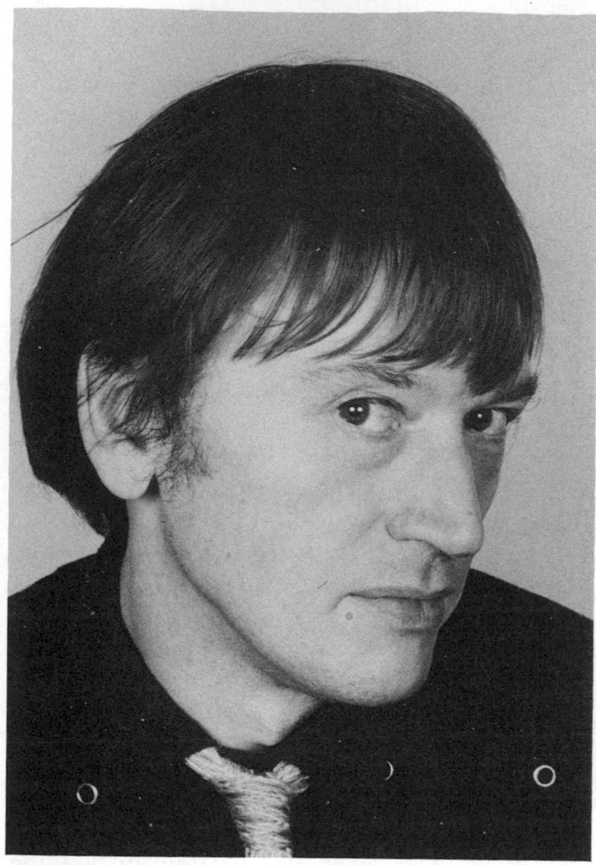

Figure 22.16 Characteristic head turn in left lateral rectus palsy.

Near 20 Δ Eso
Distant 60 Δ Eso   fixing left eye

The deviation is much greater when the patient tries to fix with the left eye, i.e. the eye with the lateral rectus palsy.

8. **Hess chart** (Figure 22.17): These charts are arrived at by placing the patient in front of a screen on which is an enlarged version of the grid on the chart. The eyes are dissociated, using red and green goggles or a mirror. Using first one eye and later the other to fix on the various points of the grid it is possible to draw in not only the underaction of an affected muscle but also any associated overaction of muscles of the other eye. This test helps to confirm a suspected weakness and provides a record against which any subsequent change can be seen.

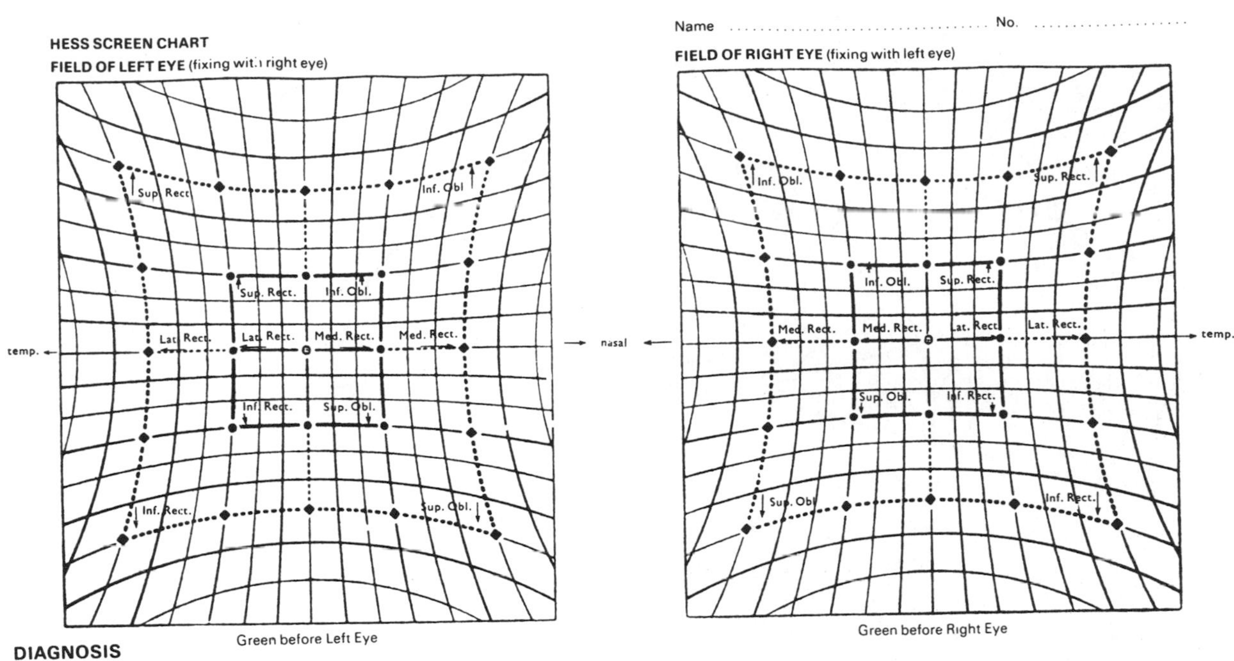

Figure 22.17 Hess recording chart.

9. **Field of BSV** (Figure 22.18): This chart shows the two visual fields overlapping. The patient sits at an arc perimeter with both eyes open for this test and indicates when a target becomes double.

Treatment

The patient was given a 20 Δ base-out Fresnel prism on the left lens of his glasses and reviewed fortnightly (Figure 22.19). The prism moves the image on the retina and compensates for the esotropia. This allows the patient to see single while holding his head straight.

The strength of prism used is determined by the patient; often only one third to one half of the measurement is required to produce comfortable BSV. If the patient does not wear glasses, 'planos' can be ordered or the patient's sunglasses can be used.

The palsy may recover spontaneously or require squint surgery.

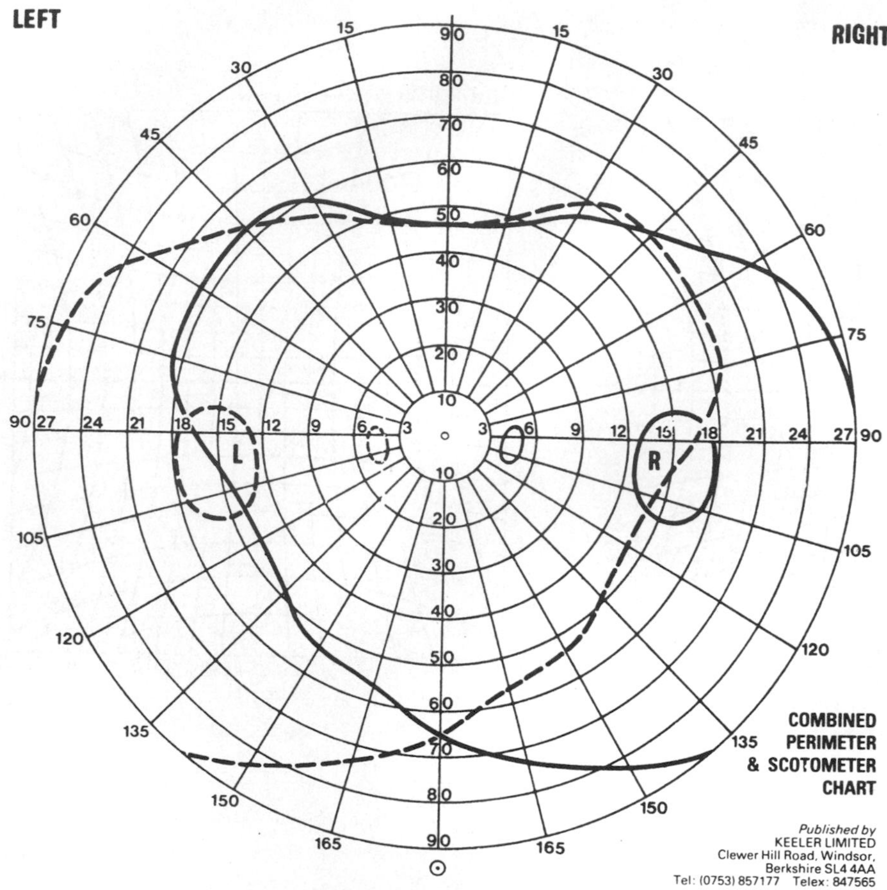

Figure 22.18 Field of binocular single vision.

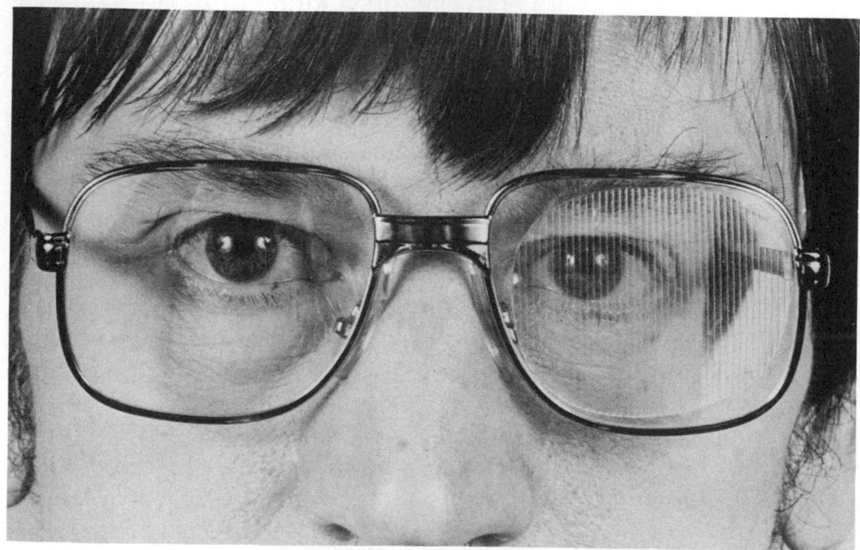

Figure 22.19 Straightening the head with the aid of a Fresnel prism.

Mechanical Deviations

These occur when there is a mechanical restriction to free movement of the globe in the orbit. They may result from injury, faulty innervation or muscle inflammation, as shown in the following three examples.

Blow Out Fractures

These usually result in limited movements, typically when looking up and down, due to a trapped or damaged inferior rectus muscle. The fracture in the floor is normally repaired within 7–10 days if enophthalmos is present and diplopia is severe.

Duane's Syndrome

This is due to a congenitally abnormal nerve supply to the lateral rectus. The globe retracts when trying to adduct. The children (usually girls) often turn their heads to avoid the limited horizontal movements in this condition. Surgery is performed if the head-turn is unsightly.

Dysthyroid Eye Disease

The extraocular muscles become enlarged, due to inflammation which makes them tight and inelastic. Diplopia occurs when fusion can no longer keep the eyes aligned. Prisms are prescribed until the inflammation subsides, which can take up to 4 years. In a minority, squint surgery is indicated when the condition has stabilized. Inferior rectus recession is sometimes performed using an adjustable suture (Chapter 21).

Nursing Care

The nurse may encounter patients with ocular motility problems in many situations, either in the community or in the hospital as an inpatient or outpatient. Armed with an understanding of orthoptics, the nurse is able to help in the management of patients with ocular motility problems by carrying out the following actions:

1. describing the tests which patients are likely to undertake in the orthoptic clinic and helping to relieve any anxiety;
2. explaining the importance of regular refraction and describing the effects of the cycloplegic drops used;
3. reinforcing the need to wear glasses to correct vision and squint;

4. explaining the effect of wearing Fresnel prisms;
5. congratulating children seen wearing their occlusive patches;
6. supervising occlusion while children are admitted and supporting despairing parents who have not been able to carry out this treatment at home;
7. checking that pre- and postoperative orthoptic assessment is undertaken;
8. explaining the aims and methods of squint surgery, preparing them for surgery and ensuring a safe postoperative recovery;
9. alerting medical staff if incorrect surgery is planned or if muscles become detached postoperatively;
10. ensuring that self-care is possible prior to discharge, that the patient or carer is able to instil medication correctly and that he is aware of the need to do so;
11. informing the patient or carer of how to prevent secondary infection and avoid irritants such as smoky atmospheres or swimming, especially in chlorine-treated water, for at least 3 weeks;
12. helping adults to adapt to diplopia.

23 Ophthalmic Disease in Developing Countries

John Sandford-Smith

Chapter Summary

There are several obvious differences in the pattern of eye disease in developing countries as compared to developed countries.

1. Eye diseases are more common in developing countries, and blindness is a much more common disability. In most developed countries about one person per 1000 is registered as blind. In developing countries the prevalence of blindness may be as much as one person per 100.
2. Some diseases, such as trachoma, xerophthalmia and onchocerciasis, are common in developing countries but are rarely seen elsewhere.
3. The patients often do not seek help until their disease is very far advanced. They may be totally blind from cataract or glaucoma. It is not unusual to see penetrating eye injuries, burns and severe infections that have been neglected.
4. The eye is an external organ and so its diseases are very much influenced by the climate and the external environment. Therefore the pattern of eye disease may vary greatly from one area to another in, for instance, central Africa. Just south of the Sahara Desert the climate is very hot and at certain times of the year flies are numerous. There is a high prevalence of trachoma, which is spread by flies. There is also a high prevalence of pterygium and corneal degeneration caused by solar radiation and irritation by sand. Further south in the savanna grassland these diseases are much less common. However, this is the area where onchocerciasis or river blindness is found. Still further south in the

tropical rain forests the incidence of blindness is much less, though fungal infection of the cornea and loisis may occur.

Not only are the diseases very different, the role of the ophthalmic nurse is also different. In all developing countries the medical services are inadequate to meet the needs of the community. This is especially true in rural areas, far away from the major cities, where there may be no medical services at all. This greatly affects the work and responsibility of the ophthalmic nurse. The following are some examples of the type of extra work an ophthalmic nurse may need to do in developing countries besides providing nurse care:

1. **primary health care and particularly health education**: this is a major challenge in most developing countries, especially to make local communities aware of what they themselves can do to keep their eyes healthy; the ophthalmic nurse is usually the most appropriate person to organize primary health care, which is unfortunately often neglected in developing countries;
2. **clinical work**: seeing patients often without medical supervision and often taking full responsibility for their clinical care, in the absence of any qualified ophthalmologist;
3. **surgery**: the responsibility given to the nurse will depend on the circumstances; the ophthalmic nurse is often responsible for routine postoperative care and in some situations nurses may be trained to carry out minor or even major surgery with or without supervision;
4. **other**: the nurses may be involved in management roles such as stock-keeping and maintaining records; there are often no opticians, so the nurses may be involved in dispensing simple spectacles for presbyopia and aphakia.

Obviously, any nurse working in developing countries must be a very resourceful and adaptable person. Modern medical care is often expensive. Much of the equipment taken for granted in the West is very sophisticated and technologically advanced. In developing countries, neither the patient nor the government can usually afford to pay very much for medical care and there may be no-one available who can service and repair sophisticated equipment. Therefore, medical care in developing countries has to be both cheap and simple. It is one of the challenges of working in developing countries to try to provide good-quality care at a reasonable cost.

Most of the blindness in the developing countries is preventable. Blindness can be divided into three basic groups

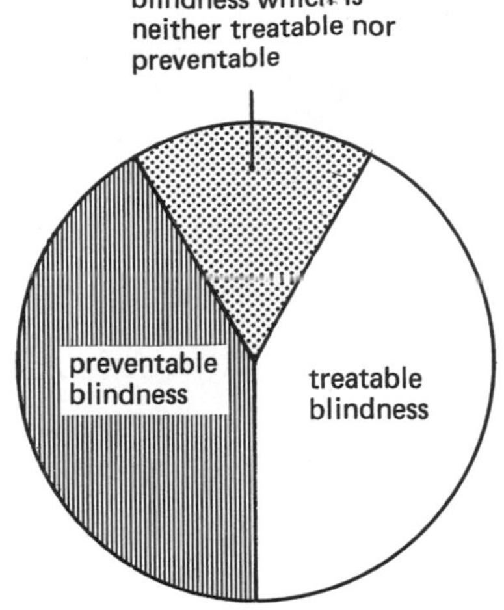

Figure 23.1 Categories of blindness in the developing world.

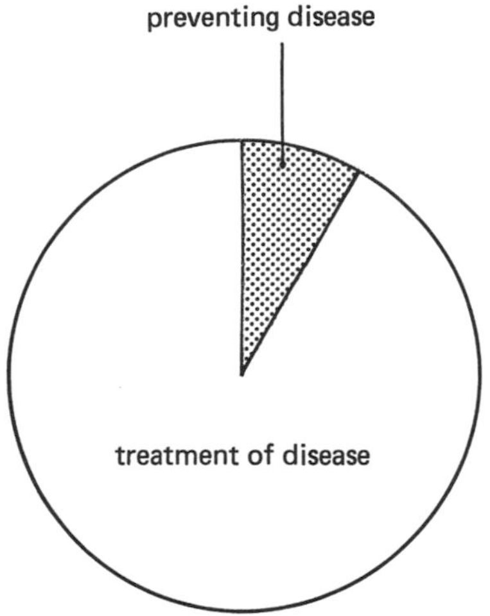

Figure 23.2 Resource allocation for ocular health in the developing world.

(Figure 23.1). First, there is blindness which can neither be treated nor prevented. Second, there is blindness which can be cured by treatment and third, there is blindness which cannot be cured but which could have been prevented.

Most blind people in the developed world have diseases in the first group. They are usually blind from congenital disorders, like retinitis pigmentosa, or degenerative conditions, like senile macular degeneration, for which at present there is no effective treatment.

These same diseases are of course found in developing countries, but there are also many blind people who have treatable or preventable blindness. By far the most important treatable cause of blindness is cataract. This is common everywhere but it appears to be more common in hot climates, where people are affected at a younger age.

Preventable blindness, however, is a big problem; the most important causes are trachoma, xerophthalmia, glaucoma and onchocerciasis. The World Health Organization (WHO) has identified these four conditions, plus cataract, as being the five main causes of blindness in the world. Note that three of them, trachoma, xerophthalmia and onchocerciasis, are really only found in developing countries.

Throughout the world medical resources are mostly used for treatment rather than for prevention of disease. Community health and preventive medicine is unfortunately often the 'Cinderella' of health care and is neglected both by governments and individual health workers (Figure 23.2). Three of the five major causes of world blindness are preventable, and therefore preventive medicine, although often neglected, is even more important in developing countries.

Medical and surgical treatment is usually carried out in hospitals and clinics but preventive medicine is usually carried out in the community. This vital work is often done much better by nurses than other health workers because so much of the nurse's training and orientation is towards the community and the patient, not just the disease. In particular, the incidence of trachoma and xerophthalmia could be dramatically reduced if simple, cheap and appropriate action was taken in the community.

It is obviously not possible in one chapter to describe all the different eye diseases which can occur in developing countries. Trachoma, xerophthalmia and onchocerciasis obviously must be considered in detail. Leprosy and vernal conjunctivitis are also described; leprosy because it frequently involves the eyes and vernal conjunctivitis because it is a very common and often disabling condition in developing countries.

Trachoma

Trachoma is an infective disease of the conjunctiva and cornea caused by a micro-organism called *Chlamydia trachomatis*. Chlamydias are bacteria with particular features which can only survive inside living cells. Fortunately, like other bacteria they are sensitive to some antibiotics. Trachoma is common in all developing countries but especially in dry, hot climates where flies are very common, such as the Middle East and Africa. It is always associated with poor hygiene and bad living conditions.

Symptoms and Signs

The disease starts as a mucopurulent conjunctivitis. After about 2 weeks the specific signs of an active trachoma infection are seen:

1. The tarsal conjunctiva hypertrophies so that to the naked eye its surface appears rough and velvet-like rather than shiny, and the underlying subconjunctival blood vessels cannot clearly be seen.
2. Follicles, which are little patches of lymphoid tissues, can be seen in the conjunctival fornix and especially on the upper tarsal conjunctiva. It is necessary to evert the upper eyelid to assess a patient with suspected trachoma.
3. There is a superficial keratitis on the upper part of the cornea and blood vessels can be seen growing down from the upper limbus on the surface of the cornea.

Eventually the infection will heal and just a few scars are left on the upper tarsal conjunctiva. The scars appear as faint irregular white lines of fibrous tissue running just under the conjunctival surface. There is also some faint superficial scarring of the upper part of the cornea. This is called trichiasis. Sometimes the whole of the eyelid becomes deformed and contracts so that all the eyelashes rub against the cornea (upper lid entropion). The lower eyelids may also be similarly affected. In these more severe cases the corneal scarring may also be much more dense and widespread, causing eventual blindness in adult life. Both the lacrimal passages and meibomian glands may also be affected.

Epidemiology

There has been a lot of research in recent years to try to discover why trachoma is sometimes a severe disease and in other situations is quite mild. The disease is usually spread from person to person by direct contact, sharing the same piece of cloth to wipe the eyes. In the areas where trachoma is common most young children have the active form of the disease. They recover, but immunity to trachoma does not develop and they often become reinfected. The dry, sandy atmosphere of the desert irritates the eye and provokes excess conjunctival secretions, thus making the inflammation worse. Other forms of conjunctivitis like adenovirus and *Haemophilus influenzae* infections cause further damage to the surface of the eye, and spread from person to person in the same way. If the eye is infected only once or twice it heals with minimal scarring, but repeated infection causes more serious scarring. Once trichiasis and entropion have developed the eyelashes constantly irritate the cornea, producing corneal abrasions and ulcers. Each time the corneal scarring becomes more dense and opaque and finally the patient goes blind. Women go blind more often than men, probably because they are in close contact with young children, who are the biggest source of active infection. Doctors and nurses, however, who examine many patients with trachoma rarely catch the disease themselves simply by obeying a few simple rules of hygiene. It is usually only spread when living conditions and personal hygiene are poor.

Chlamydia may also live in the genital tract and may spread, particularly in the Western world, by sexual contact, causing urethritis in men and cervicitis in women. In particular, newborn babies can develop eye infections with *Chlamydia* if the mother is carrying the organism in her genital tract (see also Chapter 15).

TREATMENT

Chlamydia trachomatis is sensitive to tetracycline, erythromycin and sulphonamides. Because the organism lives in the body cells it is protected from the action of the antibodies, so the treatment needs to be prolonged. Topical treatment is probably as effective as systemic, and has fewer side effects. The usual recommended dose is tetracycline eye drops or ointment four times a day for 6 weeks, though compliance is often poor. Surgical treatment may be necessary to correct trichiasis and entropion. This should be done as soon as possible, otherwise the eyelashes will rub against the already damaged cornea, causing progressive scarring. The eyelashes may be removed by electrolysis or cryotherapy or an operation may be performed to realign them.

The Prevention of Blindness from Trachoma in the Community

This is most important because in certain communities almost the entire population has trachoma. Most preschool children will be active carriers of the disease and most adults will show some scars from previous infection. Fortunately, the scarring will usually be mild but up to 2% of the community may have a significant visual handicap from trachoma.

The following methods will all help in the prevention of trachoma blindness in the community:

1. Encourage personal and community hygiene, with the disposal of rubbish and faeces to prevent flies breeding. Provide facilities to wash faces and clothes. Young mothers and school children should also be taught the basic rules of hygiene.
2. The mass use of local antibiotics in young children with active trachoma treats individual cases and also limits the number of carriers for the disease in the community. It may be effective against secondary bacterial conjunctivitis as well. Intermittent doses of antibiotics are presently recommended by the WHO for mass community treatment. Either drops or ointment are given twice daily for one week each month for 6 months.
3. Surgery for patients with trachoma is often the last chance of intervening before eventual blindness develops. However, it is a real challenge to cope with large numbers of people with trichiasis and entropion who need appropriate surgical treatment.

Xerophthalmia

Xerophthalmia is a disease of children caused by vitamin A deficiency. Vitamin A keeps all epithelial tissues healthy and helps in the production of mucus. The conjunctiva and cornea are more susceptible to vitamin A deficiency than any other epithelial tissues. The word xerophthalmia literally means 'dry eyes'. It is strictly not an accurate term because tear production still occurs. In fact there is a deficiency of mucus in the tears so that the tears will not wet the conjunctiva and cornea properly and they therefore appear to be dry. Eventually, severe corneal ulcers develop, leading to blindness. Other factors contribute to these ulcers as well as vitamin A deficiency, in particular measles and protein energy malnutrition. Therefore xerophthalmia is sometimes more generally called 'nutritional corneal ulceration'. The World Health Organization estimates that each year 200 000 children suffer from nutritional deficiency worldwide, of whom half will die and a quarter will be left blind or partially sighted.

Vitamin A is a fat-soluble vitamin called retinol which is stored in the liver. There are two main sources of dietary vitamin A.

1. **Plant foods**. Most plant foods contain orange pigments called carotenes which the body converts to retinol. Green leafy foods such as spinach, some root crops such as carrots, and coloured fruits such as mangoes, papayas and tomatoes are good sources of carotene. Red palm oil is an excellent source, whereas starchy white foods like rice and cassava contain virtually none.
2. **Animal foods**. The liver is obviously a very good source of retinol; dairy produce and eggs are also rich in it.

Vitamin A also helps in the production of rhodopsin, the pigment found in the rods of the retina that are responsible for night vision; consequently 'night blindness' may be a feature of vitamin A deficiency.

Signs of Symptoms of Vitamin A Deficiency

The first signs are in the conjunctiva; there is drying, thickening and increased pigmentation of the conjunctiva. Often, foamy material is found at the lid margins. One characteristic sign is a Bitot's spot, which is a cheesy-looking deposit near the limbus in the interpalpebral fissure.

Next, the cornea becomes involved and also appears dry; finally corneal ulcers appear, usually in the exposed lower two thirds of the cornea. These may progress very rapidly, with the whole cornea appearing to dissolve away. This is called keratomalacia. If the child survives, the end result will be a total corneal scar, phthisis bulbi or staphyloma (Figure 23.3). If the disease is arrested at an earlier stage there may be complete recovery or a smaller corneal scar.

Other Causes of Nutritional Corneal Ulceration

There are other factors beside vitamin A deficiency which are also significant in causing these severe ulcers. Most children who are vitamin-deficient have other dietary deficiencies as well and are also prone to many infections. The most important of these factors are as follows.

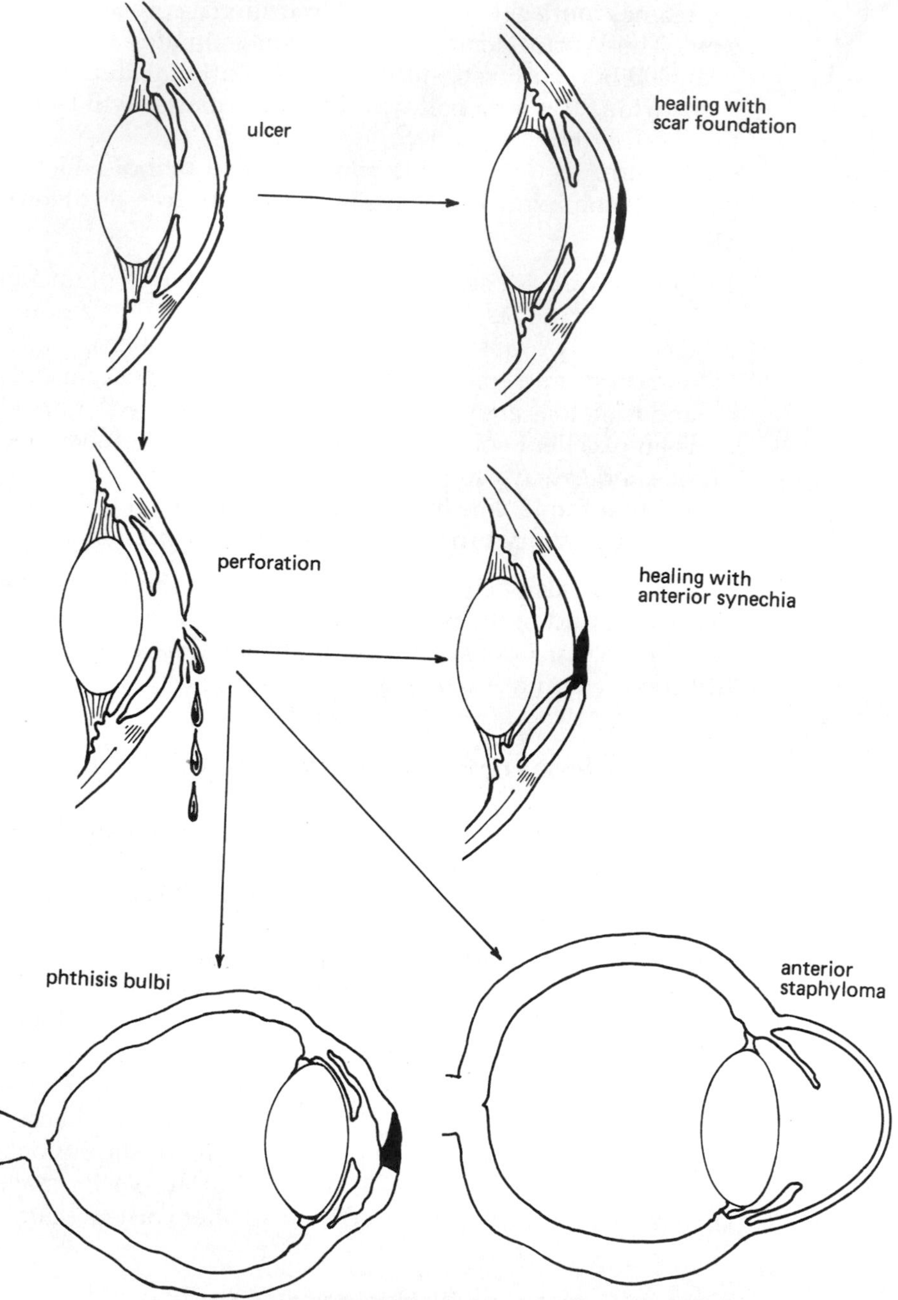

Figure 23.3 Possible consequences of corneal ulceration.

1. **Protein energy malnutrition**: this lowers the child's resistance to disease. In particular it will lower the synthesis of retinol-binding protein in the liver and therefore prevent the transport of retinol to the tissues.

2. **Measles and other infections**: measles in particular is a very important cause of nutritional corneal ulceration, especially in Africa. Measles involves the conjunctival and corneal epithelium, causing a keratoconjunctivitis. Measles and malnutrition also depress the cellular immunity of the body, so that herpes simplex virus (HSV) may infect the cornea.
3. **Exposure of the cornea**: many sick children, especially if they become dehydrated, may not close their eyes properly so that the exposed cornea first becomes dry and then ulcerates.
4. **Secondary bacterial infection** may occur once corneal ulcers have developed.

Treatment

Many of these children are desperately ill and need intensive general treatment. Specific treatment of the eye is as follows:

1. Vitamin A by mouth: the WHO recommends the following doses: 11 mg immediately, then the following day and 2 weeks later.
2. Protect the cornea of sick children from dehydration and exposure. This usually means teaching mothers to keep their sick children's eyes shut.
3. Give antibiotic drops or ointment prophylactically every few hours to prevent ulceration, or intensively every hour if ulceration has already occurred.
4. Antiviral agents – acyclovir or idoxuridine ointment – applied hourly to the eye are indicated for any ulcer which could possibly be caused by HSV.
5. Nutritional advice and education for the mother. The treatment for nutritional diseases is much more complicated than just giving out tablets and injections and eye drops. In most cases malnutrition is the root cause of the disease and the mother must be taught and encouraged to feed her child properly.

Prevention

Many of these children die. Many are blind and irreversibly handicapped when first seen. Some recover with good vision and a very few may have their sight restored with major surgery (corneal grafting). However, the only proper solution to this tragic disease is prevention.

Economic, political and cultural factors may all underlie malnutrition and poverty. However, there are some specific ways in which nutritional corneal ulceration can be prevented.

1. Encourage the community to cultivate and eat the right foods. In areas where vitamin A deficiency is worst (South India, Bangladesh and Indonesia) green leafy vegetables abound. Mothers should be taught how to provide nutritious and cheap weaning foods for their children.
2. Provide vitamin A capsules for pregnant and nursing mothers and young children.
3. Fortify specific foods with vitamin A at factories where they are made.
4. Vaccinate children against measles.
5. Health education: every opportunity in child health clinics, maternity clinics, schools and community meetings should be taken to emphasize the dangers to young children of nutritional corneal ulceration and how it can be prevented.

Onchocerciasis

Onchocerciasis is a disease of the eye and skin caused by the filarial worm *Onchocerca volvulus*. The worm is transmitted from person to person by various species of biting blackfly, in particular *Simulium damnosum*, the buffalo gnat.

This fly breeds near fast-flowing rivers and streams and the disease is most common near such rivers, hence the name of 'river blindness'. It is found in central Africa and the Yemen; it also occurs in Central America.

The adult worm lives under the skin, forming pea-sized nodules. The female worms survive for many years (up to 20) and produce large numbers of larvae called microfilaria. These live for about one year and migrate through the skin, and in and around the eye. If a fly bites a person who has living microfilaria in the skin they may be ingested by the fly, where they develop further and are then transmitted to another person.

It is the microfilaria which damage the tissues in onchocerciasis. If the person is heavily infected, large numbers of microfilaria are found in the skin and eye. When they die, their death causes a localized inflammatory reaction.

Symptoms

Changes in the Skin

At first there is severe itching and a papular rash. After some years the skin atrophies. There may be depigmenta-

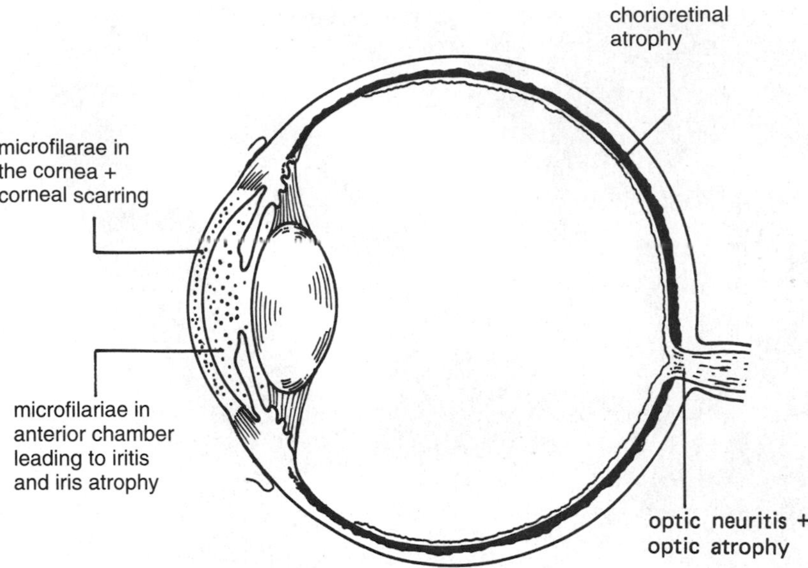

Figure 23.4 Involvement of the eye in onchocerciasis.

tion, particularly of the shins, and chronic oedema of the groin.

Changes in the Eye

Most parts of the eye can be affected (Figure 23.4).

1. **Cornea**: microfilaria are found in large numbers in the cornea (and anterior chamber) but can only be seen with a slit-lamp. When they die a localized inflammatory reaction develops and after many years the cornea becomes scarred, starting at the periphery in the exposed interpalpebral fissure.
2. **Iris**: there is a mild chronic iritis. Eventually, iris atrophy occurs in heavily infected patients.
3. **Retina and choroid**: chorioretinal atrophy eventually occurs in heavily infected patients. This usually starts on the temporal side of the macula and spreads to involve the whole posterior part of the retina and macula.
4. **Optic nerve**: inflammatory changes develop around the optic nerve head, causing optic neuritis and ultimately atrophy.

Visual Loss in Onchocerciasis

This only occurs in people who are heavily infected, and takes many years. The loss of vision may be caused by

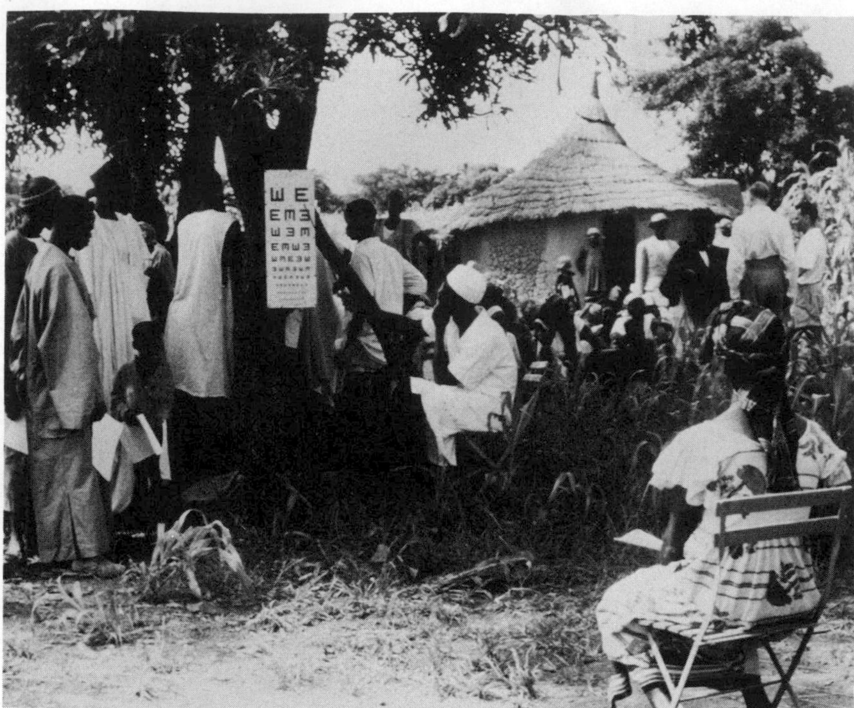

Figure 23.5 Eye testing in a village in an onchocerciasis zone.

corneal scarring, iritis and glaucoma, optic atrophy or chorioretinal degeneration. In areas where onchocerciasis is endemic both the prevalence of infection and blindness vary greatly from place to place and even between villages. In badly affected areas the entire community will have some infection and up to 10% of the adults may have serious visual loss (Figure 23.5).

Diagnosis

Diagnosis is best made by demonstrating living, moving microfilaria in the skin. A tiny fragment of skin from the iliac crest or a lateral canthus is placed in saline and examined under a microscope. After a few minutes the microfilaria will be seen actively moving the saline.

Treatment

Until recently there was no effective treatment for onchocerciasis. It is still not possible to restore the sight of people who have already gone blind with onchocerciasis, but treatment is now available for people who are heavily infested with microfilaria but can still see.

Ivermectin is a drug which appears to prevent the adult worms producing the microfilaria. There is therefore a gradual fall in the numbers of living circulating microfilaria. It only seems necessary to take the drug once a year or every 6 months. It should not be given to pregnant or nursing mothers, young children or people who are seriously ill. It is available from the makers, Merck Sharpe & Dohme, free of charge to those who will use it carefully and responsibly.

PREVENTION

At present the mass use of ivermectin in the community seems to be the most promising way to prevent onchocerciasis. If the number of the people in the community with onchocerciasis can be reduced then the disease will not spread so easily. There is also a place for attempts to reduce or eliminate the fly, *Simulium*, which causes the disease. In order to do this the rivers and breeding grounds of the flies must be sprayed with an appropriate biologically acceptable insecticide.

LEPROSY

Leprosy is caused by a bacterium called *Mycobacterium leprae*. It mainly affects the skin and the superficial nerves, causing skin changes and loss of function of the nerves. Leprosy is a very complex disease because the body can react to the organism in different ways. It may show very little reaction so that the organisms multiply and are found in large numbers. This is called 'lepromatous' leprosy or multibacillary leprosy. Alternatively, there may be a marked tissue reaction to the organism so that there are many inflammatory cells but very few micro-organisms. This is called 'tuberculoid' leprosy or paucibacillary leprosy. In between these extremes are various types of intermediate or 'borderline' leprosy.

Eye care in leprosy is important for two reasons. First, changes in the eye may be the means of diagnosing leprosy. Secondly, known leprosy patients should have their eyes checked regularly for any complications because leprosy quite often affects the eyes and may lead to blindness. The following changes may be seen.

1. The eyelashes and the eyebrows may be missing, especially the lateral end of the eyebrows. This is called madarosis.
2. There may be a partial or complete facial palsy so that the eyelids will not close properly.

3. Thickening of the corneal nerves or inflammation of the corneal stroma may occur. Loss of corneal sensation is an important feature. The combination of a facial palsy and an anaesthetic cornea can very rapidly progress to blindness due to corneal ulceration.
4. There may be nodules on the iris and chronic iritis, so the pupil becomes very constricted, or an acute iritis. Secondary glaucoma and all the other complications may develop.

The two complications of leprosy that commonly cause blindness are corneal ulcers and iritis.

Treatment

Leprosy can be treated with several drugs. The standard treatment is to give dapsone, rifampicin and clofazimine. It may be necessary to continue treatment for many years and this is usually carried out by a doctor with a special interest in leprosy. If facial palsy or corneal anaesthesia occur great care must be taken to prevent corneal ulceration. The eyes should be inspected frequently and lubricant drops such as methylcellulose should be applied by day and antibiotic ointment at night.

The palpebral fissure should be narrowed with a tarsorrhaphy, or a more sophisticated tendon transplant operation can be done to restore eyelid closure. If the facial palsy has developed recently the patient is given systemic steroids. Acute iritis should be treated in the usual way.

Vernal Conjunctivitis

Vernal conjunctivitis or spring catarrh is an allergic type of keratoconjunctivitis occurring in children and young adults. It is a manifestation of atopic disease and often occurs with asthma and eczema. For some reason it is extremely common in most hot and tropical countries and is therefore mentioned here. The characteristic symptom is itching of the eyes, which may be persistent and annoying. There is often a stringy, mucous discharge from the conjunctiva. The exposed conjunctiva around the limbus in the palpebral fissure becomes pigmented, giving the eye a darker appearance. The conjunctiva may proliferate and become thickened and inflamed, either at the limbus or on the upper tarsal plate. Occasionally, shallow central ulcers develop. These become lined with a plaque of mucus and will not heal easily until this plaque is removed. The disease usually subsides as the patient gets older. Fortunately the vision is very rarely affected unless a corneal ulcer has developed.

The treatment is difficult. Local steroid drops are very effective in relieving the symptoms but unfortunately the patients or their relatives may use these excessively without supervision and the complications of local steroid treatment may be seen. Sodium cromoglycate drops applied four times a day also have some effect in relieving the symptoms.

Further Reading

For anyone who is seriously involved in ophthalmic nursing in developing countries this chapter is only an introduction. The following literature might be helpful.

Sandford-Smith, J. (1989) *Eye Disease in Hot Climates*, 2nd edn, John Wright, Bristol.

Teaching Aids At Low Cost (TALC). This organization produced excellent and cheap teaching aids on many subjects relating to health care and eye diseases in developing countries. (Address: Institute of Child Health, London, WC1N 1EH.)

WHO manuals: *Xerophthalmia*, *Leprosy* and *Blindness Prevention*.

Appendix

Ophthalmic Books Widely Available for Reference

Dodd, A. (1993) *Rehabilitating Blind and Visually Impaired People: A Psychological Approach*, Chapman & Hall, London.

Eagling, E. M. and Roper-Hall, M. J. (1986) *Eye Injuries – An Illustrated Guide*, Butterworths, London.

Kanski, J. J. (1990) *Synopsis of Ophthalmology*, 6th edn, John Wright, Bristol.

Miller, S. J. (1984) *Parson's Diseases of the Eye*, 17th edn, Churchill Livingstone, Edinburgh.

Newell, F. (1986) *Ophthalmology – Principles and Concepts*, 6th edn, C. V. Mosby, St Louis, MO.

Spalton, D. J., Hutchings, R. A. and Hunter, P. A. (1984) *Atlas of Clinical Ophthalmology*, Churchill Livingstone, Edinburgh.

Vaughan, D. R., Astbury, T. and Riordan, E. (1992) *General Ophthalmology*, 13th edn, Appleton & Laing, London.

INDEX

Page numbers appearing in **bold** refer to figures and page numbers appearing in *italic* refer to tables.